Yoga in Britain

Yoga in Britain
Stretching Spirituality and Educating Yogis

Suzanne Newcombe

eⵇuinox

SHEFFIELD UK   BRISTOL CT

Published by Equinox Publishing Ltd
UK: Office 415, The Workstation, 15 Paternoster Row, Sheffield, South Yorkshire S1 2BX
USA: ISD, 70 Enterprise Drive, Bristol, CT 06010

www.equinoxpub.com

First published 2019

British Library Cataloguing-in-Publication Data
A catalogue record for this book is available from the British Library.
ISBN-13 978 1 78179 659 7   (hardback)
          978 1 78179 660 3   (paperback)
          978 1 78179 661 0   (ePDF)

Library of Congress Cataloging-in-Publication Data
Names: Newcombe, Suzanne, author.
Title: Yoga in Britain : stretching spirituality and educating yogis /
    Suzanne Newcombe.
Description: Bristol : Equinox Publishing Ltd., 2019. | Includes
    bibliographical references and index.
Identifiers: LCCN 2018042548 (print) | LCCN 2018056236 (ebook) | ISBN
    9781781796610 (ePDF) | ISBN 9781781796597 (hb) | ISBN 9781781796603 (pb)
Subjects: LCSH: Yoga. | Great Britain.
Classification: LCC BL1238.52 (ebook) | LCC BL1238.52 .N49 2019 (print) | DDC
    613.7/0460941--dc23
LC record available at https://lccn.loc.gov/2018042548

Typeset by Witchwood Production House

Contents

Illustrations

A Brief Note on Vocabulary

The majority of vocabulary specific to yoga comes from the Sanskrit language. Some anglicisation has inevitably occurred in the English-speaking world, although practitioners are generally keen to preserve the punctuation and spelling. Variations in print are usually a matter of whether these foreign words should be set in italic, whether they should be capitalised, and whether they should make use of the diacritic marks as specified by the International Alphabet of Sanskrit Transliteration (IAST). (The latter was devised to allow for an unambiguous reading of Indic text using the Latin alphabet.)

For the purposes of this title, I have adhered to the IAST transliterations where possible and italicised, mostly avoiding capitalisation. The exceptions are those words that enjoy such widespread popular use that such treatment now seems pedantic: these include 'asana', 'pranayama' and, of course, 'yoga' itself. The capitalisation of 'Bhakti Yoga', 'Ashtanga Vinyasa Yoga', 'Hatha Yoga', etc. either derives from their usage in the literature of the twentieth-century yoga milieux being discussed or because they are used as proper nouns, identifying modern movements or 'schools'.

Acknowledgements

The central question that started this research was 'How can this thing called "yoga" that is apparently Indian now be such an unremarkable activity in Britain?' The more I researched the subject, the more layers I uncovered of the history and contemporary practice of the variety of things called 'yoga'.

I first began looking at yoga with the eyes of a social scientist under the guidance of Professor Eileen Barker at the London School of Economics and Political Science: her mentorship for my MSc degree and later for my work at Inform has afforded me an invaluable apprenticeship in how to approach the world with critical curiosity. Her modelling of how to conduct participant observation, interviews, and reconsider assumptions based on empirical evidence has been transformative and challenging, and I am very grateful for the encouragement and support she has given me over many years.

Much of the research for this book was conducted during my time as a PhD candidate in the Faculty of History at the University of Cambridge (2003–2007). During this time, I was financially supported by a scholarship by the Evan Carroll Commager Fellowship from Amherst College and an UK Arts and Humanities Research Council (AHRC) postgraduate award for PhD study. At Cambridge, my supervisor Simon Szreter was a constant source of support and encouragement, as well as offering critical critiques on my historical research skills and writing style. His input has immeasurably improved the rigour of the research and the clarity of explanation. Elizabeth de Michelis and the research community at the Dharam Hinduja Institute of Indic Research (DHIIR) at the Faculty of Divinity at Cambridge University provided invaluable collegial discussion and inspiration. I am particularly grateful for the opportunity to collaborate with Elizabeth de Michelis and Mark Singleton with the Modern Yoga Reading Group at Cambridge in 2004, a 2003 Workshop on Modern and Global Ayurveda and a 2004 International Conference on Modern and Global Ayurveda under the DHIIR. These were formative experiences in my understanding of the history and contemporary context of yoga practice; I am very grateful to have been a part of this unique research environment. My doctoral examiners Dominik Wujastyk and Alistair Reid provided invaluable critical comment and suggestions which I hope were addressed in this significantly revised version.

Acknowledgements and gratitude are also owed to the many others who provided friendship and moral support and influenced my thinking while I was studying at Cambridge. These important people include Rachel Berger, Taylor Sherman, Jennifer Black and Dagmar Wujastyk. I would like to thank Rudolf Elliott Lockhart whose collaboration in creating and running Workshops on the Interdisciplinary Study of History (WISH) at Cambridge's Centre for Research in the Arts, Social Sciences and Humanities (CRASSH) was a source of great fun and provoked an expansion of my thinking. Conversations with fellow researchers Véronique Altglas, Karel Baier, Philip Deslippe, Elliott Goldberg, Beatrix Hauser, Anne-Cécile Hoyez, Cathryn Keller, Anne Koch, Séverine Desponds Meylan, Klas Nevrin, Liina Puustinen, Matti Rautaniemi, Benjamin Richard Smith, Julian Strube, Raphaël Voix, Maya Warrier and many others greatly enriched my understanding of yoga and related subjects.

I would also like to acknowledge some of the people who, earlier in my life, inspired me to research and write. Crucially, Martha Sandweiss nurtured and encouraged my first forays into historical research, and Janet Gyatso consistently challenged my assumptions and improved the clarity of my thinking and analysis at Amherst College. Susan Fleming Tate was also very instrumental in giving me initial coaching in the art and discipline of writing.

During many of these years I was working at Inform, then based at the London School of Economics, an organisation that provides information on new and minority religious movements. I am grateful for having had the opportunity to work in an environment that considerably broadened my understanding of the large number of new and minority groups that incorporate yoga into their beliefs and practices. I am grateful to my colleagues at Inform for their support and encouragement over many years; in particular, thanks are due to Amanda Van Eck Duymaer van Twist, Sarah Harvey, San Kim, Silke Steidinger, Jane Cooper, Sibyl McFarlane, Nick Parke, Rebecca Catto, Susannah Crockford and Shanon Shah, and to many of the other interns and researchers, as well as the enquirers, who have also enriched and deepened my understanding.

My colleagues in the Ayuryog project have been an invaluable source of inspiration and support. Without the support and encouragement of Dagmar Wujastyk in particular this project may not have been completed. The good humour and encouragement of Christèle Barois, Jason Birch and Jacqueline Hargreaves has also been very much appreciated. My colleagues at the Open University have also been a source of unflagging support; in particular, I would like to thank Hugh Beattie, Graham Harvey, John Maiden, Stefanie Sinclair and Paul-François Tremlett for their encouragement and empathy in the final stages of writing.

To all those who were so generous with their time, and with their personal archival material found in closets, shoeboxes and in distant memories, I am extremely grateful. This book could not have been researched without the assistance of so many people. Simon Ertz provided excellent professional help in the Hoover Archive at Stanford University which holds extensive material relating to Sir Paul Dukes. Radha Mohan Das and Gauri Das have been very helpful with regard to the history of ISKCON. Particularly generous were Geraldine Beskin, Ken and Angela Thompson, Kenneth Cabral and Yasmin Benson, Muz Murray, Mina Semyon, Satyar Atnananda Saraswati, Swami Tripurananda, Kailash Puri, Indar Nath, Jim Pym, Ernest Coates, Claire Buckingham, John and Ros Claxton, Chris Tobler, Judy Tobler, Hector Guthrie, John Bradford, John Roycroft, Stella Cherfas, Vi Neale-Smith and Lorna Walker: their help and enthusiasm were extremely encouraging. Many of those I interviewed have kept in touch with me to correct my misunderstandings; any remaining errors are my own responsibility and I continue to be open to corrections where necessary.

Some of the chapters of this book draw on material previously published. This material has been re-used with permission of the publishers. Much of the material used in Chapter 3 first appeared as 'The Institutionalization of the Yoga Tradition: "Gurus" B.K.S. Iyengar and Yogini Sunita in Britain', in Mark Singleton and Ellen Goldberg (eds.), *Gurus of Modern Yoga* (Oxford University Press, 2014): 147–67, used with permission from Oxford University Press. Some of the material in Chapter 2 first appeared in 'Magic and Yoga: The Role of Subcultures in Transcultural Exchange', in B. Hauser (ed.), *Yoga Traveling: Bodily Practice in Transcultural Perspective*

(London: Springer, 2013): 57–79, reproduced with permission from Springer. Finally, subjects covered in Chapter 4 were first covered in 'Stretching for Health and Well-Being: Yoga and Women in Britain, 1960–1980', *Asian Medicine* 3(1) (2007): 37–63, reproduced here courtesy of Brill.

The editors and reviewers at Equinox Publishing have been very professional and helpful in the process of getting this book into print. I would especially like to thank Janet Joyce and Valerie Hall at Equinox; Matthew Clark for his invaluable review of the book manuscript; and Dean Bargh of Witchwood Production House for the copyediting and typesetting.

Much-needed personal support and inspiration has been offered by my friends and family, including in particular Ruth Galinsky and Olivia McCannon Glazebrook, who over the years have both responded to my moaning with encouragement. I am particularly grateful for the patience and support of all kinds and the love extended by my ever-supportive parents Jim and Susan Hasselle. My biggest debt of gratitude in writing this book goes to my husband Alaric and my daughters Ayesha and Kansas – thank you for making my life joyful and vivacious, and for putting up with me during my research and writing process. Without your love and support this project would have been impossible.

The initial research for this book was supported by an Arts and Humanities Research Council (AHRC) postgraduate award for PhD study. Further research and revision of this manuscript was undertaken while supported by the Ayuryog project which was made possible through funding from the European Union's Horizon 2020 research and innovation programme under grant agreement no. 639363.

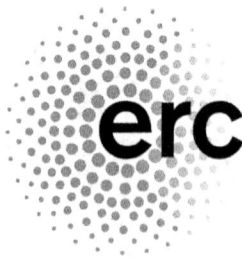

erc

European Research Council

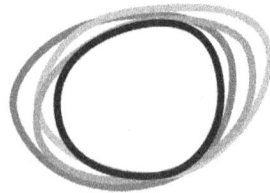

Arts & Humanities
Research Council

Prologue

Rethinking Yoga

Over 200 million people, it has been estimated, participate in 'yoga' globally, including over 100 million in India (Tangali 2016). In 2016, active yoga practitioners in the United States were estimated to number 36 million individuals who spend over $16 billion on classes, clothes and other yoga accessories (Yoga Alliance 2016), while in the United Kingdom more conservative estimates (Jarvis 2014; Carter 2004) suggest that about 500,000 participate in a yoga class every week. Yoga practice is also increasingly to be found in other locations such as South America, Africa and Japan. Its popularity has been undoubtedly influenced by the Indian Prime Minister Modi's proposal to the United Nations to instigate International Yoga Day, which was first celebrated on 21 June 2015, an event that marks a growing trend towards an increasing acceptance of something called yoga. While practices going by the name of yoga have been becoming more socially acceptable and popular since at least the mid-nineteenth century, much of the rapid growth has been very recent, with millions becoming aware of the practice only in recent decades. What we now see as yoga, spreading in popularity across the globe, represents a flexible and multifaceted group of related traditions.

'Yoga' does not mean the same thing to each of its 200 million adherents. For some, yoga is primarily a physical exercise offering better health and well-being; for many Indians, yoga represents union with the ultimate reality at the spiritual heart of their religious understandings. As such, it is unsurprising that the growth in popularity has been accompanied by a crisis in authenticity among practitioners. In particular, yoga in a post-1980s, neoliberal context has demonstrated a diversity of 'brands' and a focus on selling products, as well as a number of high-profile scandals revealing the unethical behaviour of teachers in what might be regarded as primarily an ethical discipline.

In justifying their participation, some practitioners align themselves with a narrative of belonging to ancient traditions; some
emphasise pragmatic mental and physical benefits; some point to
a lineage of teachers and techniques; while others focus on ethical
and spiritual development as the measure of their discipline. Where
an understanding of history is absent, various fundamentalisms can
rush in to fill out the narrative. By fundamentalisms, I mean stories
of origin or a 'true essence' of yoga based on over-generalisations,
stereotypes and other unempirical assumptions about the nature of
others' experience and practices.

Over the course of the twentieth century, the myriad ways in
which yoga was studied, popularised and practised have led to the
kaleidoscope of different understandings of yoga we have today.
Most of the key popularising individuals had their own sense of
authenticity; some voices became more powerful and influential than others; but all those who had an enduring influence on
the popularisation of yoga were searching for something deeply
meaningful on a personal level. Most had genuine interest in and
respect for the Indian traditions from which yoga originated.
Yet there were immense variations in how these understandings
were articulated and how their ideas shaped practice. All those in
this story are imperfect humans, who at times behaved less than
ethnically and brought their own biases and limitations to their
teaching of the subject. It is legitimate to criticise interpretations of
yoga that may have later proved harmful to specific individuals, or
perpetuated unwanted general cultural assumptions, e.g. colonial,
postcolonial, and/or neoliberal biases. But it is also important to
appreciate the multiplicity of practices and beliefs associated with
yoga and seek to understand what the practitioners are doing in
their own terms.

Yoga consists of embodied practices and ideas about the meaning of those practices. It often comes with an expectation that it
should be explained and defined. A standard narrative might
touch on Indus Valley seals, ascetic practices in the first century
BC, the codification of Patañjali's sutras, various tantric and haṭha
developments, and go on to include an accommodation with current scientific world-views. Writing a linear introduction to define
yoga is often unavoidable. But such a standard piece of writing
places the researcher in an ideological position that may obfus-
cate other aspects of critical observation. An essentialist, linear

narrative at once legitimatises and de-legitimises the variety of political positions held by actors involved with yoga globally. Unspoken assumptions and essentialist understandings of yoga often lead to different traditions speaking at cross-purposes, unable to engage in dialogue, or actively antagonistic towards one another.

As often mentioned by yoga enthusiasts, the etymological root of yoga is *yuj*, which means 'to join' or 'yoke'; and many contemporary yoga practitioners will explain that 'yoga' means the joining of the self to God, or the finite to the infinite (Whitney 1997: 132). However, a vast diversity of meanings, practices and associations are attached to the word 'yoga', with interpretations as diverse as 'skill in work', 'desire-less action', 'acquisition of true knowledge', 'indifference to pleasure and pain', 'addition' (in arithmetic) and 'conjunction' (in astronomy)' (Banerji 1995: 44). As the scholar David Gordon White has famously summarised, '"Yoga" has a wider range of meanings than nearly any other word in the entire Sanskrit lexicon' (White 2012: 2).

An important part of its appeal in Europe has been its practical benefits in association with an ancient (i.e. legitimate) spiritual tradition: the roots of yoga, it is sometimes claimed, go back as far as 2500 BC.[1] Although usually associated with Hinduism, the techniques of yoga have been used by Buddhists, Jains and Sikhs while maintaining their own metaphysical beliefs (Bronkhorst 1981, 1998; Eliade 1954, 1963; Sarbacker 2005, 2008; Mallinson and Singleton 2017). The philosophical tradition of yoga was traditionally understood as a technique for realising the nature of consciousness (*puruṣa*) unfettered by the real empirical world (*prakṛti*) and codified in Patañjali's *Yoga Sūtras* written some time between 374 and 425 AD (Woods 1914; White 2014; Maas 2013). The first evidence we have of the variety of meditation techniques that have become associated with yoga dates from around the time of the Shakyamuni Buddha (c. 400 BCE).[2] But the first records we have of physical postures now associated with yoga (Haṭha Yoga) were recorded by groups of

1. Dhyansky (1987). For an example of a British claim, see 'Means Better Than the End?', *Yoga: Journal of the British Wheel of Yoga* 11 (1972), p. 12: 'The Yoga of bodily posture and breath-control, even in its classical form is but a particular specialized technique within a wider discipline that goes back ... nearly a thousand years before Christ.'

2. See Diamond (2013) for material culture evidence of yoga practices.

renunciants in northern India and can be dated to around 1100 AD (Mallinson and Singleton 2017: xx–xxi). Traditionally, instruction in yoga was imparted in a pedagogical relationship between teacher and student and not by the solitary reading of texts (Mallinson and Singleton 2017: 48–9). It has therefore been difficult to trace accurately the development of yoga traditions through the centuries, although important work in this regard for the medieval period has recently begun (Mallinson and Singleton 2017; Birch 2011, 2018).

I therefore concur with several colleagues in asserting that yoga can only be studied in a particular context (Burger 2013; Jain 2015: xiv–xvii). It is important to offer more complicated definitions of yoga – understanding yoga in non-essentialist, but rather in instrumental, situational terms. It is only by considering yoga in precise locations that statements about its significance and effects can have any meaning (Newcombe 2018). This book aims to describe one such location: twentieth-century Britain. As such, it contributes to a small but growing literature on the development of yoga traditions in both India and beyond. Key literature in this regard includes works by Joseph Alter, Keith Cantú, Philip Deslippe, Elizabeth de Michelis, Elliott Goldberg, Mark Singleton and Julian Strube, which have demonstrated that periods of colonialism and *fin de siècle* exchange caused a reframing of the yoga tradition within India in response to European thought and culture (Alter 2004a; de Michelis 2004; Goldberg 2016; Singleton 2010; Deslippe 2018, Cantú 2016a, 2016b; Strube 2017, forthcoming). The popularisation of yoga in Britain is but one recent chapter in thousands of years of a fluid and responsive practice of things called yoga.

While this book attempts to create a narrative of how yoga was popularised in Britain during the twentieth century, it must be understood as incomplete and partial in its account; my research is most comprehensive for the period between 1945 and 1980. Aspects of the popularisation of yoga in the first half of the twentieth century are outlined in the first chapter of this book. Karl Baier, Henrik Bogdan, Gordon Djurdjevic and Julian Strube have done some good initial exploration of the overlaps between yoga and various esoteric milieux (Baier 2009, 2012, 2016a, 2016b, 2018; Bogdan 2006, 2010, 2013; Djurdjevic 2014). There is quite a lot more research to be done on how yoga began to be practised in Europe during the late nineteenth and early twentieth centuries.

This book deals only very lightly with elements of transformations and popularisation after the 1980s; more contemporary developments in yoga have been covered with a variety of social science perspectives in recent academic literature.[3] The chapters in this book might be best understood as vignettes, or windows into an understanding of how yoga became a popular and acceptable leisure activity in Britain during this period. Future research will undoubtedly uncover more windows offering different views.

Reductionist narratives about neocolonial oppression or cultural appropriation are seen to be unsustainable considering the multiplicity of actors and motives involved in the popularisation of yoga and in the face of the empirical, historical evidence. Popularisers of yoga were both Indian and British by ethnicity. Ankur Barua (2016) has pointed out that the architects of modern, independent India 'often critically interrogated, rejected, and appropriated specific aspects' of the British colonial frameworks for what they perceived as their country's most pertinent and genuine needs. Likewise, those who investigated, interrogated and taught yoga traditions in the twentieth century were usually attempting to respectfully explore a tradition which might meet present needs. A great many of those popularising yoga in Britain were Indians by birth, but a number of other influential individuals were not.

Of enduring influence, but not directly discussed in this narrative, is the influence of Swami Vivekananda's presentation of yoga, the significance of which has been argued by Elizabeth de Michelis (2004; see also Beckerlegge 2000, 2004). Although also of crucial importance, a social history detailing the activities and influence of the Theosophical Society in Britain has yet to be written.[4] These themes form an important back-story to what is discussed in this book. During the twentieth century, Vivekananda's categories and presentation on yoga are demonstrably influential by virtue of their reiterations and re-presentations by other yoga teachers.

This narrative considers the practices commonly pursued under the title of 'yoga'; it looks at who participated in these practices, and what were the perceptions of their purpose. Attention will focus on the groups that were most significant in establishing yoga as a

3. Some relevant recent works include Beaman and Sikka (2016), Hauser (2013), Horton and Harvey (2012), Jain (2015), Schnäbele (2010) and Singleton and Byrne (2008).

4. But for the European context see Baier (2009, 2012, 2016a).

widespread social activity in Britain, and whose historical record is recoverable. In the twenty-first century, economic imperatives have moved the teaching of yoga from an educational context and into the consumer high street. However, the aims and motives of contemporary practitioners are still deeply influenced by the groundwork and narratives created during the twentieth century. In Britain, yoga was popularised in a way that suited a centralist, adult-education context which emphasised physical safety and health over enlightening transformations. This emphasis on safety exists in tension with the potential for transformation, paradigm shifts and radical re-evaluation of an individual's sense of meaning-and-purpose in life. The regulated educational or therapeutic context does not absolutely exclude the potential for such experiences, but perhaps it does make them less likely.

During the twentieth century Britain was a Christian country experiencing a secularising of public space; the British public became increasingly sceptical of religious language, but not necessarily uninterested in religious aims. Around the middle of the century, religious beliefs were increasingly being relegated from public discourse into individuals' private consciousness. But that does not mean that spiritual quests were absent from the individual practitioners' minds as they approached a largely physical practice. The educational syllabuses and public forums in which yoga became popularised in Britain transformed it into a product that could be transmitted globally and which did not need to rely on a few charismatic teachers and their direct students. The methods and literature produced in twentieth-century Britain have been globally influential on how yoga is practised – and on assumptions about how it should be practised. These assumptions have at times filtered back to the Indian subcontinent, even as competing narratives about the place of yoga in Indian culture and heritage continue to evolve.

In presenting the stories in this book, I hope to complicate the stereotypes inherent in considering others' practices and bring more nuanced history into the discussion. The way in which yoga was popularised in Britain provides an important background to an understanding of how and why it enjoys such contemporary popularity – which cannot be explained simply by reference to some of its current, neoliberal forms. It is my hope that the scholars and practitioners reading this volume will discover a more multifaceted narrative about what yoga has represented for various people in the twentieth century. By appreciating how yoga practitioners were educated in the last hundred years, we educate ourselves to face the future – not necessarily with clear answers, but hopefully with fewer erroneous assumptions, less prejudice and more empathy.

Chapter One

The Literary Elite: Booksellers and Publishers

If you wanted to find out about yoga in early-twentieth-century Britain, you would most likely turn to a book. The people with access to such literature in the early twentieth century were, largely, middle- and upper-class eccentrics who read widely. Some of these also undertook exercises related to concentration and relaxation in the privacy of their own homes or with small groups of interested friends. Indian texts on yoga had been imported from India since the late nineteenth century, becoming more available via cheaply produced English translations sponsored by the Theosophical Society. In the late Victorian period, interest grew in alternatives to the Church of England, especially among the educated elite. Explorations at the edge of a scientific understanding of religious phenomena and into human psychic abilities were subjects of educated fascination, as science for the first time was equal to the task of addressing these areas. Many such interested parties found their way into the networks of the Theosophical Society or the Spiritualist Society. These organisations were more eclectic than dogmatic, and their bulletin boards gave details of newly published books and dates of public lectures on esoteric subjects.

Printed books on yoga came out in a slow trickle; no more than twelve new titles a year on the subject are found in British copyright libraries before 1963. But this accelerated in the 1960s, assisted by the advent of paperbacks and by the increasing visibility of Indian yoga teachers in Britain. After 1963 the number of yoga titles published annually grew to reach a peak of 49 new titles in 1978. Following the Beatles' well-publicised association with the Maharishi in 1968, interest became even more widespread. Although the number of new titles levelled off in the 1980s, they were still being produced at more than double the 1960 rate. Yoga was a regular feature on television from 1972 onwards, with cheap paperback books to accompany the series. The print media publishers and sellers exerted a major influence on how yoga was received in Britain throughout the twentieth century, even while yoga was being popularised in new venues during the post-war period.

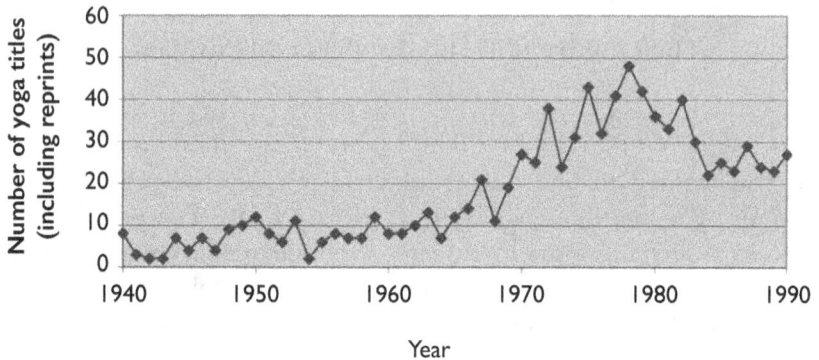

Fig. 1.1 Number of titles on yoga published each year. All books including the word 'yoga' in the title held in the British copyright libraries published in each year between 1940 and 1990.[1]

However, yoga was not confined to the printed word: throughout the twentieth century, social networks connected the largely independent readers and their solitary practices. The networks nonetheless consisted of the booksellers and publishers who traded in esoteric subjects such as Indian religions and set the agenda of how yoga was presented and defined. Their choice of materials was often based on personal experience of the practices and on general knowledge of esoteric religions. Notwithstanding commercial objectives, British booksellers and publishers were also concerned about their reputations for quality. Only a handful were active in this field, so a small number of individuals wielded significant influence in endorsing teachers or books. Perhaps the most influential hub in this network was to be found in Watkins Bookshop in central London.

1. I was not able to find any concise source for numbers of books bought, published or printed in Britain on a particular subject. However, one copy of each book printed in Britain is required to be deposited within the Consortium of Research Libraries (CORL). Searching their online catalogue was an efficient way of estimating numbers of books published on yoga in a given year. Although additional holdings of the same book in different libraries were excluded, reprints and second editions of previously published books were included when they appeared in a new year.

Watkins Bookshop

Watkins Bookshop had its origins as a Theosophical distributor; the founder of Watkins Bookshop, John Maurice Watkins (1862–1947) was a personal friend and secretary to Theosophical Society founder Helena Petrovna Blavatsky (1831–1891).[2] From 1893, John Watkins began distributing Theosophical Society books, largely published at the Theosophical Society's headquarters in India, to subscribers in England from stock lists (Gilbert 2004).[3] Watkins Bookshop became independent from the Theosophical Society in 1896 and the list expanded to encompass a wide variety of specialist religious, esoteric and occult titles. From 1901, Watkins Bookshop operated from a shop front in Cecil Court off Charing Cross Road (Gilbert 2004).[4] Its central London location and specialist expertise made Watkins a gathering point for those interested in esotericism, unusual religions and 'rejected knowledge'.[5] John Watkins fostered an atmosphere of comfortable discussion, serving tea in his office to regular visitors in the interwar period, among whom were prominent esoteric and cultural figures such as William Butler Yeats, George William Russell (who wrote about Celtic mysticism and Irish nationalism under the pseudonym Æ), Aleister Crowley, G.R.S. Mead and A.E. Waite (Gilbert 2004). From 1919, Watkins Sr was joined in running the bookshop by his son, Geoffrey 'Nigel' Watkins (1896–1981).

The bookshop was sometimes described as an 'event', with browsers networking to share information about spiritual teachers and techniques. Writing near the end of his life, the popular writer on Buddhism and Eastern spirituality, Alan Watts (1915–1973), described the role of Watkins Books in his early self-education. According to Watts, Nigel Watkins:

> runs the most magical bookshop in the world, and is the most unobtrusively enlightened person I have ever known . . . He sells books on Oriental philosophy, magic, astrology, Masonry, meditation, Christian mysticism, alchemy, herbal medicine, and every occult and far-out subject under the sun. But he himself has, if you will take his own advice, perfect discrimination in what one should read, for he knows

2. Personal interview with Jim Pym (7 July 2015).
3. For Theosophical history, see also Campbell (1980), Dixon (2001) and Godwin (1994).
4. In New York City the major source for esoteric books was Weiser's Bookstore, established in 1926 on Fourth Avenue.
5. For more on this subject, see Gilbert (2009).

that much of this literature is superstitious trash . . . Nigel not only became my bibliographer on Buddhism, comparative religion, and mysticism, but also my trusted advisor on the various gurus, pandits and psychotherapists then flourishing in London (Watts 1972: 107).

In Geoffrey Watkins' obituary frequent visitor and Blake scholar Kathleen Raine remembered:

From all over the world seekers converged upon the bookshop in Cecil Court where in the back office (where books not on sale to the public at large were kept) first old Mr Watkins, and later young Mr Watkins, held court under the scrutiny of a faded but magisterial photograph of H.P.B. [Blavatsky] herself . . . Geoffrey Watkins was a mine of accurate information about all those esoteric groups, societies and individuals who were concerned with the Western esoteric tradition (Raine 1982).

Thus, Watkins Bookshop was an important location for information about a wide variety of alternative religious and spiritual traditions. As one of the few specialists in sourcing books on yoga, patrons of Watkins included some early members of the British Wheel of Yoga, which would become one of the most influential networks for promoting yoga in Britain from the 1960s onwards.[6]

Watkins Jr took sole control of the bookshop in 1947 and was a well-known figure among those interested in unusual forms of religion and spirituality. He was understood by many to be a 'book guru', suggesting 'perfect' books on subjects that included yoga and Indian spirituality. Jim Pym, who worked in Watkins Bookshop as assistant manager, specialising in second-hand books, recalled Nigel Watkins:

He just was an incredible fount of knowledge for everything spiritual. I remember many times someone at the till with a book, and Geoffrey saying, 'No you don't want that, try this one . . .' 'Well, okay,' they might reply, 'but I still want this one . . .' Then, later they would come back and say, 'No, you were right: I didn't want that book.' Geoffrey was a guru who taught you by pointing out the right books. And he did this with loads of people. He wouldn't claim any special ability – just saying 'I'm a bookseller, I can pick the right books' – but he was,

---

6. Personal interview with Jim Pym (7 July 2015). For example, in *Yoga: Journal of the British Wheel of Yoga* 20 (Summer 1974), p. 24, there is an advertisement for 'Watkins Bookshop. The Mystical Bookshop, for all books on Yoga, Mysticism, Comparative Religion, Healing and allied subjects'.

he was more than that ... and just to be with him was a wonderful experience.[7]

This personal assistance in the search for esoteric religious knowledge made Watkins Bookshop a place frequented by those pursuing a variety of spiritual quests. Under Nigel Watkins the bookshop expanded from its roots in Theosophy and spiritualism into a wider variety of 'rejected knowledge' (Gilbert 2004). In the late 1970s and early 1980s, Pym remembered Watkins Books as 'in the heart of everything. Spiritualism, psychology, yoga, Christian meditation, Buddhism, it was all around that whole thing'.[8] By the mid-twentieth century, Watkins Books was an established and well-connected source of information for all kinds of esoteric knowledge, not merely books.

But in this specialist field, Nigel Watkins was more than a guide to consumers of esoteric books: he also advised publishers. As the premier esoteric bookseller in Britain, Nigel Watkins was well positioned to identify and influence the popularity of any particular esoteric field. As the above quotes testify, Watkins was widely considered a source of accurate information about the various esoteric groups and activities in London and his advice in both these capacities was solicited by British publishers interested in esoteric materials: both Penguin and Allen & Unwin publishers had occasion to directly or indirectly consult Watkins about yoga. This placed Nigel Watkins in a uniquely important role in determining how yoga was received in Britain. In 1956, A.S.B. Glover (1895–1966), Senior Editor at Penguin and well known for his encyclopaedic memory, approached Watkins with the idea of commissioning a book on yoga (Lane 1966).[9] This shows Glover's significant regard for Watkins: Glover was himself a Buddhist and also interested in Theosophy and other religious groups, and thus would have already been aware of the field of potential authors (Lewis 2005: 237).

---

7. Personal interview with Jim Pym (7 July 2015).
8. Ibid.
9. See also 'Yoga: Ernest Wood', DM 1107/02.0448 2, Penguin Archives. In a letter dated 8 November 1956 from Nigel Watkins to A.S.B. Glover of Penguin Books: 'Many thanks for your letter concerning the publication of a Penguin book on Yoga. Of course I shall be delighted to see you and give you any help I can. In the meantime I will continue to peruse another line, which I started when Christmas Humphreys first approached me in the matter ...'

Penguin Yoga

Penguin had established a reputation for affordable paperback
books with a wide readership by buying up publication rights for
out-of-print and uncopyrighted classics. Since 1935 Sir Allen Lane
sold 'six-penny copies of high quality fiction' in established bookshops, newsagents, and even from dispensing machines (called
'Penguincubators') at popular railway stations.[10] Penguin's Pelican
imprint was launched in 1937 with commissioned books designed
to educate as well as entertain; its subject matter encompassed a
wide remit of both new commissions and non-fiction classics in
low-cost paperbacks. Penguin was a highly influential and profita-
ble business. By 1968, the Penguin Publishing Company, Ltd could
boast over 3,000 titles in print and a wide distribution throughout
the English-speaking world; it had around 600 employees and an
annual turnover of over £4 million.[11] While the educated reading
public still constituted a minority of the British population, the cheap
and accessible Penguin books served to widen this population.

With their inspired and disciplined eye for marketing, Penguin
staff had identified a market for books on yoga by July 1956. One
travelling representative reported that a Penguin bookseller in
South Africa:

> showed me a number of expensive books on Yoga and advised me
> that there was a considerable interest in this subject. He was unable to
> obtain any cheap editions on Yoga and suggested that we might very
> well include a book dealing with this in our series.[12]

This representative also read that Indian booksellers were antici-
pating high sales for a new yoga book and thought Penguin might
be able to profit from this market.[13] The Penguin employee continued in his memo, 'I believe it was at one time our intention to
publish a book on this subject and perhaps you would advise me

10. For an early history of Penguin publishing, see Penguin (1960, 1985) and
Baines (2005).
11. 'Buckmaster & Moore, Penguin Publishing Company Ltd Stock Report',
1968, DM 1819/11/6, Penguin Archives.
12. From RAD to ASBG 'Memo', in 'Yoga: Ernest Wood', DM 1107/02.0448 2,
Penguin Archives.
13. '"Yoga Asanas Simplified": New Popular edition will make sales history! By
Sri Yogendra', in *The Book Lover Everyman's Literary Guide*, 3/22 (June 1956), back
cover, in 'Yoga: Ernest Wood', DM 1107/02.0448 2, Penguin Archives.

of the present position.'[14] This question was quickly addressed by the editorial committee and, by September 1956, a letter was written to Christmas Humphreys (1901–1983), founder and president of the Buddhist Society, asking for suitable candidates for a commissioned book on yoga.[15] Glover had first approached Humphreys as an author for the Penguin book on Buddhism for this new series in March 1948.[16] This commission on Buddhism related to an already established Penguin project of publishing books on each of the 'world religions'. In 1948, titles on Islam, Judaism and Christianity were also commissioned for Pelican.[17] Penguin settled for an adaptation of Humphreys' 1928 pamphlet 'What is Buddhism?' for its book *Buddhism* published in 1951.[18] The first print run for *Buddhism* was for 38,500 paperback copies, of which about 26,000 were sold on subscription before publication.[19]

Brainstorming with Glover in search of an author for a Pelican title on yoga, Nigel Watkins suggested former Theosophist Ernest Wood (1882–1965).[20] Wood was born in Manchester, left school at sixteen and, having become involved with the Theosophical Society, pursued correspondence courses for university qualifications. From 1908–21, Wood worked for the Theosophical Society in India, studying Indian religions and administering schools and colleges. After the Second World War, Wood settled in the United States where he served as dean and president of the American Academy of Asian

14. From RAD to ASBG 'Memo', in 'Yoga: Ernest Wood', DM 1107/02.0448 2, Penguin Archives.

15. Letter from Penguin to Humphreys, 27 September 1956, in 'Yoga: Ernest Wood', DM 1107/02.0448 2, Penguin Archives. The personal and networking connections between Buddhism and yoga studies in pre-war London would be a fruitful area for more research.

16. Glover to Humphreys, 3 March 1948, in 'Buddhism by Christmas Humphreys', DM 02.0228 5, Penguin Archives.

17. Glover to Humphreys, 30 September 1948, in 'Buddhism by Christmas Humphreys', DM 02.0228 5, Penguin Archives.

18. Humphreys to Glover, 9 March 1948, in 'Buddhism by Christmas Humphreys', DM 02.0228 5, Penguin Archives. According to Humphreys, the leaflet 'has sold steadily for twenty years and we are now selling rather faster than we did twenty years ago'.

19. Glover to Humphreys, 9 April and 15 May 1951, in 'Buddhism by Christmas Humphreys', DM 02.0228 5, Penguin Archives. The latter missive reports that 3,000 of these copies were shipped to the USA and 2,500 to Australia.

20. Humphreys to Glover, 16 October 1956, in 'Yoga: Ernest Wood', DM 1107/02.0448 2, Penguin Archives.

Studies during the 1950s.[21] Although published in popular edition,
the 1959 Pelican book is densely written and omits any illustrations
of yoga asana, although some photographs of Swami Vishnudevananda were tentatively suggested by the author.[22] It would have
been very hard for an uneducated reader to wade through its philosophical analysis and descriptions of concentration and breathing
exercises. Nevertheless, at least two readers were inspired to write
to Penguin asking for the author's address in pursuit of further
instruction in yoga.[23] The title sold well; *Yoga* was reprinted in 1962,
1965 and 1970.

Penguin also published a translation of the *Bhagavad Gītā* in
1962, making the work easily accessible to all with an interest in
Indian religions at an affordable price: it was a standard book on
the Wheel of British Yoga reading list.[24] The translator, Juan Mascaró (1897–1987),[25] had already published and translated selections
of the Upaniṣads in 1938 with the well-established publisher John

21. Autobiographical sources on Ernest Wood include Wood (1936, 1959). Louis
Gainsborough, a devotee of Aurobindo, founded the American Academy of Asian
Studies in 1951; its current successor is the California Institute of Integral Studies.
As far as I am aware, a history of this interesting organisation has yet to be written,
but see Kripal (2007) and Goldman (2012).

22. Wood to Penguin Editorial Department, 11 January 1958, 'Yoga: Ernest
Wood', DM 1107/02.0448 2, Penguin Archives: 'As regards illustrations, I am not
in favour of these being very prominent as they must of necessity refer to the infe-
rior and more physical aspects of the subject. I am enclosing some small sketches
made under my direction by an artist here, and also some copies of poses by Swami
Vishnudevananda, whom I know personally, and from whom I have permission to
use and reproduce them, with due acknowledgement in the introductory notes, if
they are used.' Swami Vishnudevananda was one of the most popular exponents
of Swami Sivananda's teachings in Canada. The file also noted that original prints
(which were not provided by Wood) would have been needed to reproduce the
images and that it would increase the cost of production considerably.

23. 'Yoga: Ernest Wood', DM 1107/02.0448 2, Penguin Archives.

24. For instance, these translations are specifically mentioned in Chris Stevens's
'Bookstall' on the back cover of *Yoga: Journal of the British Wheel of Yoga* 4 (Summer
1970).

25. Juan Mascaró was born in Majorca and became interested in the occult as
a teenager. Wanting to understand the original sources of what he read, he was
inspired to study Sanskrit. Mascaró read modern and Oriental languages at Down-
ing College, Cambridge and was for some time a Professor of English at the University of Barcelona. Returning to Cambridge after the Spanish Civil War, Mascaró
worked on his translation of the *Bhagavad Gītā*, as well as supervising and occasionally lecturing on languages and religion at Cambridge. 'The Bhagavad Gita', DM
1107/044 121 2, Penguin Archives. See also autobiographical material in Mascaró
(1999).

Murray in their 'Wisdom of the East' series, under the title of *The Himalayas of the Soul* in 1938.[26] Penguin bought the rights to reprint *The Himalayas of the Soul* and brought it out under the title of *The Upaniṣads* in 1965.[27] Sections of the Upaniṣads had been available in English from the early nineteenth century, although they were printed in India. The first easily accessible English translation was Max Müller's, published by Oxford University's Clarendon Press in 1879. The transition from the Upaniṣads availability only in distinguished hardback copy in 1928 to its appearance as a popular paperback in 1965 is illustrative of the change in popularity and accessibility over the twentieth century.[28]

Penguin's aim was to deliver popular literature with decent standards of scholarship. However, there is no evidence in the Penguin archive that any other Sanskrit scholar was consulted about the accuracy of Mascaró's translation.[29] A few years later Professor Ninian Smart, who had studied Sanskrit at Yale and was pioneering the secular study of comparative religion at Birmingham and Lancaster Universities during the 1960s, wrote to complain that Mascaró's translation of the Upaniṣads and *Bhagavad Gītā* were 'very

---

26. John Murray began the 'Wisdom of the East' series from 1905 and published a wide range of titles, including *The Sayings of Lao Tzu* (1905), *The Teachings of Zoroaster and the Philosophy of the Parsi Religion* (1905), *Brahmana Knowledge: An Outline of the Philosophy of Vedanta* (1907), *A Feast of Lanterns: An Anthology of Chinese Poetry* (1916), *The Secret Rose Garden of Sa'd ud din Mahmud Shabistari* (1920), *Anthology of Ancient Egyptian Poems* (1925) and many more, including selections from the *Ṛg Veda*, the *Panchatantra*, and the *Bhagavad Gītā*. Archives relating to John Murray publications up to 1920 are held at the National Library of Scotland and some materials are still held privately by the John Murray family.

27. Mr A to D.L. Duguid Esq., Penguin Books, dated 29 April 1961, writes: 'The current interest in Eastern philosophy and "religion" seems waxing rather than waning; and in light of the degree of success that has attended Penguin's Buddhist efforts, I should imagine there need be little fear of not finding an adequate market for a selection of the Upanishads.' In 'The Upanishads', DM 1107/044 163 8, Penguin Archives.

28. Additionally, the Theosophical Society produced translations of the Upaniṣads in 1896, 1894, 1918 and 1920.

29. The single anonymous reviewer for Penguin commented: 'I think it is fair to say that he is the only translator I have come across who has managed to present the Upaniṣads, or a part of them, in decent, readable, literary English; and as far as I am able to judge – which can only be by comparison to other translations, since I have no Sanskrit, to do so without distortion of their context or meaning . . .' 'The Upanishads', DM 1107/044 163 8, Penguin Archives.

poor and we should find substitutes'.[30] But, within limits, accuracy at Penguin was secondary to sales, and Mascaró's translations sold well and were reprinted several times.[31]

From the correspondence in the Penguin files, it appears that Mascaró maintained a strong personal interest in his publications. He wrote to Penguin when they requested permission to reprint his earlier translation of the Upaniṣads: 'I am glad that they become well known as I am certain, I think I know well, that the Upaniṣads are amongst the greatest conceptions and visions of man on our earth.'[32] There was much correspondence regarding approval of his proofs, and one of Penguin's internal memos remarks:

> I have had Juan Mascaró on the phone from Cambridge worry [sic] about his proofs . . . I think we should let him have is way, as this means so much to him, and he has a true mystic's obstinacy, if he is opposed he will pay you a long visit and charm you into agreeing with him . . .[33]

Regardless of his accuracy as a translator, Penguin ensured that Mascaró's translations reached a wide audience: as mentioned above, both Mascaró's Upaniṣads and *Bhagavad Gītā* regularly featured in the reading lists and on the book stalls of the British Wheel of Yoga's journal *Yoga* and remain in print.[34]

Hari Prashad Shastri and the Shanti Sadan

The Penguin series on world religions also commissioned a book on Hinduism but it proved rather difficult for Glover to find an appropriate author. In 1948, Humphreys suggested a Dr H.P. Shastri 'who has an enormous following, is a genuine scholar and is a very fine lecturer'.[35] Hari Prashad Shastri (1882–1956) was at this time teaching a particular form of Indian philosophy, Advaita Vedānta, and meditation in London under the name of the Shanti Sadan

30. Memo from RH to JV dated 18 March 1969, in 'The Upanishads', DM 1107/044 163 8, Penguin Archives.

31. 'The Upanishads', DM 1107/044 163 8, and 'The Bhagavad Gita', DM 1107/044 121 2, Penguin Archives.

32. 'The Bhagavad Gita', DM 1107/044 121 2, Penguin Archives.

33. Ibid.

34. For example, see: 'Chris Stevens' Book Stall', *Yoga* 3 (Spring 1970) and *Yoga* 11 (Spring 1972), back cover.

35. Humphreys to Glover, 23 October 1948, in 'Buddhism by Christmas Humphreys', DM 02.0228 5, Penguin Archives.

(Peace Temple). It is likely that it was Shastri who wrote a book for Penguin that was not considered suitable; the title appears to have been dropped until an alternative author was found and *Hinduism* came out under Pelican in 1961.[36] Despite the disapproval of the Penguin editorial staff, Shastri had developed a small but influential following among the intellectual elite.

Shastri arrived in London in 1929 and was initially engaged to lecture at the Theosophical Society's meeting in Holborn (central London) for a period of a few months. Theosophical politics eventually terminated this arrangement, perhaps because Shastri was clearly promoting his own teaching. But this association lasted long enough for a nucleus of interested students to become established. Shastri has been described as a charismatic speaker who mixed erudition with clarity; the current president of the Shanti Sadan remembered Shastri as embodying a quality of 'genuineness', and described him as a speaker who did not try to manipulate his audience.[37]

By 1935, Shastri had built up enough of a following in London to start a newsletter. During the second half of the 1930s, around twenty to thirty people regularly attended the weekly worship (called Satsang). Shastri gave public lectures on the Upaniṣads, the *Bhagavad Gītā*, Buddhism, Taoism and comparative religion and philosophy. Some of these were held at the centre's headquarters, others at Caxton Hall. Occasionally, Shastri lectured out of London.[38] During the 1930s, the Shanti Sadan occasionally took out advertisements in *The Times* for lectures in 'Yoga or Spiritual Training' or 'Eastern Philosophy and Mysticism'.[39]

36. Penguin to A. Basu, 20 September 1954: 'We have had for some time a book on Hinduism written several years ago, more or less at our suggestion but which on receiving we did not feel was all together quite suitable for its purpose. At the same time its existence has rather restricted us from making enquiries in other quarters.' After approaching several academics, Penguin finally settled on a manuscript written by K.M. Sen (the grandfather of the Nobel Prize economist Amartya Kumar Sen who had recently completed his PhD at Trinity College, Cambridge). In 'Hinduism by K.M. Sen', 02.0515, Penguin Archives.

37. Personal interview with Dr A.M. Halliday, President of the Shanti Sadan (13 September 2006).

38. For examples see the *Shanti-Sadan Bulletin* (1935–41) and *Shanti Sevak: A Quarterly Magazine* (1942–49). For a while there were study groups outside of London, but these dissolved; London remains the only continuous location of group meetings.

39. Classified ads, *The Times*, 3 March 1938, p. 1, col. B, and 14 January 1944, p. 6.

According to autobiographical and hagiographical accounts, Shastri was born into a Brahmin family in the United Provinces and took a doctorate in Sanskrit at the university in Varanasi (Benares). Although exact details are unclear, he apparently held a number of academic positions teaching philosophy and eventually accepted teaching positions at the Imperial University and Waseda University in Tokyo between 1916 and 1918. According to the Shanti Sadan, Shastri then accepted an invitation from Dr Sun Yat-sen, the founder and first President of the Republic of China, to live and work in that country between 1918 and 1929.[40] After the death of his Chinese patron in 1925, political instability probably led Shastri to leave China for London.

While still living in the United Provinces, though exactly when is not clear, Dr Shastri was accepted as a disciple by a man known as Shri Dadaji Maharaj, born Narayana Prasad (1854–1910). This guru maintained a regular job as a clerk on the Indian railways, was married and had children. However, Shri Dadaji, or 'Shri Dada', was seen as an enlightened saint, and groups of disciples would form around him as he moved from city to city with his employment. Shastri wrote a detailed account of his guru's life in *The Heart of the Eastern Mystical Teaching* (1948), where he recounts that Shri Dada's teachings included a kind of leitmotif claiming yoga's spiritual affinity with Britain: for example, according to Shri Dada, 'There is only one country in the West which is fit to attain eminence in the realm of spirituality and it is Angala Desha [Britain]' (Shastri 1948: 268). Apparently, Shri Dada felt a personal 'call' to Britain; Shastri reports that his guru was overheard praying to Shiva thus:

> '. . . Yet the supreme task which Thou has given me still awaits fulfil-
> ment. The only Adwaita, based on the traditions of Manu and Iksh-
> waku, is not yet transmitted to Angala Desha, where many of Thy
> daughters and sons are to incarnate and to have the privilege of being
> pioneers in the spiritual field . . . but if my wishes are worth being
> listened to, I would remain in an obscure spot near Anupashar on the
> Ganges and sing out the remaining breaths of my life in Thy praise . . .'
> (Shastri 1948: 105).

Shastri's understanding was that, among the British population, there could be found reincarnated Indians ready to receive the

---

40. Shastri was appointed Professor of Philosophy at Nankwan College and also served as dean of the Foreign Department of Hardoon University at Shanghai.

teachings of Advaita Vedānta. This belief would have encouraged his resolve to teach in Britain and also fortified the confidence of his new British followers. Shastri also claimed to have been a disciple of Swami Rama Tirtha (1873–1906) and wrote an alternative hagiography of Tirtha's life which was highly critical of Tirtha's main disciples who remained in India (Shastri n.d.; Rinehart 1999: 34–5).

Shastri's teaching offered a particular appeal to the well-educated British middle classes.[41] Shastri tells a British devotee that the 'Truth' will be conveyed in Britain 'without any show, without any drum-beating', commanding him to 'practice spirituality in obscurity' (Shastri 1948: 262–3). This idea that spirituality is properly a private matter fitted in well with middle-class English sensibilities. This attitude would have been advantageous for Shastri in finding sponsors in Britain and would have encouraged more Britons to consider taking Shastri's teaching seriously. There was a certain similarity to some of the patrons of the Theosophical Society, of which well-educated women of independent means were particularly active supporters. The second president of the Shanti Sadan, Marjorie Waterhouse, had graduated in 1930 from Girton College, Cambridge. In 1943, an elderly woman with a long-term interest in meditation endowed a house in Ladbroke Grove, London for the use of the organisation.

The yoga Shastri taught was not focused on asana, but on concentration exercises contemplating the nature of reality as defined by Advaita Vedānta.[42] Shastri's somewhat idiosyncratic interpretation explains that the essence of Advaita Vedānta (non-dualist soteriology) as taught by the eighth-century philosopher Adi Śaṅkara is embodied in the couplet:

> *Brahman sattyam jagan mithya*
> *Jivo Brhamaiva na parah.*

Which Shastri translates as:

41. For example, there is a photograph of Shastri in the Shanti Sadan with Sarvepalli Radhakrishnan, the first Spalding Professor of Comparative Religions at Oxford who later became President of India. The Shanti Sadan's emphasis on great ideas may have alienated those who were not confident of their intellectual abilities.

42. Shastri's interpretation and translation of Adi Śaṅkara is at variance with contemporary scholarly understandings: for example, Potter (1981). For a more contemporary assessment published by the Shanti Sadan publishing house, see Alston (1980–89).

> God is real, the world is illusory
> The individual soul and God are one and the same (Shastri
> 1957: 21).

Contemporary translations of this couplet would stress that Brah-
man is an impersonal divine without attributes, whereas translating
it as 'God' implies an equivalence with Judeo-Christian ideas of a
divine with a particular personality. For Shastri, the goal of yoga,
and human life, is to experience this statement as truth; he recom-
mends his students meditate on his translation of this statement, or
an equivalent statement such as 'Know that Allah is nearer than the
neck-vein' from the Quran (Shastri 1957: 41, 45). This knowledge,
embodied, frees the individual from all fear and sorrow as well as
the cycle of rebirth assumed in Indian culture. For his practical programme of yoga, Shastri suggests an hour's practice first thing in
the morning. There are several parts to the recommended practice:
reflecting on a scriptural text, concentration on a light in the middle
of the body and repeating the word 'om' as a mantra 108 times.
Shastri suggested breathing exercises, or pranayama, to assist with
relaxation and concentration. Initially, he recommended that the
interested reader commit to this programme for six weeks to test its
effect (Shastri 1957: 59–60). For members of the Shanti Sadan, meditation exercises might be modified in personal consultation.

Besides these practical techniques, Shastri taught understanding
and tolerance between religion and cultures. According to Shastri's presentation, Advaita Vedānta asserts that all paths of religion
point towards the same ultimate reality. In *Yoga,* he presents the
life stories of three 'yogis', his two personal teachers Rama Tirtha and Shri Dada as well as Kōbō-Daishi (774–835), also known
as Kūkai, the founder of the 'True Word' tradition of Buddhism
in Japan. Shastri reports of Shri Dada explicitly teaching that all
lovers of God are on the same path and should be respected. This
theology is described as 'universalism' by the current president of
the Shanti Sadan. Therefore, Shanti Sadan members who wanted
to remain Christian could still incorporate the practical techniques
into their lives and test their effects. In 1943, *The Times* (London)
found this universalism unusual enough to comment on the language used in an unveiling ceremony of a painting of Krishna at the
newly opened Shanti Sadan; the reporter noted that the unveiling
was done with prayers to the 'Inner Ruler worshipped as Krishna,

Christ and Allah'.[43] In the 1940s, Shastri gave all his students yogic (Sanskrit) names, but members did not change their names publicly. The yogic names were used within the Shanti Sadan, to symbolise how the initiate 'sheds his earthly titles on entering the Path of the ancient and Royal Science of Yoga and assumes henceforth a new Name bestowed by the traditional Guru'.[44] This combination of seriousness, culture, erudition and discretion suited at least some middle-class English sensibilities.

By the time of Shastri's death in 1956, the Shanti Sadan was well established as a small circle of individuals continuing in the tradition of quiet dedication to Shastri's articulation of Advaita Vedānta. While the Shanti Sadan still survives, it has remained numerically small. However, Shastri's *Yoga* circulated widely in the 1960s and '70s and has been kept in print by the Shanti Sadan.[45] The major London bookshop Foyles used Shastri's manuscript to publish its handbook on *Yoga* which was printed in 1957, 1958, 1966, 1974 and 1976. Shastri has maintained a quiet legacy in the domain of yoga in Britain with a small group of dedicated initiates. The yoga of this group emphasise Vedantic realisation, personal meditation exercises, and the company of like-minded ethical people.[46]

The Atlantis Bookshop and Paul Brunton

From 1922, Watkins had competition from the Atlantis Bookshop, a ten-minute walk from Cecil Court on Museum Street, near the British Museum and Library. They shared customers with a friendly sense of competition. Atlantis emphasised Western Magic in its booklists, while Watkins traditionally focused on Theosophical, Indian and other Asian movements.[47] Atlantis was founded by

43. 'Painting of Hindu Deity', *The Times*, 18 January 1943, p. 6, col. C. The article notes that 'Hindu, Moslem, and Christians' were in attendance as well as the Nepalese minister.

44. *Shanti Sevak: A Quarterly Magazine* (1942).

45. 'Dr H.P. Shastri: Obituary', *The Times*, 6 February 1956, p. 12.

46. In 2006, Halliday numbered those that regularly attend the centre at around fifty (personal interview, 13 September 2006). He notes that the Sadan's journal has a circulation of about 500 and that the internet has vastly increased the number of those interested in purchasing literature from the society. The centre in London and a small centre in Australia remain the only ones directly affiliated to Shastri.

47. The Atlantis Bookshop established its own small publishing company, the Neptune Press, in 1935 to release esoteric and occult titles. After Brunton's departure, the Neptune Press made the turn towards Western esotericism more apparent

Michael Houghton and Paul Brunton (born as Ralph Hurst [1898–1981]), who shared a flat on Tavistock Square around the time of the First World War (Hurst 1989: 44–8).[48] It appears that Brunton was the son of undistinguished working-class parents: the 1901 census lists his father as a factory hand in a margarine plant.[49] That Brunton later led his son to believe that his roots were in more select Hampstead is perhaps a reflection of the esoteric, spiritual circles of London in the 1920s and '30s, populated as it was by the cultural elite of Bloomsbury (Hurst 1989: 148). Houghton and Brunton and their friends frequented meetings of the Theosophical Society and the Spiritualist Society, the latter being particularly popular after the First World War (see Hurst 1989: 44–8). During the 1920s, Brunton was writing articles in the journals *Success* and the *Occult Review* under the name of Raphael Hurst.

During the first quarter of the twentieth century in particular, yoga and occultism had some interesting links in the esoteric milieux of Britain. Aleister Crowley (1875–1947) advertised his *Book Four, Part I* (1913), which combines reflections on the *Yoga Sūtras* of Patañjali with European, ceremonial magick, in periodicals such as the *International Psychic Gazette* which explored a variety of alternative topics.[50] The pages of this journal often featured items from Theosophists, but also about physical culture, Indian mystics, will-development courses, palm reading, 'psycho-photography' and spiritual healing; advertisements featured books from the publisher Rider & Co., Theosophical and New Thought publishing

when it published Aleister Crowley's works and also put out pagan revivalist Gerald Gardner's practical book *High Magic's Aid* in 1949 before the repeal of the Witchcraft Act in 1951. Personal interview with Geraldine Beskin (12 January 2007).

48. For esoteric circles in interwar London, see also Owen (2004, 2006).

49. The only information Brunton published about his origins was that he was born in London in 1898. However, the 1901 Census of England and Wales records the existence of a three-year-old Ralph Hurst, the name by which Brunton's first wife knew him (Hurst 1989: 128).

50. Founded by Crowley and associate George Cecil Jones around 1907, the Initiatory Order of the A∴A∴ also was based on a fusion of ceremonial magick and ideas drawn from yoga. Crowley himself learned some meditation and knowledge of Indian religions while travelling in India in 1901 from Ponnambalam Ramananathan, the Solicitor General of Ceylon who had a previous association with Allan Bennett (1872–1933), who knew Crowley, both being members of the Hermetic Order of the Golden Dawn.

houses.[51] That there were none directly advertising 'yoga courses' at this time reinforces the hypothesis that most yoga was learnt from printed material in Britain during this period. However, within the pages of this periodical can be found an advertisement for a 'Divine Healing Centre' near Victoria in London which featured interviews with 'Brother Ramananda' (with Sister Sita in attendance).[52]

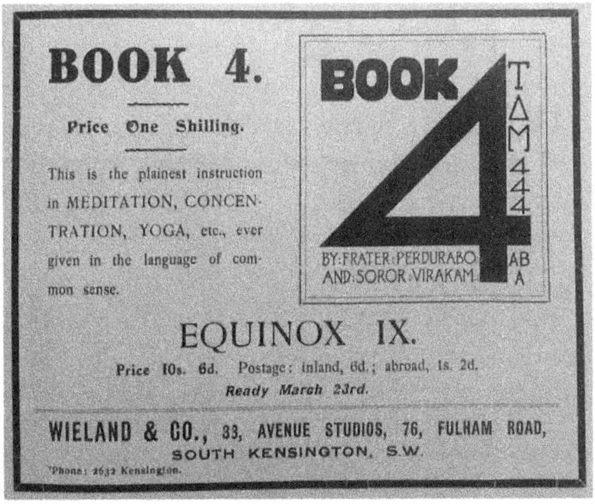

Fig. 1.2 Advertisement for Aleister Crowley's *Book 4* from the *International Psychic Gazette*, March 1913, p. 243

During the early years of the twentieth century, yoga was a subject of interest for occult initiatory orders such as the Order of Oriental Templars (OTO), and often associated with sexual magic and ideas drawn from Indian tantra.[53] In 1920, Crowley experimented with living out his philosophy in the residential setting of the Abbey of Thelma, attracting much attention from the British tabloid press. Thus yoga, as a part of the occult, became more popularly associated with wild and immoral behaviour. While repelling the majority, this also increased the curiosity of a minority. Crowley

51. In 1925, an associate of Crowley, J.F.C. Fuller, published *Yoga: A Study of the Mystical Philosophy of the Brahmins and Buddhists* with William Rider & Son, which subtly influenced understandings of yoga.

52. *International Psychic Gazette*, May 1913, p. 308.

53. It is likely that these ideas of sexual magic and tantra were introduced by Carl Kellner (1850–1905) and Franz Hartmann (1838–1912); for more detail on the origins and nature of their understandings, see Baier (2018), Bogdan (2013) and Djurdjevic (2012).

continued to lecture on yoga in the 1930s, publishing his *Eight Lec-tures on Yoga* in 1939. Crowley's teachings on Thelma and on yoga are nearly synonymous in their goals. He unites what he calls "mag-ick" – defined as 'the science and art of causing change to occur in conformity with the Will' – with an understanding of yoga as 'Union with the Absolute' (Crowley 1939: 9–10).[54] Crowley's ideas on yoga and Thelma would resurface in the 1960s as various coun-ter-cultural movements interacted.[55]

A fascinating figure called Rollo Ahmed also billed himself as an occult yoga teacher during the 1930s. Based largely in Brighton, he was also associated with Aleister Crowley, the Wiccan Doreen Valiente (1922–1999) and the popular novelist Dennis Wheatley (1897–1977).[56] However, not all yoga presentations at this time were directly associated with the occult. There may also have been a man called Sri Nandi teaching yoga in Hampstead, North London, possi-bly as early as 1939.[57] A first incarnation of a Ramakrishna Vedānta Centre also existed in London from around 1934.[58]

54. 'The principles of Yoga, and the spiritual results of Yoga, are demonstrated in every conscious and unconscious happening. This is that which is written in The Book of the Law – Love is the law, love under will – for Love is the instinct to unite, and the act of uniting. But this cannot be done indiscriminately, it must be done "under will," that is, in accordance with the nature of the particular units concerned . . .'; for the definition of magick, see Crowley (1939: 76). For more on Crowley, see Bogdan (2006, 2010, 2013) and Bogdan and Starr (2012).

55. In particular, the Atlantis Bookshop was a site where Western Magic and various ideas of yoga mingled. The journal *Gandalf's Garden* 3 (1969/70), pp. 27–9, had an article on 'Aleister Crowley Revisited' (see Chapter 5 of this volume for more on *Gandalf's Garden*). See also Urban (2006).

56. Chris Josiffe is researching Rollo Amhed's biography; from conversations with him it seems likely that Amhed could have picked up his knowledge of yoga from Yogi Ramacharaka's books, although research is ongoing. Amhed fits well into the American travelling yoga salesman 'type' described by Deslippe (2018) and is likely to have originated from this milieu (Josiffe 2017). Many of Dennis Wheat-ley's pulp-fiction novels had occult themes, e.g. *The Devil Rides Out* (book 1934, film 1968); during the 1970s, he oversaw 'The Dennis Wheatley Library of the Occult' series with publishers Sphere.

57. Clark (n.d.) and 'The Long-standing Import', *Yoga & Health* 8 (1971), p. 54. However, I was able to find no mention of yoga in the local paper, the *Hampstead and Highgate Express*, during the year of 1939; but a teacher by this name definitely appears to have been in Hampstead in the early 1960s.

58. Swami Avyaktananda who founded the centre diverged from central direc-tives. In 1948 Swami Ghananda re-founded the Ramakrishna Vedānta Centre from a flat in Belsize Park, and Swami Avyaktananda moved to Bath where he continued teaching independently. Personal interview with Swami Tripurananda (1 August 2006).

While immersed in this exploration of alternative religions Brunton first came into contact with yoga and Indian religiosity. In the early 1930s, he travelled to India and wrote a travelogue of his experience in seeking spiritual enlightenment. The resulting manuscript was published as *A Search in Secret India* (1934) under the name of Paul Brunton and it was by this name, or the initials 'PB', that Brunton was known for the remainder of his life. In 1935, the Atlantis Bookshop established its own small publishing company, the Neptune Press, to bring out esoteric and occult titles. Some time after Brunton's return from India, Brunton and Houghton parted company.[59] Houghton retained ownership of the Museum Street bookshop and the Neptune Press, which subsequently turned more strongly towards Western esotericism, publishing Aleister Crowley's works. It was also the first publisher of pagan revivalist Gerald Gardner's practical book *High Magic's Aid* (1949). Despite this shift away from Indian spirituality, the Atlantis Bookshop continued as a networking hub for alternative spirituality, and the clientele of the Atlantis and Watkins Bookshops overlapped throughout the twentieth century.[60]

Meanwhile, Paul Brunton continued to influence understandings of yoga. *A Search in Secret India*, detailing Brunton's personally transformative meetings with mystics and holy men of India, was extremely popular, being constantly reissued in the 1950s and '60s, and remains in print today.[61] In 1971, the popular magazine *Yoga & Health* claimed that Brunton's books 'probably turned more people onto the path of Yoga than any other books of their kind'.[62] *A Search in Secret India* develops the idea of the spiritual 'quest', a kind of twentieth-century *Pilgrim's Progress* for middle-class seekers. It culminates with Brunton's encounter with Ramana Maharshi (1879–1950), who lived on a hill near the south Indian city of Tiruvannamalai. Brunton is widely credited with bringing the Maharshi

59. This parting was reportedly precipitated by Brunton's refusal to publish some of Houghton's poetry in his book. Personal interview with Geraldine Beskin (12 January 2007).

60. Around 1962, Wally Collins, a friend of Houghton, assumed ownership of the bookshop and Michael Houghton died not long afterwards. The Collins family reinvigorated the stock and set the shop on a firmer financial footing, according to Collins's daughter Geraldine Beskin who took over management of the shop after her father died. Personal interview with Geraldine Beskin (12 January 2007).

61. It was reissued in 1955, 1957, 1964, 1965, 1970 and 1983.

62. *Yoga & Health* 6 (1971), p. 46.

to the attention of spiritual seekers worldwide.[63] However, Brunton's ultimate conclusion is that the 'true guru' is the 'inner guide' or 'higher self'. Brunton also corresponded with some readers and encouraged them to treat him as a guru figure. He travelled in India during the 1940s and published several more influential books on yoga. He developed a small following of disciples, but remained a largely distant figure living with sympathetic supporters in New Zealand, America and Switzerland.[64] His books were re-popularised in the 1970s when excerpts appeared in the journal *Yoga & Health* and he regularly appeared on the Wheel of Yoga reading lists.

Allen & Unwin and Gerald Yorke

Publishers Allen & Unwin played an important part in popularising yoga in Britain, with perhaps their most significant title being B.K.S. Iyengar's *Light on Yoga* (1966). Elizabeth de Michelis argues that *Light on Yoga* 'played a major role in raising postural practice standards to higher levels of performance' and became 'the acknowledged point of reference in the sense that no modern postural yoga practitioner or school could afford to ignore its existence' (de Michelis 2004: 211). As will be described later, *Light on Yoga* helped convince the Inner London Education Authority to allow yoga as an approved subject in the capital's adult education syllabus.

The best-known story of how *Light on Yoga* was 'discovered' by Allen & Unwin relies on serendipity and an implicit concept of God's grace. B.K.S. Iyengar was initially brought to London as personal yoga teacher to the violin virtuoso Yehudi Menuhin. According to an oft-repeated story, two of Menuhin's personal friends

---

63. For more on the Ramana Maharshi, see Forsthoefel (2005: 37–53). For example, British Wheel of Yoga founder Wilfred Clark started a correspondence with Jim Pym based on their mutual interest in this figure (personal interview with Jim Pym, 7 July 2005). B.K.S. Iyengar lists him along with Ramakrishna Paramahamsa, Swami Ramdas of Maharashtra, Jñāneśvar and Kabir as a sage who 'evolved straight into kaivalya (freedom) without experiencing all the intermediate states of life or the various stages of yoga' (B.K.S. Iyengar 1993a: 4).

64. There are two published sources about the life of Paul Brunton, one by his son Kenneth Hurst (1989) and another within the autobiography of Jeffrey Moussaieff Masson (2003 [1993]). Hurst's biography is reverential, respectful and full of gratitude towards his father. In a direct challenge to this account, Masson described the painful disillusionment he experienced having grown up with Paul Brunton as his family's guru. Masson is better known for his anti-psychiatric bestseller *Against Therapy* (1989).

and Iyengar's yoga students, Angela Marris (1916–2007) and Beatrice Harthan (1902–1998), accompanied the Menuhin family during their annual stay in Gstaad, Switzerland, where Menuhin had founded and oversaw an annual month-long music festival. During this festival, Menuhin employed Iyengar's services for a daily yoga class.[65] Iyengar showed these women two chapters of a book he was planning on writing, 'to help all his pupils during the eleven months of each year' when he was in India. In their free time, Ms Harthan and Ms Marris offered to type the manuscript out to make it more presentable. As the women found European typewriters difficult for accurate touch-typing, Beatrice Harthan put a copy of her manuscript into her briefcase to re-type on her return to London.[66] Returning from the airport in London, Harthan 'paid an unpremeditated visit to [the] Buddhist Society Summer School' and, arriving late, took one of the few empty seats, which happened to be next to Gerald Yorke, who worked for Allen & Unwin publishers sourcing India and esoteric books.[67] Yorke reportedly whispered to Harthan that he was looking for a new book on yoga to replace Theos Bernard's work, *Hatha Yoga,* which had been in circulation for fifteen years (Bernard 1939, 1950).[68] During the break, Harthan produced Iyengar's manuscript at which Yorke 'became at once most excited about it'.[69]

The true story may be less serendipitous. Yorke was known to have attended the Buddhist Society's summer school and had been working for Rider publishers sourcing books on Hinduism and Buddhism throughout the 1950s.[70] It is therefore likely that Hart-

65. Sponsored by Menuhin to teach him during this festival, Iyengar also taught the Italian musician and future yoga teacher Vanda Scaravelli and Jiddu Krishnamurti for several summers (personal interview with Angela Marris, former secretary of Menuhin's Asian Music Circle in London, 30 June 2005).

66. Personal interview with Angela Marris (30 June 2005).

67. For more on Gerald Joseph Yorke (1901–1983) and his overlaps with occult networks, see Newcombe (2013), Richmond (2011) and Verter (1997: 175–98).

68. For more on Bernard's life and influence, see Hackett (2012) and Love (2010).

69. B. Harthan, 'A Great Teacher of Yoga', *Bhavan's Journal,* August 1975. In the archives of the RIMYI, Pune.

70. Letter from Mr Gerald J. Yorke to Mrs Eileen Pearcey, 30 August 1964: 'Your 22 August. Please forgive delay in replying as I have been at the Buddhist summer school . . .' and letter from Mr Gerald J. Yorke to Philip Unwin, 25 February 1964: 'I come up to London from Forthampton normally once a month for a meeting of the Council of the Buddhist Society . . .' 'Yorke, G', AUC 856/20, Allen & Unwin Archives. Rider, now an imprint of Random House, has not kept any archival

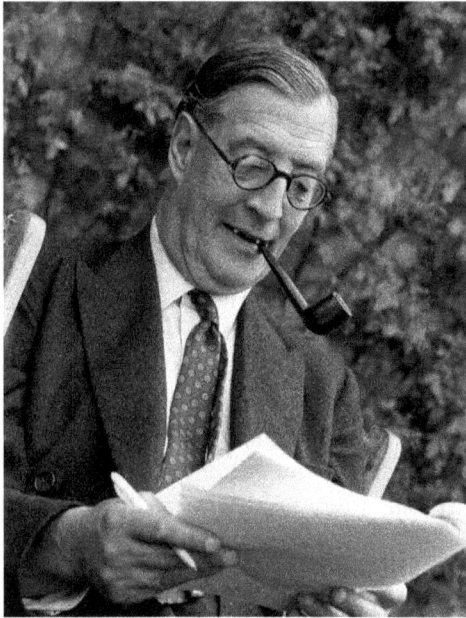

Fig. 1.3 Gerald Yorke (Bodhi) reading a paper in his favourite chair on the verandah with his iconic pipe in his mouth (late 1960s). Photograph courtesy of Michael Yorke.

han, armed with Iyengar's manuscript, sought him out at this venue in 1962 (Taraporewala 1978: 197).[71] Allen & Unwin correspondence about B.K.S. Iyengar begins in April 1964, when Yorke wrote to Philip Unwin about the 'extensive revision' of 'A Projected book on Hatha Yoga by BKS Iyengar', suggesting that Yorke had seen an earlier draft manuscript.[72] Iyengar's student, B.I. Taraporewala (1978: 195–6), reported that Iyengar had been working on the book since 1960. According to Taraporewala, a legal journalist in Bombay, it was rumoured that an unnamed Bombay publisher was interested in producing a book of asana instruction; Taraporewala first showed photographs of his teacher to this publisher in 1956.[73] This

material relating to titles on yoga for the pre-war period (personal correspondence with Jean Rose, Library Manager, Random House Group Archive & Library).

71. 'In 1962 I made contact with the late Gerald York [*sic*] who was the reader at various publishers, including Allen & Unwin and Ryder [*sic*]. The result was that he strongly recommended 'Light on Yoga' to Allan & Unwin [*sic*] as a much needed masterpiece on the philosophy and practice of Yoga'. B. Harthan, 'The Beginning of the Iyengar Movement in Britain', typewritten manuscript in the archives of the Iyengar Yoga Institute, Maida Vale.

72. Letter from Yorke to Unwin, 20 April 1964, in 'Yorke, G', AUC 856/20, Allen & Unwin Archives.

73. Letter from Yorke to Unwin, 29 July 1964: 'I am so glad that you are going to make an offer for *Light on Yoga*. I have written to Iyengar urging him to accept the 50

was the year that Yogendra's *Yoga Asanas Simplified* was reissued in India in an affordable 'popular' edition with expectations of attracting large numbers of middle-class Indian book-buyers.[74]

Taraporewala claims to have developed the format used in *Light on Yoga* in dialogue with this unspecified Bombay publisher. In contrast to other books on asana, 'it was decided that some text had to be written to show the technique of performing the asana by describing the intermediate stages whereby one reached the final pose' (Taraporewala 1978: 196).[75] Additionally, it was decided that further information on each pose was to be presented in a specific format:

> First the name of the asana was explained and a brief note given about the personality or legend connected with the name. Next, the technique was described in numbered paragraphs step by step in a language as simple as possible. Last, the benefits of the asana were stated (Taraporewala 1978: 196).

The process of composition, according to Taraporewala, was collaborative, although it was always clear it was Iyengar's book:

> Every few weeks Iyengar would come to Bombay [from Pune] with handwritten notes ... Every Saturday evening after the asana sessions, Iyengar, a friend or two, my wife and I would proceed to the flat of Smt. Martha Wartenburger, one of Iyengar's oldest pupils, with our papers and files. There, after refreshments ... we would read the typescript prepared by me. Martha would ... tell me that I should yield to the words selected by Iyengar for after all it was his book and not mine and I would hold on to the view that the word did not

---

advance, which will disappoint him as apparently he spent 200 on getting all the 600 odd photographs taken . . .' in 'Yorke, G', AUC 856/20, Allen & Unwin Archives.

74. The headline that caught Penguin's attention was '"Yoga Asanas Simplified": New Popular edition will make sales history! By Sri Yogendra' in *The Book Lover Everyman's Literary Guide* 3/22 (June 1956), back cover, in 'Yoga: Ernest Wood', DM 1107/02.0448 2, Penguin Archives. For more on Yogendra, see Goldberg (2016: 2–74), Rodrigues (1982) and Singleton (2010).

75. Also letter from Gerald Yorke to Philip Unwin, 3 November 1964, 'Yorke, G', AUC 856/20, Allen & Unwin Archives: 'Moreover it [*Light on Yoga*] is the first book to illustrate in photographs how to get into the final position, instead of merely an illustration of the final position, for all asanas etc. dealt with. Since the more complicated postures nearly always start from the final posture of a simpler exercise, there are, through the cross-referencing, up to ten illustrations for any given posture – a unique feature.' However, S. Sundaram wrote a book in 1928 entitled *Yogic Physical Culture or The Secret of Happiness* which also contains intermediate stages of yoga asana and a similar format to *Light on Yoga*.

correctly reflect what was in Iyengar's mind . . . (Taraporewala 1978:
196–7).

Taraporewala was also responsible for referencing Iyengar's
asana to the personality or legend associated with the name. For this
he used a variety of traditional source books including the *Haṭha
Yoga Pradīpkā,* the *Gheranda Samhitā,* the *Śiva Samhitā,* the *Bhagavad
Gītā* and the Upaniṣads, Patañjali's *Yoga Sūtras,* and other standard
books on Indian philosophy (Taraporewala 1978: 196).[76] Officially,
Iyengar employed the services of Taraporewala to 're-English' the
manuscript and Taraporewala eventually received £250 of Iyengar's royalty money as payment for his work.[77]

Both Iyengar and Taraporewala have written that Gerald Yorke
made a major contribution in fine-tuning the English in *Light on
Yoga.* Iyengar later admitted that 'Though I was a teacher with thirty
years' experience, I had never attempted to write even an article on
yoga. Also my English in those days was not good' (B.K.S. Iyengar
1993a: xx). Iyengar reflected further on Yorke's influence:

> In his admonitions about my style, Mr Yorke was as forceful as my
> guru, Sri T. Krishnamacharya, was about my yoga . . . His encourage-
> ment was my touchstone, spurring me to express my thoughts in as
> exact and precise a form as possible. Since then [the editing of *Light
> on Yoga*] I hold him to be my 'literary guru' (B.K.S. Iyengar 1993a:
> xx–xxi).

As Taraporewala later reflected:

---

76. It is not clear whose idea it was to include explanations of the names and
legends of yoga postures. However, it is likely that Taraporewala did the research
and Iyengar and Yorke were responsible for the final form. Iyengar had wanted to
include a bibliography of these books in *Light on Yoga,* but Yorke felt that the bibliography presented was inadequate and unnecessary. Yorke to Unwin, 16 November 1964: 'P.S. I have turned down Iyengar's bibliography for the Light on Yoga as
not being adequate', in 'Yorke, G', AUC 856/20, Allen & Unwin Archives.

77. Letter Yorke to Unwin, 29 July 1964, *Light on Yoga by Iyengar,* 'He [Iyengar]
wants 7½% of his 10% royalty himself and the balance of 2½% to be paid to Mr B
I Taraporewala of Bombay . . . This is to pay Taraporewala for re-Englishing the
book . . . I have about a week's work in finely polishing the English and inking in
my pencilings', and Yorke to Unwin, 12 August 1964: 'I have had a minor flood of
letters from Mrs Harthan and Iyengar and a Photostat of the suggested contract
. . . the point is that Iyengar insists 25% of *all* royalties, but excluding *any* advance
royalties, should go to Taraporewala until the latter has received 250', in 'Yorke, G',
AUC 856/20, Allen & Unwin Archives.

His [Yorke's] command over the English language and his ability to condense and clarify are uncanny, and with a few excisions and revisions, he can improve what one has written . . . immeasurably (Taraporewala 1978: 197).

Light on Yoga owes its success partly to the considerable contribution of Gerald Yorke of Allen & Unwin in presenting Iyengar's concept to an English audience. Although the introduction outlined the religious/philosophical context of yoga, *Light on Yoga* delineates practical benefits without reference to anything overtly magical or religious. The result was a book that was often referred to as the 'Bible' of asana practice.[78]

After publication was agreed, Philip Unwin discussed with Yorke the best ways to publicise *Light on Yoga*. Iyengar had appeared on television in 1963 with Yehudi Menuhin and there was an attempt to arrange another appearance to publicise the new book. However, there appeared to be a problem with potential presenters' time as well as a refusal on Iyengar's part to appear next to yoga teachers unknown to him. In a letter sent to Yorke, Iyengar wrote:

It was suggested to me that I should take part with other yogis. As I was not known to them, nor I knew their practices, I did not like to involve my name or Mr Menuhin's name with them.[79]

Although no promotional television appearance materialised, the book launch was well publicised. They sent the book to major papers in India and to the BBC; leaflets were sent to British yoga groups and were also distributed at Iyengar's 1966 demonstration at the London Commonwealth Institute.[80] Exporting books to India was relatively problematic, involving import quotas and local politics. But Philip Unwin was confident: 'There is no doubt however that the book is going to India all the time in small quantities.'[81] Watkins Bookshop also continued to serve as an information centre

78. For example, 'BKS Iyengar being the author of what is virtually the Yoga Bible, "Light on Yoga" as well as being Yoga teacher to Yehudi Menuhin' (Tuft 1971).

79. Yorke to Unwin, 8 June 1966, in 'Yorke, G', AUC 856/20, Allen & Unwin Archives.

80. Wendy Harthan [*sic*] to Gerald Yorke, 11 May 1966, in 'Yorke, G', AUC 856/20, Allen & Unwin Archives.

81. Unwin to Yorke, 23 May 1966: 'Light on Yoga has made an excellent start and our own sales are approaching 2000 apart from the 1500 to Schocken Books New York. The Indian position is most tantalizing and we continually prod our agents there to agitate for the issue of further import licenses. Much seems to depend upon

for those in London who wished to purchase the book.[82] Although issued in a comparably expensive hardback edition with over 200 high-quality black-and-white plates, *Light on Yoga* was a commercial success for Allen & Unwin.[83]

Gerald J. Yorke was personally involved in introducing the first three major books circulating on 'hatha yoga' to the British public: Bernard's *Heaven Lies Within Us* [*On Yoga*] (1941) and *Hatha Yoga* (1950), Yesudian and Haich's *Yoga and Health* (1953), as well as *Light on Yoga* (1966). Both *Hatha Yoga* and *Yoga and Health* were considered very successful in terms of profit margins and sales figures. In recommending the publication of *Light on Yoga* to Allen & Unwin, Yorke wrote:

> The nearest equivalent to it that Rider have published in 1944 on my advice – is Theos Bernard's *Hatha Yoga* - 68 pp text with 37 pp. half tones and only describing 37 asana etc. but selling at 21/- has sold to date over 13,000 copies and still sells at the rate of just under 300 a year. The first imprint was 7,000.[84]

Allen & Unwin eventually settled on a first run of 5,000 copies for *Light on Yoga* and the final publishing price was a rather expensive £3.15s. in 1965.[85] However, Allen & Unwin's trust in Yorke's judgement wasn't only on account of Bernard's book. In 1952, Yorke read a revised manuscript of Selvarajan Yesudian and Elisabeth Haich's *Yoga and Health* for Unwin.[86] This book sold very well (at least 9,500

the local position of the author concerned and his relationship with official circles', in 'Yorke, G', AUC 856/20, Allen & Unwin Archives.

82. Wendy Harthan [*sic*] to Gerald Yorke, 11 May 1966: 'I have directed many many people to Watkins, from where we get new "starters" on Yoga!!', in 'Yorke, G', AUC 856/20, Allen & Unwin Archives.

83. Yorke to Iyengar cc. Philip Unwin, Mrs Harthan, RE: Light on Yoga, 30 November 1966: 'Sales seem to have passed the 4000 mark, so many congratulations', in 'Yorke, G', AUC 856/20, Allen & Unwin Archives.

84. Yorke to Unwin, 3 November 1964, in 'Yorke, G', AUC 856/20, Allen & Unwin Archives. According to the archivist for the Random House Group, which currently owns the Rider imprint, 'There is very little surviving from the early days of Rider'; and there are no surviving records for its yoga titles except for 'confidential contracts' (personal correspondence with Jean Rose, Library Manager, Random House Group).

85. There was a lot of correspondence about the price of the book; this final price is what appears on the jacket of the first edition.

86. Unwin to Yorke, 9 August 1952: 'Thank you very much for letting us see the copy of your report on *Sport & Yoga* which is returned herewith. We imagine that the MS has been considerably revised since you saw it last year – in fact, it is a fresh translation form the German made by an Englishman – and we shall therefore

in Britain by 1958)[87] and on this basis Unwin was willing to trust Yorke's advice on yoga books.[88]

From the late 1920s, Yorke corresponded with Aleister Crowley, eventually becoming an associate and providing financial support.[89] From the late 1920s, Yorke went on several retreats to practise magic and meditation, wandering in 'native garb' in North Africa for several months in 1930, as well as spending two months 'practising Yoga' in a Welsh cave in 1931 (Verter 1997: 181). Due to financial demands from Crowley, in March 1932 Yorke's father presented his son with an ultimatum: he must place his funds in a trusteeship or resign from the family businesses and sever all relations with the family.[90] When an opportunity appeared for Yorke to travel to China as a newspaper correspondent, Yorke agreed to place his funds in a trust (thus maintaining his inheritance) and went to work in China as an occasional correspondent for Reuters between 1932 and 1935 (Fleming 1934; Verter 1997: 192; Yorke 1935).[91] While

---

be most grateful if you will be good enough to read it again in its present form', in AVC/577/2, Allen & Unwin Archives.

87. Unwin to Yesudian, 10 June 1958: 'Our own sales of books are as follows *Yoga and Health* approximately 9,500 and the sales continue steadily', in 'X-Z 1958', AUC 820/17, Allen & Unwin Archives.

88. Unwin to Yorke, 5 November 1964: 'After our experience with Yesudian that we are perfectly happy to proceed with Iyengar on the basis of 4,000 first printing to be published at 50s. It would appear that an absolute minimum of 3,000 is certain and it would be surprising if we did not succeed in selling at least 1,000 in the States. I had not troubled Geoffrey Watkins on this one – he is very obliging and I don't like to worry him too often. It is usually difficult for one bookseller to advise one seriously as between 3,000 and 4,000', in 'Yorke, G', AUC 856/20, Allen & Unwin Archives.

89. The correspondence between Crowley and Yorke is held at the Warburg Institute, Yorke 84/116, Yorke D2–5, and Yorke 84/115. In the summer of 1927 Yorke was reading Aleister Crowley's *Book Four*, the first half of which is a rendering of Patañjali's *Yoga Sūtras* with techniques on asana and pranayama; the second half is an introduction to magical rituals from a more 'Western' esoteric perspective. By reading Yorke's esoteric exercise book kept at the request of Crowley, Verter found that Yorke had begun to study the books on this reading list in August 1927. The recommended reading list for a 'Student', the first grade in Crowley's system, included Vivekananda's *Rajah Yoga*, the *Śiva Samhitā*, the *Haṭha Yoga Pradīpikā*, Daoist teachings by Kwang Tze, as well as Crowley's works to date. See Crowley (1913) and Verter (1997: 181).

90. Verter (1997: 192), based on correspondence at the Warburg Institute.

91. See also 'British Correspondent Arrested', *The Times*, 11 March 1933, p. 9, col. C.

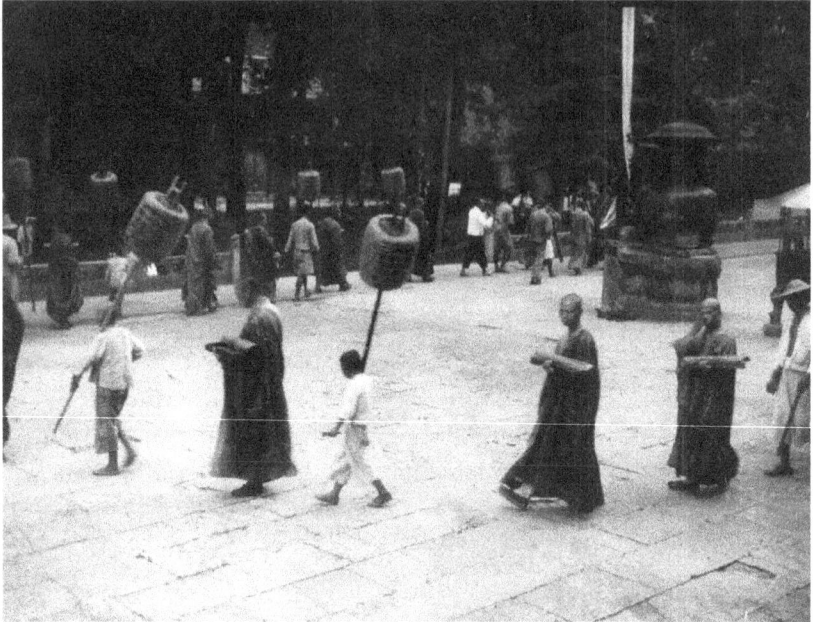

Fig. 1.4 Photograph taken by Gerald Yorke of an event at a monastery on his travels in China in the early 1930s. Photograph courtesy of Michael Yorke.

there, Yorke took the opportunity to experience life inside Buddhist monasteries.[92]

When he returned to Britain, Yorke adopted the expected lifestyle of the oldest son of an upper-class landowner.[93] However, Yorke still made use of his personal experience with, and continued interest in, esoteric religions by advising publishers on manuscripts.[94] By the late 1950s, Yorke had a formal arrangement as regular

92. 'I knew that he [Gerald] had lately been living in a Buddhist monastery outside Hangchow, and R and I set out to comb these establishments for traces of an old Etonian . . . At once it was admitted that there had been an Englishman staying there, who claimed that in his native country he was a member of Parliament. (This was new if rather apocryphal light on Gerald.) At another he was known, but had recently departed, leaving no clue as to his whereabouts save the address of a Buddhist organization in Shanghai' (Fleming 1934: 163). Peter Fleming and Gerald Yorke did eventually meet in China and travelled together for some time.

93. On his return in 1936, Yorke settled down to work in the family firm, married the daughter of a major general and developed hobbies in family genealogy and Gloucestershire topography (Verter 1997: 195).

94. He was already in contact with Rider when Theos Bernard's manuscript was presented around 1943 (Yorke to Unwin, 3 November 1964, in 'Yorke, G', AUC 856/20, Allen & Unwin Archives).

advisor for Rider's list of books on Buddhism and Hinduism.[95] In 1964, when the Hutchinson's group decided to either sell the Rider list or 'run it down', Yorke offered his services on a freelance basis to Phillip Unwin at Allen & Unwin Publishers.[96]

It is important not to overstate Yorke's influence on the publishing of yoga books in Britain. Books on the subject found their way to publishers without being sourced by Yorke, and many that Yorke turned down were published elsewhere.[97] But Yorke's influence on the selection of titles was substantial, and he was gifted with an ability to change Asian authors' writing into smooth English prose. Yet Yorke's influence may help explain, in part, why the publications of the disciples of Swami Sivananda (1887–1963) were not more influential in Britain. From a global perspective, Sivananda has been one of the most influential proponents of yoga: the young Mircea Eliade (1907–1986), the influential Romanian scholar of comparative religions and yoga, studied under him in the early 1930s.[98] By 1936 Sivananda had enough followers to establish the Divine Life Society as a more formal organisation, which published books and pamphlets promoting the society and its guru. Swami Vishnudevananda (1927–1993) was 'sent' by Sivananda to popularise yoga in the West and was considered a specialist in yoga asana (Krishna 1995). Vishnudevananda made his home in Quebec from 1959 onwards and opened many Sivananda Vedanta Centres in Europe (particularly in Germany) and North America; the first Sivananda Yoga Centre

95. Yorke to Unwin, 25 February 1964: 'I want to remain free to choose the Rider List at a fixed salary in the event of Lusty selling Rider as a going concern to a reputable publisher. Having chosen the Rider list since 1957, I have an obligation to and affection for the imprint', in 'Yorke, G', AUC 856/20, Allen & Unwin Archives.

96. Letter from Yorke to Unwin, 29 January 1964: 'Lusty has informed me that Hutchinsons will either sell Rider as a going concern (has already approached you in the matter) or allow the Rider List to run down. I am not therefore allowed to accept fresh material for publication by Rider. Books on Buddhism and Hinduism are slow selling in the main and do not fit in with the rest of the Group's activities ... [I would like to discuss] the possibility of my transferring my position as a "literary adviser" to your firm and syphoning your way good quality Hindu and Buddhist books, as I have been doing for Rider', in 'Yorke, G', AUC 856/20, Allen & Unwin Archives.

97. For example Alain (1957: x) (the author's real name was Max Alain Schwendiman). Reader's Report on 'Yoga for You', AURR 1/4/14, Allen & Unwin Archives.

98. For more of Sivananda's influence on Mircea Eliade as well Eliade's reception in Europe, see Bordas (2011, 2016).

in London was established in 1971, being taken over more centrally by Swami Vishnudevananda's organisation in 1972.[99]

Sarah Strauss has argued that the worldwide promulgation of Sivananda's English-language publications helped create an

> imagined community in Anderson's sense – a global community of people who, though they are rarely acquainted in the face-to-face sense, nevertheless feel themselves connected through their shared interest in and practice of yoga (Strauss 2005: 40, referring to Anderson 1983).

However, Gerald Yorke was not impressed with Sivananda's pamphlets and did not assist in the creation of this particular 'imagined community' of yoga practitioners in Britain. Writing in 1964 to Philip Unwin, Yorke reflected:

> Sivananda has about 100 books and booklets to his credit, none of which will sell much over here. Refused to publish him with Rider. He blows his own trumpet continuously . . . I mistrust him.[100]

Most of the publications from the Sivananda organisation were published by Sivananda's own Divine Light Society press and thus did not undergo the rigorous stylistic polishing that Yorke provided for his chosen manuscripts. Another early illustrated guide to asanas was Sivananda's disciple, Swami Vishnudevananda's *Yoga Asana,* which was published by the large British publisher Thorsons in 1959.[101] Sivananda's disciples maintained a more overtly religious focus than some yoga authors, taking religious vows and founding ashrams. Thus, Gerald Yorke may have had a significant personal influence on the relative lack of popularity in Britain of Sivananda's yoga.

While anticipation of popular demand was an important consideration, booksellers and publishers often had a personal interest in the subject matter of yoga and esoteric religiosity. The few teachers

---

99. But evidence of the limitations of its influence is provided by the school's absence from Stephen Annett's 1976 guide to 'Spiritual Groups and Growth Centres in Britain' under its 'Eastern Oriented Groups'. Yoga groups associated with Sivananda's disciples Swami Satyananda (the Bihar School of Yoga) were also influential in Britain from the 1970s onwards.

100. Yorke to Unwin, 12 March 1964, in 'Yorke, G', AUC 856/20, Allen & Unwin Archives.

101. Thorsons is now an imprint of HarperCollins. I have not been able to locate an archive, neither have I received a reply from HarperCollins itself as to the status of any relevant materials.

in Britain that were actively offering instruction on yoga were well known to the booksellers and publishers, who were in a position to promote at their own discretion those teachers they valued. As such, the former played an important role in identifying and determining the forms of yoga that were to become integrated into British culture.[102]

The readership of books on yoga and other esoteric religions comprised a subculture within British society. However, booksellers and publishers were not agents of a counter-cultural project: their purpose lay in expanding the interest in yoga to enlarge their market. The introduction of the paperback format, particularly by Penguin, also increased yoga's accessibility as a subject to general readers: the rise in the number of yoga titles published from the 1960s onwards implies an expanding market. This access to printed material likewise stimulated more interest in the subject, creating a ready-made market for the local education authority evening yoga classes that began to appear in this period.

---

102. For more on British esoteric networks before 1939, see Owen (2004, 2006) and Farnell (2005).

Chapter Two

The Self-taught Yogis, Adult Education
and the Wheel of Yoga

By the late 1960s, yoga in Britain was being practised in groups by several thousands of people.[1] This community arose first through networks of magazines and postal courses, then, in the post-war period, in the framework of adult educational evening classes which were heavily subsidised by local government.

There were some mail-order courses on yoga in the interwar period, one important one being advertised in physical culture journals such as *Health & Strength,* which also featured articles on yoga. These articles began to appear in the context of physical culture in the early 1930s and continued into the 1950s. Many of the postures that are now in the repertoire of asana-focused yoga classes in the twenty-first century were also part of the physical culture exercises of this period, especially those for women.[2] The basic message of the physical culture movement was one of perfecting the body and making it as healthy as possible, although it was not simply about glorification of the physical body: for example, an article by 'Sheikh Iftekhar Rasool' enjoined readers to look after their body because it is a vehicle of the soul. He wrote: 'the living body is the instrument used by the mind for the soul's expression; and the finer the instrument the more brilliant will be the results of its activities', before going on to describe the importance of *prana* and effective control of breathing,[3] although Rasool did not provide many details about how to master *prana*. Readers must have nonetheless expressed an interest in the subject as, in 1933, a series of five articles by Cameron Hannah appeared, on "Introductory Health Wisdom of the East", which, as Mark Singleton has described, fit in well with 'the

1. Personal estimate of Wilfred Clark in a letter to Ken Thompson, 16 March 1967, collection of Ken Thompson.
2. *Heath & Strength,* 2 January 1932, p. 5.
3. *Heath & Strength,* 15 June 1932, p. 740.

magazine's staple weekly advice on holistic health, hygiene, and personal morality' (Singleton 2010: 155). The articles by Hannah focus largely on pranayama and the importance of physical and mental control.

Concomitantly, Indian physical culturists such as K.V. Iyer and Ramesh Balsekar, both of whom also had associations with yoga, regularly featured in photographs in *Health & Strength* in the inter-war period, placing Indian physical culturalists on an equal footing with such icons as Prussian-born Eugen Sandow (1867–1925) who popularised bodybuilding on global tours and in the *Sandow's Magazine of Physical Culture* from 1898. Sandow relocated to London in 1906 thanks to the generosity of a wealthy Indian-born Parsi who attributed his return to health to Sandow's physical culture regime.[4] London had a well-established physical culture scene: *Health & Strength* magazine was first published in 1898, and there was a physical school at Ludgate Circus near the City of London as early as 1902. The physical culture creed was more than just the pursuit of the 'body beautiful': early literature emphasised the importance of exercise as preventative medicine, especially in cases of 'consumption' (pulmonary tuberculosis), and as a means to a better life. An instructor at the Health and Strength School was interviewed in *Vim* magazine in 1902:

> in athletics what is one man's meat is another's poison. From further observations, which he made quite spontaneously, I was to gather that, though a professional exponent of physical culture, he was well aware that physical exercise ought to be merely a means to an end, and not itself the end and aim of existence.[5]

As the British government were recruiting for the Second Boer War (1899–1902), they discovered that a surprising proportion of the population (up to 60%) was unfit for military service due to their poor levels of physical fitness. This resulted in a government-led Committee on Physical Deterioration, which produced a report emphasising the importance of improving the health and fitness of the general population (FitzRoy 1905: 6–7).

---

4. For more on Iyer and Balsekar, see Goldberg (2016), Singleton (2010) and Newcombe (2017).

5. 'The Health and Strength School', *Vim: A Magazine of Health and Beauty* 1/1 (15 December 1902), p. 12.

An association between physical culture and yoga continued in *Health & Strength* from the 1930s into the 1950s. For example, in 1956 Bennoy Chowdrey wrote a series of articles on 'Yoga for Women', and the nineteen-year-old Hazel Cleaver, who won the 1954 Health & Strength League 'Miss Britain' title, partially attributed her physique to the practice of yoga, which had been taught to her by a former professional dancer, Tom Wheeler.[6] Although in the pages of this magazine yoga was promoted as something suitable for women to engage in, it was not an exclusively female activity. The virtues of good posture, diet and self-control were moral imperatives for all involved with the Health and Strength League. The idealised male bodies in photographs conformed to the muscular ideal of the global physical culture movement.

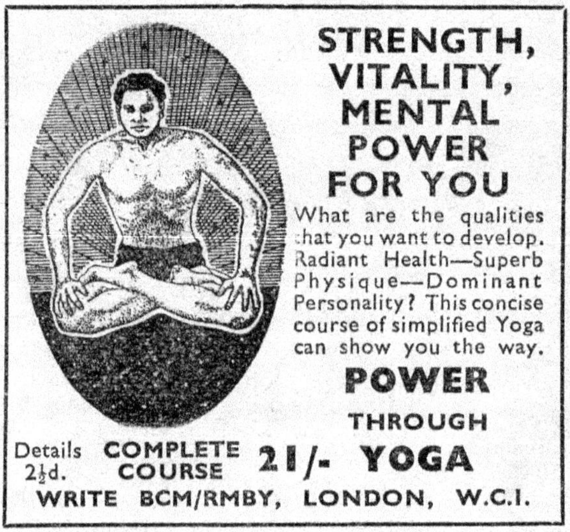

Fig. 2.1 Advert for a course in yoga from *Health & Strength*, 1956.

Advertisements in *Health & Strength* occasionally included yoga correspondence courses as well as yoga books on sale alongside others on physical culture, mental control, diet and judo. Physical culture was perhaps a minority interest, but improving the health of the population was seen as both an individual responsibility and a national imperative in the early twentieth century. Eugenics was

6. Mendes, 'We're Proud of Wally and Hazel', *Health & Strength*, 17 March 1954, pp. 11–12.

still a widespread preoccupation, the belief being that healthier adults would transfer their physical prowess to their offspring and create a healthier nation or race. However, improving one's health and fitness, for example in association with the Heath and Strength League, was still largely a leisure-time activity: a luxury for those whose lifestyles and incomes allowed it.

Sun salutation exercises (*sūrya namaskār*) were first popularised in Britain in 1936 – not in association with yoga but in the context of the physical culture movement. In this year, Bhawanrao Pant Pratinidhi (1869–1951), the Raja of Aundh, travelled to London to promote a film screening at the British Film Institute which documented his family's promotion of *sūrya namaskār* exercises in schools within their jurisdiction. Bhawanrao Pant had long been interested in physical culture and promoted *sūrya namaskārs*, as well as yoga asanas, gymnastics, wrestling and other sports in the compulsory and free schools in Aundh which he established in 1923. In 1928, he published *Surya Namaskars* (1928), a step-by-step English-language guide to the exercises (Alter 2000: 94).

Pratinidhi gave lectures at the British Film Institute and was interviewed at the Savoy Hotel by the American-born journalist Louise Morgan (1886?–1964), who had relocated to England.

Morgan had advertised Rajah's film in the *News Chronicle* with the headline 'Surya Namaskars – The Secret of Health: Mothers Look Younger Than Daughters – Rajah's Way to Banish Age and Illness' and ran a four-part series of articles in the same newspaper from 30 July 1936 providing a step-by-step guide to *sūrya namaskār*. Her upbeat lifestyle advice prompted much correspondence along the lines of 'told me of remarkable cures, of the restoration of faith and hope . . .' (Morgan in Goldberg 2016: 284). Morgan edited and introduced Bhawanrao Pant Pratinidhi's *Ten Point Way To Health* (1938), which had photographs of Bhawanarao Pant's son Apa Pant illustrating the postures.

During the mid-1930s promotion of *sūrya namaskārs* was not aimed only at women: in December 1937, Indian R.S. Balsekar graced the cover of the British bodybuilding magazine *Superman,* with an article detailing the 'World's Oldest P.C. [Physical Culture] System' – which was revealed to be *sūrya namaskār* (a second part in the following issue described yoga asanas). Although Pratinidhi's book and the practice generally faded from public attention during the Second World War, Apa Pant resurrected the concept with the publication of his *Surya Namaskars: An Ancient Indian Exercise* (1970) while he was the Indian High Commissioner in Britain (see Goldberg 2016: 285–319).

Desmond Dunne: Yogism, Relaxation and Mind Control

In the late 1940s, a Briton by the name of Desmond Dunne (b. 1913) taught something called 'Yogism', and later taught under the aegis of the Insight School of Yoga. In the 1940s and '50s, Dunne emphasised the suitability of the mental aspects of yoga for Westerners, claiming the physical aspects to be of historical interest only (Dunne 1951: 15).[7] Dunne paid the British social research organisation Mass-Observation (MO) to interview 'a representative cross-section of the

7. Dunne includes a chapter on 'traditional yoga' asana which he says is lifted from the Geranda Samhita [*sic*] and is presented with the following warning: 'Many of the historic poses are quite unsuited to Western use. The list below is given solely for its historic interest.' Dunne mentions a translation by Vasu (i.e. Rai Bahadur Srisa Chandra Vasu) published in Madras in 1933. In fact, this translation was first published in 1896 possibly at the behest of the Theosophical Society, which would have ensured its circulation among its Western followers. This book is a Vaishnava text focusing on haṭha yoga, conventionally dated 1675 although the first extant manuscript is actually dated 1805, according to Mallinson (2004).

public in a London district about their reactions to life' and reported the responses in his book *Yoga for Everyman* (1951).[8] The MO questions focused on discovering what proportion of the general population was affected by 'a lack of energy, frustration, the sense of purposelessness' – problems which Dunne believed could be alleviated through his system of Yogism. According to Dunne's report of the survey, 47% of the general population felt that they did not have enough energy, 56% reported that they were either definitely not or doubtful that they were 'getting what they want out of life' (Dunne 1951: 18). In Dunne's view, the afflictions of civilised life are a 'lack of energy, frustration, [and] the sense of purposelessness' (Dunne 1951: 19).

However, Dunne believed that the public was neither looking for a 'spiritual' solution nor was familiar with the term 'yoga'. When asked 'What does the word *Yoga* mean to you?', 44% admitted they had no idea what the word meant and another 20% offered that it was something foreign. However, a minority of respondents had specific ideas, suggesting that yoga was 'a religion or religious man' (26%), 'a system of exercise' (16%) or 'a system of mental and physical control' (4%). As a self-appointed expert on yoga, Dunne concluded:

> that the average person does feel the need of some stimulus to happier living, but is ignorant of Yogism as a solution. He looks instead for some new physical or material boon that might help him redress his impediments (Dunne 1951: 22).

Considering that late 1940s Britain was still very much recovering from the war, and that rationing lasted into the early 1950s, this dismissal of the importance of material comfort was perhaps somewhat idealistic. While Dunne was not emphasising the religious or spiritual elements of yoga, he recommended that his readers consult the books of Paul Brunton, 'who has written the best English books on traditional Yoga' (Dunne 1951: 106).

Dunne taught primarily by means of correspondence course from an address in Surrey. There were also overseas branches in France, Belgium, Switzerland, Morocco, New Zealand, Norway and the USA. By 1956 he was promoting his mail-order 'School of Yoga'

8. A Mass-Observation archivist was unable to find any record of this research in the MO Archive at the University of Sussex, noting that they only have incomplete records dating after 1949 when the organisation began taking private commissions.

in the pages of the US-based *Mystic Magazine* and appears to have had success in publishing his later books first in the United States.[9] At this time, he was charging £4 for the twelve-lesson course (equivalent to about £88 in 2018), which implied a correspondent with a certain amount of disposable income and some commitment to the course.[10]

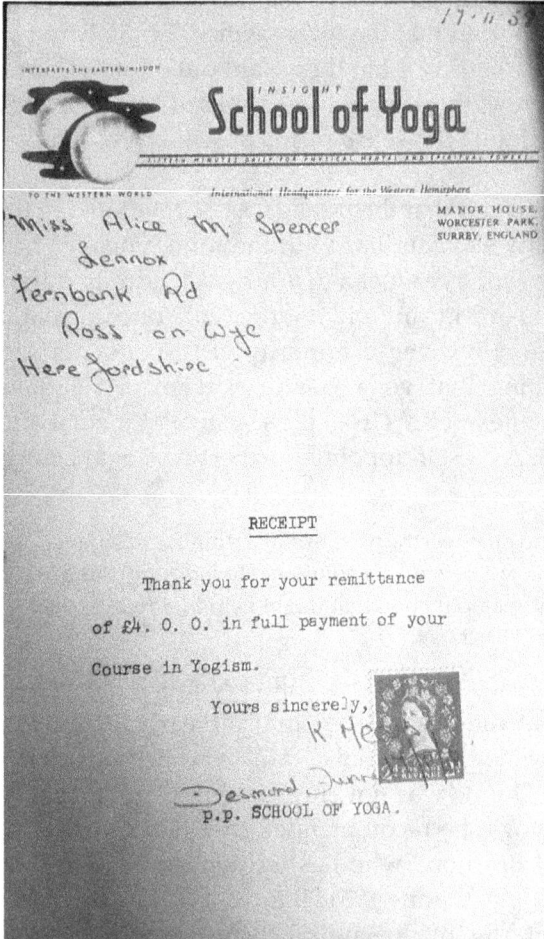

Fig. 2.3 Insight School of Yoga receipt, 1958.

9. *Mystic Magazine* 3 (1956). This reference is courtesy of Philip Deslippe.

10. Desmond Dunne's physical location in 1958 is not yet clear, nor are the date and place of his death. I have in my possession a postal course sent from the Insight School of Yoga from Surrey to Hay-on-Wye in 1958, but a K. Mears signs for Dunne, and it is not clear where Dunne was signing his pre-typed standard letters.

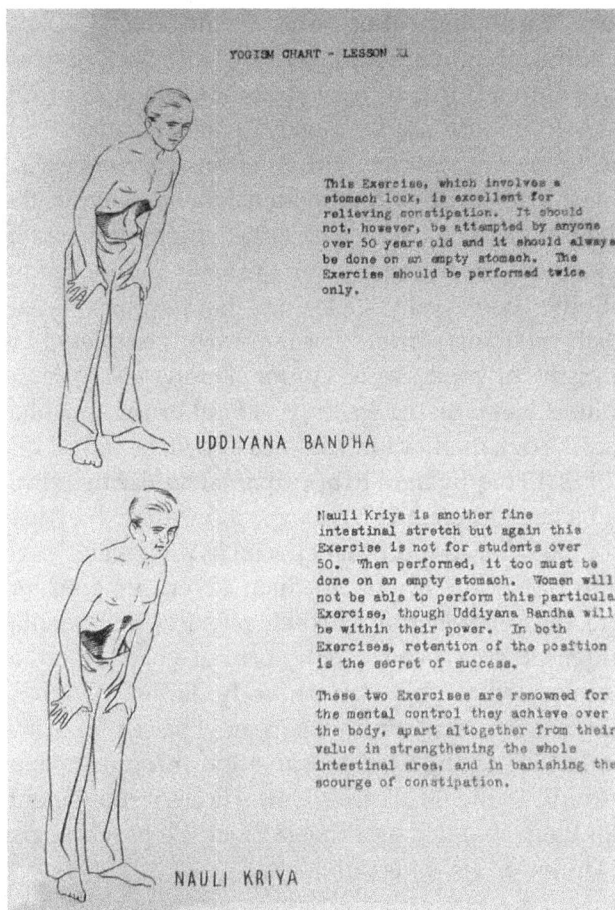

Fig. 2.4 Dunne's Lesson XI: *Uddiyana Bandha* and *Nauli Kriya*.

The correspondence exercises taught by Dunne focus on 'Deep Relaxation' by progressively concentrating on relaxing every muscle for a period of ten minutes, followed by a period of 'Deep Contraction' or conscious stretching, followed by six deep 'Revitalizing Breath[s]'. The second lesson teaches specific breathing exercises, specifically 'The Cleansing Breath' (*kapalabhati*), 'The Bellows Breath' (*bhastrika*) and 'The Saturation Breath' (*ujjayi*). Later lessons focus on aspects of good hygiene, 'Dynamic Concentration' and positive thinking for 'mind control'. Dunne encouraged regular correspondence with his students, sending out questionnaires with the weekly lessons and publishing various testimonials from satisfied customers. A few physical postures are introduced in Lessons 5 and 6, including shoulder-stand (*sarvangasan*), back arching (*bhujangasan*), and bending forward over straight legs while sitting (*pashimatanasan*). A few more asana, mostly seated positions, are introduced in the following lessons, with a 'cleansing exercise' of *uddiyana bandha* and *nauli kriyā* recommended for those under the age of fifty. In a later book, *Yoga Made Easy* (1962), first published in the USA, Dunne includes more yoga asana, probably influenced by the popularity of other books on yoga asanas that had been circulating in the English-speaking world.[11] For those who completed his twelve-lesson Yogism correspondence course, Dunne also offered an 'Advanced Course' based on the writings of Paul Brunton, which promised 'advanced Yoga meditation routines and steps to full Initiation' for a fee of £1.10 (equivalent to approximately £22 in 2018).

Dunne also had a keen interest in hypnosis, publishing *The Manual of Hypnotism* in 1959.[12] A connection between hypnosis and yoga is also evidenced in *Health & Strength*, in which advertisements and articles emphasise the relationship between physical and mental control. Dunne attempted to create a new form of yoga which he believed was more suited to the Western body, largely by combining themes of mental control and relaxation. What Dunne calls 'Yogism' has similarities to the idea of 'salvation through relaxation' which was found in the *fin de siècle* New Thought movement, the books of 'Yogi Ramacharaka' and the work of the psychologist William James.[13] Dunne advises his public that:

11. Bernard's *Hatha Yoga* (1950) was in particularly wide circulation.

12. Dunne was very interested the inspiration for William Braid's development of hypnosis, which was the 'human hibernation' and burial of Indian yogis, including Hari Das in 1837. See Baier (2009, 2016b).

13. For an exploration of 'salvation through relaxation' in the context of twentieth-century yoga, see Singleton (2005); for a detailed exploration of New Thought, see Satter (1999), Jackson (1975) and James (1983 [1899]). Yogi Ramacharaka was one of several pseudonyms used by the American William Walker Atkinson (1862–1932), a prolific writer in the early twentieth century. He was associated with 'New Psychology', 'The Arcane Teaching' and the 'New Thought' movement. He probably picked up his knowledge of yoga largely from Baba Premananda Bharati, an early Hindu missionary to the United States who was in Los Angeles in the early twentieth century. Not only did Atkinson's pseudonymous books circulate widely in the USA and Europe, the are also often found on Indian reading lists of yoga titles in the mid-twentieth century. For more on Atkinson and his influence, see Deslippe (2011).

> The first thing, then, to be done by any Westerner contemplating the study of Yoga is to abandon the idea of practicing it in traditional form. Since it is evident that there is no one 'authorized' system of Yoga – on the contrary, there are many conflicting traditional versions – why not have a modern system adapted to present-day Western needs? This is exactly what I myself evolved and have taught with success to several thousand students . . . (Dunne 1951: 101).

Much of Dunne's advice concerns dietary and moral matters, largely in parallel with Edwardian 'how to live life' manuals[14] and the physical culture movement. Dunne was also reading books on naturopathy or 'Nature Cure' – which was also an interest of Mahatma Gandhi – recommending many titles of this nature in his correspondence course.[15]

Dunne argued that his Yogism was a solution to the general public's dissatisfaction with their material conditions. However, his yoga students report more simply that they simply found their lessons helpful. Dunne claimed his students reported specific mental and physical benefits, elaborating:

> at the early and middle stages of Yogism trading, the most frequently mentioned physical benefit of the Yogism exercises was the feeling of relaxation or refreshment which they induced. Towards the completion of the Course, however, these effects seem to be superseded by the sense of greater physical alertness, fitness and suppleness (Dunne 1951: 24).

Dunne's yoga was neither mystical, nor particularly spiritual. He concluded that his Yogism made people feel 'more energetic, purposeful and happier' (Dunne 1951: 22–23).

Adult Education in Britain

In the early 1960s, yoga practitioners began to make use of local education authority (LEA) adult education evening classes. LEAs typically put yoga classes into the physical education department and encouraged yoga teachers to concentrate on physical exercises promoting health and relaxation. While LEAs were responsive to public demand for courses, they also felt that they had a duty to uphold

---

14. For example, Hall (1903a,b, 1908) and Aldrich (1904). Hall was a vicar who also wrote on biology and reincarnation.

15. For example, Lesson 6 (1958), copy of Miss Alice M. Spencer of Ross-on-Wye (author's collection). On Gandhi's interest in naturopathy, see Alter (2000).

standards of quality education for their populations. The LEAs demanded assurances from yoga teachers that they were qualified to teach, stimulating professionalisation among yoga practitioners. Initially, this was achieved simply by issuing certificates but soon training courses developed along educational frameworks. Yoga's integration within the institution of adult education was an affirmation of, rather than a challenge to, British middle-class values. Yoga was received into British culture as a continuation of an established tradition of autodidactic study which had recently become institutionalised as adult education evening classes. As we have seen, prior to the LEA system, autodidactic study of yoga included physical cultural journals and correspondence courses (both academic and personal) in addition to formally published books.

Education in Britain was a private initiative until the late nineteenth century: the idea that all children should be educated for basic literacy was only established with the 1870 Education Act (Sutherland 1990: 119–69). Before then, Victorians had established a variety of private institutions for the education of working-class adults and children (see e.g. Talbot 1852). Whereas the wealthy could study privately in their own homes, the working classes needed pooled resources of study materials and facilities. In London, the Recreative Evening Schools Association was founded in 1885, which encouraged schools to widen 'the curriculum (on a self-supporting basis) by introducing subjects like cookery, wood-carving, physical training and music' (Maclure 1990: 68).

Both the working and middle classes had a long history of autodidact study. Adult education relied on the motivation of working men and women to educate themselves. Sometimes with an implicit socialist or Marxist ideology, workers ran mutual improvement societies from the late nineteenth century onwards. These associations encouraged the government to provide funding for non-political adult education (Rose 2001: 58–91, 237). In 1903 the Workers' Educational Association (WEA) was formed with the late-Victorian ideal of providing both vocational and 'liberal' education for those denied such an education in their youth (Rose 2001: 256).[16] The WEA became a powerful lobbying and organising force for both the

---

16. Matthew Arnold (1822–1888) is one of the thinkers strongly identified with this ideology (see Arnold 1964).

technical and liberal education of adults and was seen as offering an appropriately un-Marxist curriculum (Rose 2001: 256–7).

The 1906 Education Act allowed local authorities to spend government funds on higher education. Councils often provided support for a variety of private educational initiatives and university extension programmes. In some areas there was no shortage of organisations promoting adult literacy and education. For example, by 1920 Staffordshire had 'some 40 organizations including miners' classes, tutorial classes, co-operative societies and working men's clubs' promoting classes in adult education (Lowe 1970: 275). According to Lowe, while many of the working men's groups promoted an explicitly socialist agenda, the WEA 'and those involved in university extension work, were opposed to such developments and worked to achieve social harmony in the belief that education was of value for its own sake' (Lowe 1970: 263).[17]

The 1944 Butler Education Act made it a statutory duty for LEAs to provide for adult education (Chitty 2004; WEA Working Party 1960). While some LEAs already supported adult education institutes, across the nation the legislation provided an influx of money and enthusiasm for further education as the economy recovered after the end of the war. By 1960, adult educational institutions were attended by 2.25 million people of all ages, from school-leavers to the retired (WEA Working Party 1960: 2).[18] In dedicated adult education buildings, there were courses on dressmaking, bookkeeping and car maintenance as well as subjects such as Esperanto, 'great books' and physical fitness. The formation of the Open University in 1970, specifically designed for mature and distance-learning students, was an extension of this already well-developed further education movement.[19]

While LEAs saw it as their duty to promote the acquisition of useful and employable skills in their populations, the ethos was

17. See also County Borough of Burton upon Trent Education Committee, 'Creative Leisure: A Summary of Organizations Catering for Adult Interests' (1950) in the William Salt Local Studies Library, Stafford.

18. A comparison of attendance at the evening institutes c. 1960 with the 1949 government social survey shows the following changes, broken down by social class (categories I through VII). a) I–II: 1949 government social survey 7.4%, WEA students c. 1960 7.9%; b) III–V: 63.7% vs. 59.4%; c) VI and VII: 28.9% vs. 32.7% (WEA Working Party 1960: 69).

19. *The Open University* (1969). William Salt Local History Library, Stafford.

not necessarily one of quantifiable results; as a 1969 HM Inspector Report on Dressmaking courses in Birmingham reflected:

> Some members attended the class for reasons other than dressmaking but the creation of attractive clothes and the fact of belonging to a congenial group must surely contribute to their personal development and wellbeing. The warmth of the atmosphere in a very large proportion of the classes is especially noticeable. The social benefits are unmistakable while the good integration of immigrants . . . is particularly commendable.[20]

Here, HM Inspectors argued that, while a particular skill was being taught, other benefits were also important. In quite a different way, Staffordshire's Pendrell Hall offered subsidised weekend residential courses on such diverse subjects as 'Machines in our Society, The Buildings of Staffordshire, Choral Singing, Photography for Beginners and Holiday for over 60s – National Trust Houses in the Midlands'.[21] In many of these classes it was not so much the acquisition of a particular skill but an enrichment of life that was being supported 'on the rates'.

After rationing, which continued long after the Second World War, finally ended, material prosperity was a novel experience in the 1960s for the majority of Britons (Benson 2005; Kynaston 2007; Zweiniger-Bargielowska 2001). In 1960 the WEA commissioned a report on the state of adult education in Britain, which described a country increasingly becoming what American Sociologist John Kenneth Galbraith described as an 'affluent society' (1958).[22] The 1960s represented an optimistic time in British history when the possibilities of technological progress made, for instance, a four-day working week seem a real possibility in the near future (Munrow 1966). But the WEA report argued that the increasing importance of leisure made adult education more rather than less important, and also noted that the increased affluence had led to less rather than

---

20. HM Inspectors, 'Report on a Survey of the Teaching of Dress in the Birmingham Institutes of Further Education Conducted During 1965–1966', found in the City of Birmingham Further Education Committee Minutes Vol. 5 (9 June 1967–3 May 1968), Birmingham Central Library Archives Department, BCC/BH 21/1/1/5, Birmingham Central Library.

21. Pendrell Hall, 'Prospectus Spring–Summer 1964', pbox C/6, William Salt Local Studies Library.

22. 'We live in a society where many people find it increasingly difficult to focus social purpose and where domestic social abuses are certainly less obvious than they were in the past' (WEA Working Party 1960: 17).

more leisure time available for educational pursuits. The authors wrote:

> Houses with gardens and the more widespread ownership of cars impose new leisure responsibilities, while the 'do-it-yourself' movement, one of the most important recent trends in the use of leisure time, has limited the amount of time available for all kinds of non-domestic activities (WEA Working Party 1960: 8, 17).

During the 1960s, those attending adult educational institutes were much more affluent and less associated with political radicalism than those who had been attending before the Second World War.

Although the adult educational constituency for non-vocational courses still numbered a million in 1960, adult education's role in society was changing (WEA Working Party 1960: 2, 69). The 1960 WEA report concludes that 'about 57% of the total number is going to classes from a vocational motive, sometimes as a compulsory condition of their employment' and that 'about 43% go to classes of a non-vocational kind' (WEA Working Party 1960: 2). A social class comparison using the national statistics in this report shows that adult education participants mainly reflected the social demographics of the population as a whole (WEA Working Party 1960: 2). However, the WEA report also implied that the middle classes enrolled more in the liberal education courses while the working classes were disproportionately represented in the vocational ones, possibly as a requirement of employment (WEA Working Party 1960: 4). An over-representation of the middle classes was also remarked on in 1973 in the journal *Adult Education,* which was aimed at professionals within adult education: 'People think that LEA adult education consists of bingo substitutes for the middle classes' (Wegg 1973: 185).

State-funded education was revolutionised with the 1944 Butler Education Act, which attempted to equalise opportunity by ensuring every child a full-time education up to the age of fifteen. The new educational system was designed to 'equally' reward achievement. However, critics charged it with ignoring the structural elements that gave middle- and upper-class children greater opportunities outside of school hours to support their learning. Historians generally concede that the restructuring of the educational system in 1944 did more to reinforce class divisions than alleviate them (Lowe 1988, 1997; Clark 2004: 283–5). Compounded class divisions in conditions of prosperity created a situation in which the middle classes were positioned to benefit from non-vocational courses, while those in full-time working-class jobs were more interested in vocational courses to improve employment prospects (Chitty 2004; WEA Working Party 1960). Additionally, those whose backgrounds were ones in which learning and education were valued, and had already completed more than the minimal amount of schooling, were more interested in accessing the non-vocational resources of adult education. The expanding middle classes, with education being valued within their homes, were much more likely to see learning as a lifelong process and attend non-vocational evening courses for personal enjoyment. This explains why the middle classes attended LEA evening classes for leisure in venues originally designed for working men's self-improvement.

LEAs varied greatly in the organisation of their adult education courses. London had several independent adult education centres including the Mary Ward Centre in Bloomsbury, the City Literary Institute in Covent Garden and Moseley College in Waterloo. In some areas, such as Manchester, further education was almost completely devoted to ensuring their school leavers had employable skills and employment placements in the local community.[23] The term 'institute' often referred to a geographical area and not necessarily to a full-time building dedicated to adult education. Often, an 'institute' consisted of a 'principal' who coordinated and negotiated the times and venues of evening classes with the head teachers of day schools and other premises.[24] For example, Manchester adult education was divided into four cardinal institutes, each with its own 'principal'. Occasionally, these 'area principals' rented church halls or other venues for courses. In Birmingham and London buildings were dedicated to specific aspects of adult educational interest, e.g. physical education.[25]

23. Manchester Education Committee Minutes 1960–1979, Manchester Central Library Archives. For a particular instance, see Manchester Education Committee Minutes 1960–61 26A, 429.

24. This was the case in Birmingham as well as Manchester. Manchester Education Committee Minutes 1960–1979 and City of Birmingham Education Committee, Further Education Sub-committee Minutes, 1956–1972.

25. Provision for adult education demonstrated a lot of local variation. Birmingham City Council assumed authority for the Birmingham Athletic Institute, solely dedicated to physical education, which opened in 1892, while Manchester only acquired a single dedicated institute for general adult education, not further

Because adult education was stipulated in the allocation of government funds to specific local authorities, classes were offered at subsidised rates. LEAs were allowed much autonomy in determining how these funds should be spent within their particular area. The fee system was often based on a scale, which offered every class additional to the first at a substantially reduced cost.[26] The principal of the Birmingham Athletic Institute noted that many women attended two and sometimes three classes on the same evening.[27] This system made it easy for the curious but as yet not committed to try a yoga class. While yoga classes were available to all, it appears that the middle classes were particularly well positioned to take advantage of these non-vocational courses.

The British Wheel of Yoga and Wilfred Clark

Yoga's dissemination as a subject throughout Britain's adult education network was largely on account of south Birmingham resident Wilfred Clark (1898–1981). A working-class autodidact himself, Clark became involved in adult education as part of the Army Training Corps in the Second World War. Thenceforth he combined a personal interest in yoga with his professional work as an adult education tutor and local journalist. In 1963 Clark and Margaret Ward founded the Birmingham Yoga Club, expanding it to become the Midlands Yoga Association in 1964, and renaming it the Wheel of British Yoga in 1965.[28] Now known as the British Wheel of Yoga, Clark's organisation continues to be an important influence in the

education specifically, in 1948. Waterman (1992) and College of Adult Education, Manchester 1944–1990, M698/1/12003/35, Manchester Central Library Archives.

26. For example, in the academic year 1965–66, an HM Inspectors' Report on Birmingham Adult Education summarised that 'a survey of the teaching of dress in the Birmingham institutes of Further Education conducted during 1965–1966 fee charged 16/- per term under 18 5/6. Any number of classes could be attended by them and some attended more than one dress class. Principals are allowed remission of fees where they think necessary, e.g. OAP.' City of Birmingham Further Education Committee Minutes Vol. 5 (9 June 1967–3 May 1968).

27. BAI Women's Section, *Annual Report 1970–71*, MS 1468/3/1, 2, in Birmingham Central Library Archives.

28. For nomenclature, see Wheel of British Yoga *Bulletin* 25 (November 1967) and *Yoga: Journal of the Wheel of British Yoga* 7 (Spring 1971), p. 3. I have not been able to ascertain much about Margaret Ward either from written sources or interviewees. It is known that she was an associate of Wilfred Clark in south Birmingham during the 1960s. When Clark left the Wheel to found the Friends of Yoga (FRYOG) in the mid-1970s, Ward joined him and, by the late 1970s, had become more interested in

promotion of yoga in Britain. In 1995 the Wheel was recognised by the British Sports Council as the 'governing body' for yoga in Britain.[29] The Wheel changed dramatically over this time, but important aspects of its character and focus, as determined by the vision of its founder, remain.

Clark was born in Wells, Somerset, but spent most of his youth in Poole, Dorset. In the 1901 census, his Islington-born father, George William Clark, was listed with the working-class profession of a 'Coach Body Maker' and at the time of his son's first marriage in 1921, Clark Sr reported his occupation as a 'Wood Machinist'.[30] No siblings are mentioned in the census records or in any later documents about Wilfred Clark. Clark described himself in his youth as a loner, 'a virtue that was to prove a great help to me many years later when I took up Yoga practise', and added that he was 'a complete duffer at arithmetic, but by gum could [I] WRITE essays [sic]'. He reported that he came top of the borough in English when he was in technical college.[31] Subsequently, he applied for a job as a reporter with the local *Poole Herald* just before war was declared in 1914.

Clark volunteered for active duty, as soon as he was old enough, in 1916. He was introduced to his first yoga asana during his military training. When an older soldier noticed his enthusiasm for physical training without apparatus, he showed Clark a few 'Indian PT' postures he had learnt while serving in India. Wilfred Clark recalled that he did not connect these exercises with the word 'yoga' until much later.[32] His first understanding of 'yoga' was during the

---

Western esotericism and Kabbala. At this point she seems to have dropped out of yoga networks (personal interview with Ken Thompson, 28 November 2004).

29. There is some discussion in de Michelis (2004: 190–1). Upon enquiry, the Sports Council did not have any records relating to this decision.

30. National Archives, 1901 Census Online RG13, Series 2278, Piece 72, Folio 41, 259, and General Registrar's Office, Certified Copy of an Entry of Marriage for Wilfred Arthur Clark and Winifred Ada Farr, Poole, Vol. 5a, September 1921, p. 746.

31. W. Clark, 'How I Came to Yoga'. *Yoga Today* 12 (August 1987), p. 22.

32. Ibid. During his time in military service, Clark also dabbled with stage production and devised an act with a friend who was an illusionist: 'I developed in this business and became an escapologist in conjunction with my illusionist friend and also devised an act of mental telepathy' (Ibid., p. 24). Although Wilfred Clark made no association between yoga and this work, there is a traditional association between illusionists and yogis and it could not but have made the 'pranic healing' performances of his later career more impressive. For more on the association between magic and yoga, see Siegel (1991) and Shah (1998 [2011]).

First World War when he was in contact with Indian cavalrymen.[33] In retrospect, Wilfred Clark attributed his ability to live through a year and a half of fighting to the Indian soldiers' conversation on 'the True Self, equanimity and non-attachment'.[34] The parallel with Arjuna's instruction by Kṛṣṇa on the battlefield in the *Bhagavad Gītā* was important to Clark. Although he would later identify as a Buddhist, Clark claimed the Wheel of British Yoga's symbol, the *dharmachakra*,[35] represented the wheel of 'Krishna's glorious chariot' and referred to some of his first associations with yoga as inner peace on the battlefield of life.[36]

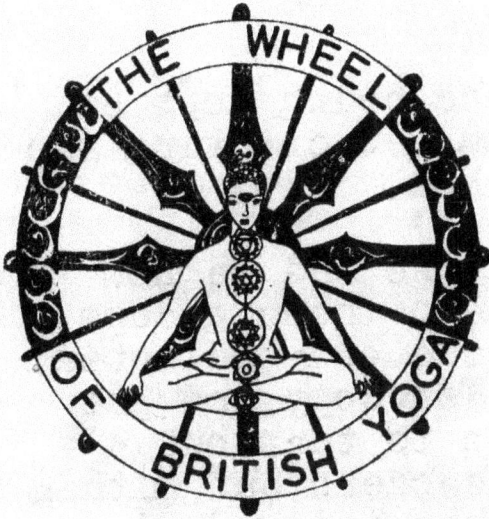

Fig. 2.5 First logo for Wilfred Clark's Wheel of British Yoga[37]

33. 'Altogether 138,608 Indian soldiers, comprising two infantry divisions, two cavalry divisions and four filed artillery brigades, saw action on the Western Front.' The two cavalry divisions remained in the war until 1917 fighting as cavalry (Visram 2002: 171).

34. Clark, 'How I Came to Yoga'. *Yoga Today* 12 (August 1987), p. 23.

35. Also a Jain symbol, the *dharmachakra* is found on the modern Indian national flag. It is often described as symbolising the passage of time and the impermanence of all phenomena (one of the Noble Truths taught by the Buddha), or the different ways in which Buddhism has been taught in different contexts, often described as 'turnings of the wheel'.

36. Clark, 'How I Came to Yoga'. *Yoga Today* 12 (August 1987), p. 25.

37. From a letterhead used by Wilfred Clark, 1968–69, in the personal collection of Ken Thompson.

According to his own account, after returning from military service in France Clark resumed his newspaper work and continued his education. He married Winifred Ada Farr on 28 September 1921 in a Congregational Church while he was working as a reporter for local newspapers.[38] According to Clark, 'I was so overworked at my job we decided that a family was out of the question, or, rather, unfair on the child' and the couple divorced some time after 1929 (Clark 1987: 24). However, during the 1920s Clark educated himself in his leisure time and developed an interest in yoga and 'Oriental philosophy'. First he read independently the works of Max Müller, then began a correspondence course on Oriental philosophy from the Oxford University Extension Society. Clark reported that he never connected the photographs of Indians 'tying themselves up in knots' with the philosophy he was learning through correspondence (Clark 1987: 24). His later writings show that he read a variety of books on yoga, mysticism and spirituality. His involvement with adult education increased during the Second World War. Too old for combat duty, Clark served in the Army Educational Corps where he reported that he tried to interest 'the troops' in yoga but gained the impression that 'the boys regarded this as "airy-fairy"' (Clark 1987: 23).

After his discharge in June 1945, Clark returned to Dorset, again working as a journalist. Here he met and married Joan Latimer, a forty-five-year-old widow. Both were very active in amateur dramatics at the time, Mrs Clark appearing under the name of Janet Latimer.[39] There is no mention of children in this marriage either. In 1948, the couple moved to Wootton Wawen, a village near Stratford-upon-Avon.[40] Wilfred Clark reported that he took employment as an assistant editor of the *Solihull News*.[41] He claimed to have risen to editorship of several local weekly papers, naming the *Sutton*

38. General Register Office, Certified Copy of an Entry of Marriage for Wilfred Arthur Clark and Winifred Ada Farr. Winifred Farr's father was employed as a gardener (domestic servant).

39. They met and wed in Taunton shortly after the Second World War (Clark 1987: 24).

40. Clark (1987) is illustrated with a photo of its author as a 'Shakespearean Actor'; Clark died at the Stratford-upon-Avon Hospital. General Register Office, Certified Copy of a Death Entry for Wilfred Arthur Clark, QBDX 692518, Stratford-upon-Avon, Warwickshire, September 1981, 31, p. 197.

41. 'Know Your Neighbour: Yoga – His Guide for Fifty Years'. *Solihull News*, 7 July 1968. Newspaper clippings in the possession of Ken Thompson.

Coldfield News and the *Erdington News* which are both Midlands weeklies (Clark 1987: 25).[42] While in Birmingham, he became well known for his amateur dramatics and became dramatic art tutor at the Hockley Heath Further Education Centre. He also taught 'the art of writing for pleasure and profit' at the Erdington Further Education Institute under the auspices of the WEA.[43]

Through his position as a part-time lecturer in these further education Institutes, Clark was in a position to present his self-taught expertise in yoga as a fit subject for these venues. According to Clark, on his WEA paperwork, he had offered 'Oriental philosophy' as one of the subjects on which he could lecture. The Coventry WEA agreed to let him give a general talk on 'yoga'. The response to these lectures was positive enough for Clark to propose the introduction of yoga classes into the further education curriculum in Birmingham.[44] Clark reported that he submitted a proposal to the LEA in Birmingham for a course on yoga early in 1962, which put him in contact with Margaret Ward, who became a co-organiser of the Wheel of British Yoga (the Wheel). Ward took the title of 'national organiser' while Clark took the title of 'honourable organiser'.[45]

In Clark and Ward's narration of the history of yoga in Britain, the influence of other individuals on the development of yoga in Birmingham has been elided: the Further Education Sub-committee reports for 1963–64 record at least five classes in the Birmingham adult education system, only one of which was run by Wilfred Clark and none by Margaret Ward. By academic year 1964–65, Yogini Sunita (who will be discussed in the next chapter) was teaching three classes at the Birmingham Athletic Institute and there were four other teachers of yoga in Birmingham who may or may not have been aligned with Wilfred Clark and Margaret Ward at this time.[46] However, Clark did not concentrate his energies on

42. I have not verified these claims with copies of the local papers.
43. 'Know Your Neighbour: Yoga – His Guide for Fifty Years' (1968).
44. Wilfred Clark 'History of Yoga in Britain', document in the personal collection of Vi Neale-Smith, and W. Clark, 'How I Came To Yoga', *Yoga Today*, 12 (August 1987), p. 25. In academic year 1963–64, Clark is recorded as teaching yoga at the Golden Hillcock Centre on Wednesday evenings from 7–9 pm. City of Birmingham Further Education Committee Minutes, 1(14) June 1963–8 May 1964, BCC/BH 21/1/1/1, Birmingham Central Library Archives.
45. *Yoga: Journal of the Wheel of British Yoga*, 1969.
46. City of Birmingham Further Education Committee Minutes, 12 June 1964–7 May 1965, Birmingham Central Library Archives.

classroom teaching but instead worked on developing a national network of yoga practitioners. Drawing on his journalistic experience, he sent in letters to local papers throughout the country asking for any individuals interested in yoga to write to him. He would file the letters, usually also sending a personal typewritten reply. Having collected a few names and addresses in proximity to one another, he would choose one and write to suggest organising group meetings. When the Wheel was more established he would publicise classes in his newsletter.[47]

Known from 1965 as the Wheel of British Yoga, Clark and Ward attempted to nationally catalogue and coordinate yoga classes throughout the country. These small cells sprouted up all over Britain, and Clark kept in touch with them through a monthly carbon-paper typewritten newsletter, the *Bulletin*, in which he suggested further reading on yoga. Coordinating correspondence, Wilfred Clark acted as the centre of the Wheel, operating out of a caravan in the garden of his Wootton Wawen home; individuals wrote to him with their interests in yoga and he helped them to form groups across the country. For example, the December 1967 Wheel *Bulletin* reports:

> Several inquiries as to the nearest class have lately come from ladies in different parts of Surrey: all have been referred to Mr. Clark by, of all people, the beauty editor of 'Women's Journal.' Why he is at a loss to know. Anyway, he has written to two county papers and hopes to get something organised in that county; the nearest classes at the moment are in London.

Clark also encouraged regular correspondence and questions from yoga students to whom he offered advice.[48] Some groups founded with Clark's help met in churches or school halls, some approached their LEA to organise a class, while others met in private homes. By 1967, Clark reported that he was regularly corresponding with at least fifty individuals throughout the country,

47. 'He [Wilfred Clark] was known and people would write to him saying "Oh, I'm starting a class somewhere, isn't that lovely," and he'd write back by return of post saying "that's fine, I wish you success. Call on me if you need any help. And then into the newsletter would go – there is a class starting in wherever. So he was the link and the newsletter was the rim of the Wheel.' Interview with Swami Satyar Atnananda Saraswati (14 July 2005).
48. Interviews with Jim Pym (7 July 2005) and Ken Thompson (28 November 2004).

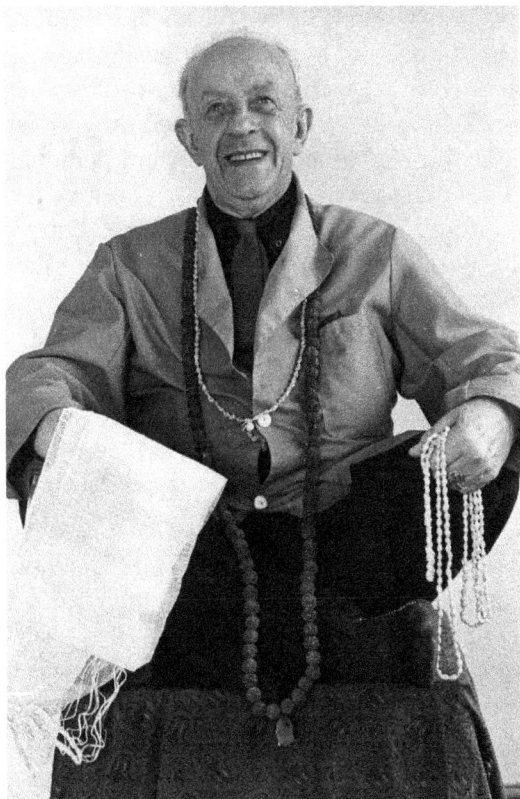

Fig. 2.6 Wilfred Clark, c. 1969. Courtesy of Ken Thompson.

many of whom were leading groups themselves.[49] With the help of Margaret Ward, this network became more formally organised and run by a committee.

In May 1967, the Wheel organised a national yoga rally attended by 'close to 200 Yoga devotees from all over the country'. The first conference had educational lectures addressing 'various aspects of the great science of good living, including an unexpected and impressive demonstration of the power of the Sacred Syllable "AUM"'.[50] By 1970 the Wheel journal *Yoga* reported that it was coordinating 'some 80 [yoga] groups, more than 100 teachers . . . [and] thousands of students' across Britain.[51] This organisational

49. Letter from Wilfred Clark to Ken Thompson, 21 February 1967. Personal collection of Ken Thompson.

50. Wheel of British Yoga *Bulletin* 20 (June 196). Personal Collection of Ken Thompson.

51. *Yoga* 2 (Winter 1970), front cover.

structure held until around 1969 when Wilfred Clark was beginning
to find that the Wheel needed to be run by a committee. In this year
the typewritten newsletters were replaced by a more professional
A5 stapled journal. Now nearly seventy, Clark stepped down from
official organisational duties but remained an important personality within the Wheel. He travelled all over the country to give lectures to yoga groups and offered 'pranic healing' sessions.[52] During
the 1970s, Clark gradually withdrew from the Wheel, although he
maintained a friendly association with it.[53]

In a tribute to Clark published on the occasion of his death, the
magazine of the Wheel, then called *Spectrum,* explained that:

> When the Wheel grew too big for him [Clark] (having confessed that
> what suited him best was a benevolent dictatorship) handed over to
> a committee. In 1972 he went off to start another one-man association
> – the Friends of Yoga.[54]

The Friends of Yoga was not entirely a one-man show. There was a
group called the Friends of Yoga (India) which Clark joined in 1972.
From this position he was asked to represent the UK on the All-In-
dian Board of Yoga and the International Yoga Co-ordination Centre (Yococen) with the purpose of establishing worldwide teaching
standards that encompassed the more spiritual and philosophical
aspects of yoga (Shringy 1977: 26).[55] Wilfred Clark travelled to India
for at least one conference and was soon issuing teacher training certificates based on the guidelines agreed at the meeting.
Although the Indian organisation changed to Yococen, Clark kept
the name of the British branch and its affiliates as the Friends of
Yoga (FRYOG). This smaller organisation continued Clark's promotion of what he felt was the 'correct' approach to yoga. As the
Wheel developed in parallel with the requests of local education

52. *Yoga: Journal of the Wheel of British Yoga,* 1969–75. Swami Satyar Atnananda
Saraswati wrote that 'Wilfred was the only pranic healer in the UK therefore people
would travel many miles to attend his sessions here at Yoga Seekers.' Personal correspondence, 6 November 2007.

53. 'Guest teachers at these seminars over the last year have included Wilfred
Clark; Alan Oakman, Westbury; Members of the 3HO Centre, London, led by John
Singh Bless; Members of the Chinmoy Centre, London; Joyce Gaines, Accrington;
Wilfred Lawler, Preston; Malcolm Strutt, Centre House, London'. 'Wales Teacher
Training', *Yoga* 20 (1974), p. 17.

54. *Spectrum,* Winter 1981.

55. The International Yoga Co-ordination Centre (Yococen) was affiliated with
the Yoga Institute of Santa Cruz, Bombay.

authorities for the issuing of certificates, FRYOG maintained the more flexible approach of the early Wheel, issuing teaching certificates both through its own teacher-training programmes and taking into account prior personal experience.[56] FRYOG however never approached the degree of success in national networking that Clark had crafted in his organisation of the Wheel of British Yoga.

The British Wheel's Yoga

The environment of Clark's Wheel of British Yoga was initially like that of the mutual education societies, where groups of individuals pooled resources and books to study a new subject together. Clark began issuing teaching certificates on behalf of the Wheel of British Yoga to those he felt had acquired adequate knowledge in the subject, by whatever means. Certificates began to be requested by LEA officials who wanted assurance that yoga teachers could be trusted as adult education tutors.[57] The first few certificates were simply issued on the basis of Wilfred Clark's personal opinion. Ken Thompson, who believes that he holds one of the first certificates (issued in 1967), remembered that he was simply given a certificate when he told Clark that his local education authority (Ilford) required one.[58] Although Clark had been running correspondence courses in yoga throughout the 1960s, by 1969 it was time to develop a more formal teacher-training programme.

After the Inner London Education Authority (ILEA)'s decision not to recognise Wheel teachers within the Inner London Adult Education classes (which will be discussed in the next chapter), Wheel members Ken Thompson, Velta Wilson and Chris Stevens put together the first 'educationally approved Wheel teacher-training course' that ran from September 1971 at the Hermitage, Brentwood

---

56. Personal interview with Ernest Coates (19 December 2004), chairperson of FRYOG at the time of the interview.

57. 'Wheel Certificates: the demand for the Wheel's certificates of proficiency for teachers has grown so enormously that the document is in danger of losing its value. It has therefore been decided to issue it only where an education authority specifically demands it. Alternatively we shall always be pleased to confirm by letter to an authority that an applicant is known to us as a fit and proper person to teach Yoga.' *Yoga* 3 (Spring 1970), p. 3.

58. Personal interview with Ken Thompson (28 November 2004).

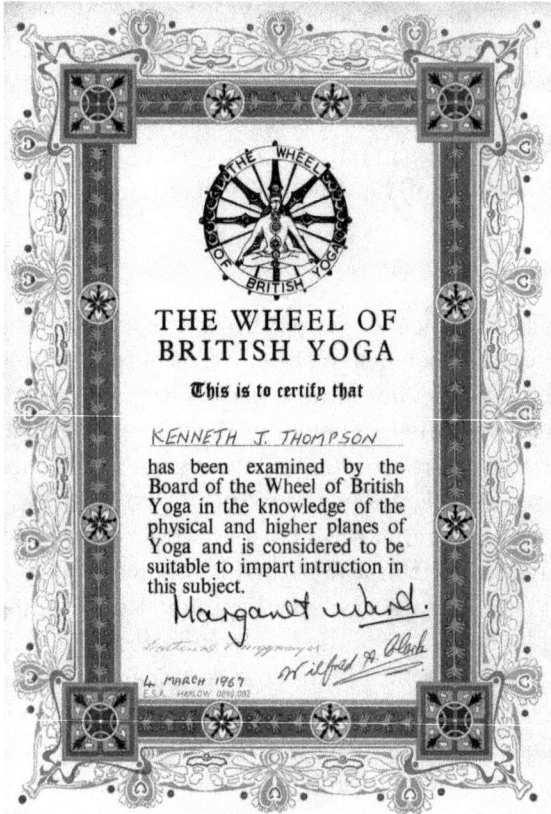

Fig. 2.7 One of the first Yoga Teaching Certificates issued by the British Wheel of Yoga. Courtesy of Ken Thompson.

Evening Institute in Essex.[59] The programme involved workshops on yoga asana and pranayama, teaching skills, and yoga philosophy. There were also other teacher-training courses that were informally approved by the Wheel.[60] Clark wrote in 1971:

> [I have] run such courses for nearly three years, covering technique in all the branches of Hatha Yoga with practical meditation and lecturing on many other forms, Raja, Gnana, Bhakti, Karma, Mantra, Yantra

59. Ken Thompson remembers that this programme was developed because the ILEA had developed a teacher-training programme with the exclusive approval of B.K.S. Iyengar. Personal interview with Ken Thompson (28 November 2004).

60. Wilfred Clark wrote in *Yoga*, Winter 1970/71, p. 3: 'For some years throughout the country established teachers of long experience have been training others to take classes and this work has been welcome having regard to the ever-increasing interest in Yoga.'

and Japa Yogs. These are enumerated to give some idea of the ground which should be covered at such courses.

In some classes – not necessarily associated with the Wheel – there is a tendency to specialise, maybe in Pranayama Yoga or postures, breathing and relaxation; it is respectfully submitted that this can only give students a restricted idea of what Yoga is.[61]

Clark's approach was based on an informal network of adult education tutoring. Yoga was presented as a subject that should be covered in breadth rather than depth, an approach that treated yoga as an adult education course, to be covered in all its aspects, in summary form.

One of the hallmarks of Clark's approach to yoga was an appreciative exploration of a diversity of yoga teachers and traditions. Such a survey of different yoga traditions fitted easily within the adult education context and did not depend to any significant extent on the personal charisma of the teacher. Clark worked hard to ensure that the Wheel of British Yoga adopted no single teacher as a guru. According to Clark, 'True Yoga' meant individual exploration towards living more ethically and more at peace; any path towards this goal was yoga – a theme that persisted after Clark retired from the Wheel.[62] Nevertheless, some of the many teachers who travelled to Britain in the 1970s were more influential on members of the Wheel than others. Generally, Indian yoga teachers who did not encourage exclusive loyalty were preferred. Teachers who found favour with the Wheel included Swami Satyananda Saraswati, founder of the Bihar School of Yoga; T.K.V. Desikachar, son of T. Krishnamacharya and teacher of what was formerly known as Viniyoga; Swami Satchidananda of Yogaville in Virginia, USA;

61. *Yoga*, Winter 1970/71, p. 3.
62. Then President of the Wheel, General D.I.M. Robbins wrote in 1977, 'all students of Yoga should try to learn at the feet of as many different teachers as they can. There are so few really good teachers, and the great masters are indeed rare. However, if you are lucky enough, and indeed deserving enough, then you will surely find more than one really good teacher in your lifetime. In this way you can be helped to achieve a balanced understanding in an unbiased awareness of what yoga really means. Then it is up to you to find the methods which best suit your one body and your one mind. This alone, through your endeavors will lead you to the ultimate and only worthwhile goal of that ever desired union between your spirit and the cosmic consciousness.' 'D.I.M. Robbins writes for us of his further Indian experiences', unlabelled article 16–17 and 21, newspaper clippings in the files of Ramamani Iyengar Memorial Yoga Institute (RIMYI), Vol. 2.

and Dr Swami Gitananda, a Canadian-born medical doctor with an Indian father, Irish mother and American wife who set up an ashram in Pondicherry in 1968.[63] The Wheel did not discuss the more sectarian International Society for Krishna Consciousness (ISKCON – aka the 'Hare Krishnas') and Transcendental Meditation in its journal *Yoga,* although it occasionally listed some of their publications.

Although there was not an official Wheel book list, several books were continually mentioned in Wheel newsletters and magazines and could be considered standard texts. In response to one enquiry about what to read on yoga, came the following 'Editor's Note' in *Yoga*:

> *Editor's Note:* Yoga literature is voluminous and growing. A small basic library might contain, in addition to translations of the Bhagavad Gita, the Upanishads and the Sutras of Patañjali, 'Fourteen Lessons in Yoga Philosophy' – Ramacharaka, 'Yoga' – Ernest Wood, 'Light on Yoga' – B.K.S. Iyengar, and 'Autobiography of a Yogi' – Sri Yogananda.[64]

During the 1970s, Wheel member Chris Stevens offered a 'bookstall' which advertised mail-order books on the back pages of *Yoga,* which stocked the advertised titles as well as many others. This allowed those who joined the Wheel to deepen their interest in what might be a difficult-to-find subject in bookshops outside central London. The books of Paul Dukes, Ernest Wood, Theos Bernard, Desmond Dunne, Paul Brunton and Richard Hittleman were widely circulated. Chris Stevens offered the Penguin editions of the *Bhagavad Gītā* and the Upaniṣads as well as the more sectarian translations by the Theosophical Society, ISKCON and the Maharishi Mahesh Yogi (Transcendental Meditation). The Penguin *Krishnamurti Reader* (1970) and Alan Watts's *The Way of Zen* (1957) also feature.[65] From the evidence of this bookstall and the letters from readers printed in *Yoga,* it appears that Wheel members were reading widely about spirituality and mysticism in Indian traditions, both Hindu and

63. Swami Gitananda and his wife Meenakshi Devi Bhavanani frequently featured in articles in *Yoga & Health* during the 1970s.

64. Wilfred Clark in *Yoga* 28 (Summer 1976), p. 29.

65. 'Two "musts" in ancient literature are "The Bhagavad Gita" and "The Upanishads"... many versions ... recommended that one go to any reasonably large booksellers and search the Penguin Classics section where both these works will be found.' British Wheel of Yoga, *Yoga Handbook* (1973), p. 9, in the possession of Vi Neale-Smith.

Buddhist, as well as exploring spirituality as presented by Far Eastern, Eastern Orthodox and Roman Catholic authors.[66]

After Wilfred Clark passed his position of 'Honourable National Organiser' over to Chris Stevens in Autumn 1971,[67] the Wheel of British Yoga became more focused on producing teacher-training certificates and international networking. The national secretary Margaret Ward wrote in *Yoga* in 1972:

> The Wheel's most important task at the moment is propagating and organizing teacher-education; a watertight and comprehensive scheme has replaced those of the past and all education authorities have been contacted, and groups have taken it up with enthusiasm.[68]

In winter 1973, the Wheel leadership decided to register it as a charity. A renaming of the organisation to the Western Yoga Federation was proposed, and there was a physical headquarters at Acacia House in West Acton, London, which ran workshops as well as serving as an administrative centre. However, at the national congress it was found that the word 'Wheel' was important to the membership and in August 1973 the organisation became the Wheel of Yoga.[69] It explained its main objectives in autumn 1973 as follows:

> The Wheel of Yoga is a co-ordinating organisation mainly operating in the United Kingdom, although having a membership in many countries overseas. It is a focal point for Yoga groups and individual devotees and its activities include public meetings, instruction seminars in all aspects of Yoga, the supervising of Yoga teacher education,

66. Titles taken from 'Chris Stevens' bookstall', a regular advertisement in *Yoga: Journal of the Wheel of British Yoga*.

67. 'Another milestone has been reached in that at last our founder, Wilfred Clark, has been able to hand over the office of hon. national organizer to a younger friend, Chris Stevens, whom we welcome to the Council. The hand over will be at the end of the year and the official ceremony at the 1972 Congress.' *Yoga* 9 (Autumn 1971), p. 2.

68. *Yoga* 11 (Spring 1972), p. 2.

69. 'One outstanding feature of the Congress thus launched in this inspiring message from across the Atlantic was the obvious desire to somehow reintroduce the word "Wheel" into the title of the organization and this is the subject of a members' ballot for which a slip is enclosed in this magazine.' *Yoga: Journal of the Wheel of British Yoga* 16 (Summer 1973), p. 3. This postal ballot was ratified at a special meeting of the Western Yoga Federation held at Acacia House on 25 August 1975. The minutes and attendance list was obtained, with gratitude to Mat Whitts, by his Freedom of Information Request to the Charity Commission (personal correspondence, 13 August 2017).

co-operating with local education authorities in Yoga tuition, and the publication of literature.[70]

While these objectives remained the same, the Wheel was looking more to Europe than India for competitive professionalisation. It was actively networking with members in

> Lebanon, Greece, Ethiopia, Africa, Germany, Holland, Belgium, France and South America, (all except Lebanon, it will be noted WEST of Suez) not to speak of others in Australia and New Zealand who are certainly not 'Oriental.'[71]

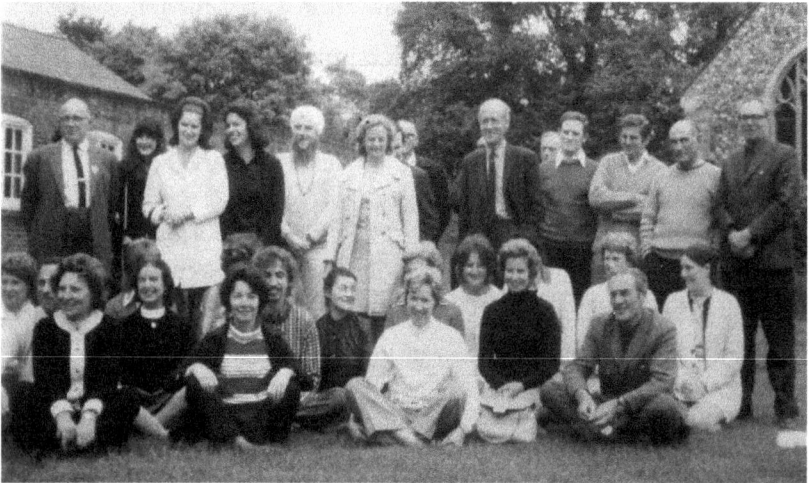

Fig. 2.8 British Wheel of Yoga event at Loughton Hall in June 1971. Photograph courtesy of Ken Thompson.

The European Union of Yoga was founded in 1972 and the first British delegation of 26 individuals attended their annual conference in 1975.[72] Having attended this conference, it was decided that a national designation was important and the Wheel of Yoga

70. *Yoga* 17 (Autumn 1973), p. 2: Charity Commission.
71. *Yoga* 14 (Winter 1973), p. 2.
72. 'Club Méditerranée 450 participants from all over Europe and some from India, Australia and South America. Professional interpreters up from Geneva turned German or French into steady clear English through one's personal headset . . . Many of the Continentals, attending for the third year and with their larger representation, were a bit surprised to meet our small group of 26 there for the first time from Britain, not that we clung together but mostly speaking only English and finding their ways foreign just made us rather noticeable.' *Yoga: Journal of the Wheel of British Yoga* 26 (Winter 1975), p. 8.

became the British Wheel of Yoga in summer 1976; it has retained this name up to the time of writing. By 1975, the Wheel had standardised these general directives into a teacher-training course with approved teacher-trainers. In this it considered itself ahead of many of the European yoga organisations.[73]

The European Union of Yoga was largely formed at the initiative of millionaire Gérard Blitz and his Club Méditerranée in Zinal, Switzerland, which served as a base for international meetings.[74] A major component of these meetings was an attempt at cross-cultural networking and sharing audiences with favoured Indian teachers. It was from these meetings that T.K.V. Desikachar's teaching began to influence the Wheel. While some of the main lectures were professionally translated from French or German into personal headsets, smaller sessions were held in the native language of the speaker without translation.[75] The annual conferences attempted to draw together some cross-cultural agreement about standards of yoga teaching and an exchangeable qualification across the continent.[76] However, the British Wheel of Yoga was sometimes lukewarm towards the European Union of Yoga, weighing the British contributions greater than the potential benefits of the continental exchange. But the desire of some Wheel members to teach on the continent and the gravitas of an international qualification has kept the Wheel actively involved with the European Union of Yoga.[77]

73. *Yoga* 28 (Summer 1976), p. 3.
74. *Yoga* 28, p. 2.
75. J. Davis, 'Zinal 1975', *Yoga* 26 (Winter 1975): 8.
76. For example, 'The purpose of Gérard Blitz's visit was to clarify the role of the EU and to discuss their proposals for a minimum programme for Teacher Training in Europe ... The Wheel's own teacher training programme began in September 1975 and we can therefore expect to be in a good position to advise on the project through our own experience. Our own Teacher Tutors will be required to examine and test the European syllabus so that a working solution can be agreed for 1978.' *Yoga: Journal of the Wheel of British Yoga* 28 (Summer 1976), p. 5.
77. '[The Wheel has been] Very involved [with the European Union of Yoga] ... Well, we came out of it at one time, because it seemed to be a waste of time and money. It costs all the federations because they have to support the EU. And they have meetings two or three times a year and decide various things ... Then after a few years ... they voted to go back in. The main reason was that however well qualified you are, unless you are a member of the European Union of Yoga, if you go to the continent to teach, you can't get a job ... So that was the main reason for wanting to be involved with them.' Personal interview with Vi Neale-Smith (17 September 2004).

Once the Wheel was established, Wilfred Clark dedicated himself to attempting to ensure that 'the whole Yoga be taught and not
merely a part of it'[78] – something that he described in the 1970s as
'True Yoga'. The early Wheel emphasised the 'spirit' of yoga over
any specific content, stressing a balance between postures, breathing, meditation, concentration exercises and philosophy. Decrying
the focus on physical postures (asana) that was popular in many
adult education classes, Wilfred Clark reiterates in the pages of
Yoga, 'Yoga is not Yoga if such factors as meditation and short philosophical talks are omitted'.[79]

In 1967, Clark recommended an asana practice primarily of sun
salutation (*sūrya namaskār*) as well as breathing exercises and quiet
contemplation. Clark emphasised that every lesson or home practice should contain 10–15 minutes of lying down and relaxing in
the dark (*śavāsana*).[80] To assist yoga practitioners in relaxation, a
variety of techniques was practised (Singleton 2005). Sometimes the
practitioner concentrated on different points of the body to relax
them; sometimes a tense–relax action was used. Other techniques
included guided imagery and counting the breath.[81] Breathing
exercises, called pranayama, were emphasised as well as a number of meditation practices. Clark suggested teachers introduce at
least one new breathing exercise to each class taught throughout
the course of an academic term.[82] For the concentration and meditation element popular exercises included concentration on a can-
dle flame, silent repetition of a word (*mantra*), counting the breath,
guided images, or trying to feel energy (*prana*) in the body.[83]

The Wheel's idea of teaching philosophy essentially consisted of
short lectures on a number of different topics. In introductory classes,
ideas of *karma* and reincarnation might have been introduced. In

78. 'Views: On the Multiplicity of Yoga Organisations', *Yoga Awareness: Quarterly Journal of Yococen* (July 1977), p. 27.

79. W. Clark, 'Means Better Than the End?', *Yoga* 11 (Spring 1972), p. 12.

80. Letter from Wilfred Clark to Ken Thompson, 16 March 1967, in the collection
of Ken Thompson.

81. 'Yoga Breathing', *Yoga* 3 (Spring 1970), p. 5.

82. Letter from Wilfred Clark to Ken Thompson, 1967, in the possession of Ken
Thompson. Examples of breathing exercises used during this period included inhal-
ing in one count, retaining the breath for four counts, and exhaling the breath for
two counts (a 1:4:2 breath) and alternate nostril breath where first one nostril and
then the other is blocked by fingers. See also Wood (1959: 85–6).

83. *Yoga,* 1969–78.

more 'advanced' groups, Clark suggested discussing ideas of 'one-ness', 'vibrations', astral planes, chakras and pranic healing. The meaning of the word 'yoga' as 'union with the divine' was a possible topic for exploration. Another topic suggested by Clark for the 'philosophy' section was outlining the various 'types' of yoga, i.e. *hatha* (focus on postures and control of the body), *karma* (focus on selfless action), *gnana* (discriminating knowledge and intellectual study), *bhakti* (devotion to God), *mantra* (use of sacred sounds) and *raja yoga* (literally 'kingly yoga' and usually referring to the eight-limbed system described in Patañjali's *Yoga Sūtras*).[84]

One woman interviewed described her first yoga class, taught by a Wheel of British Yoga member in south Wales in 1969. At the time, Vi Neale-Smith was working part-time as a medical secretary and had an eight-year-old daughter. Mrs Neale-Smith's age and situation in life was typical of those attending the LEA classes during this period. She had heard about the yoga class after expressing an interest in the subject at a church tea. A friend in her young-wives group attended a class in a nearby village and took her along to her first class.

> It was brilliant. It was fantastic. Mostly *hatha yoga* . . . mostly posture work, mostly exercises. There was a relaxation and we did sit quietly just for a few minutes at the very end. But he [Jones] didn't call it meditation. And I suppose it wasn't because it wasn't long enough really. But it was certainly a very good feeling.[85]

But this class conveyed a good enough feeling for Neale-Smith to know that she wanted, some day, to be a yoga teacher; she began attending classes regularly and taught yoga with the Wheel from 1974 onwards.[86] This first yoga class gave her a feeling of certainty comparable only to the occasion on which she first met the man who would become her husband. Neale-Smith could not articulate exactly what it was about the yoga class that she found so appealing, but she had a strong intuition that she had found something she wanted to continue.

84. Letter from Wilfred Clark to Ken Thompson, 12 April 1967. The definitions of these categories in the Wheel roughly follow those offered by Vivekananda's well-circulated books going by the same titles. See de Michelis (2004: chs. 3, 4, 5) for Vivekananda and Vivekananda (1896). For scholarly understandings of *raja yoga*, see Birch (2013).

85. Interview with Vi Neale-Smith (17 September 2004).

86. Ibid.

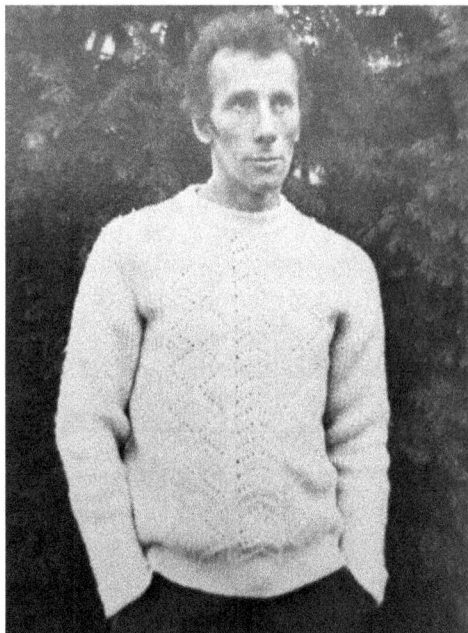

Fig. 2.9 Philip Jones.
Source: *Yoga & Heath* 2/8 (1972).

Neale-Smith's first teacher, Philip Jones, was a well-respected teacher in the Wheel. Jones had been a Welsh mining engineer whose lungs had become seriously damaged from coal dust. His yoga education was also in the autodidact tradition. According to a biographical summary:

> Then by chance, he read a book on yoga which concentrated on breath-ing techniques and decided he had nothing to lose by trying the exer-cises. He found he had a great deal to gain: his lungs gradually began to recover, his general health improved and he is now fit enough to be a full time yoga teacher. He does two hours of breathing exercises every morning and says his lungs are getting better every year.[87]

He became a committee member of the Wheel and founded the Welsh Yoga Teachers Association. Jones became well known for a distinctive and charismatic teaching, and for the emphasis on pra-nayama. Neale-Smith remembers the usual format of Jones's classes:

> And as he got us more into the classes, that [pranayama] took up quite a bit of time – maybe twenty minutes out of every lesson. Then there would be about a ten-minute relaxation and maybe about ten minutes

---

87. B.J. Smith, 'Yoga with Bagpipes', *Yoga Today* 2 (October 1977), p. 37.

meditation at the end of it. So his lessons were quite well balanced from that point of view.[88]

Wilfred Clark was very happy to champion Jones's approach to teaching yoga in preference to other teachers who focused more on the physical postures.[89]

Conclusion

The development of the Wheel of British Yoga cannot be characterised as the introduction of an alien cultural activity into Britain. Yoga was received as one subject among many that could be studied during leisure time for personal self-improvement. The yoga tradition of Wilfred Clark and the British Wheel of Yoga developed yoga as a subject within the LEA adult education evening class structure and was an extension of liberal (non-vocational) adult education. Clark designed yoga as a subject and argued that 'all aspects' should be presented in outline rather than too strict a concentration on any particular aspect. The Wheel of British Yoga believed that yoga was essentially a philosophical and spiritual subject. Yoga classes, in the early Wheel's view, should consist of asana, pranayama and meditation practices as well as short talks on important concepts for a 'well-balanced' yoga class. If individuals wanted more depth and personal instruction in one aspect of yoga, the Wheel encouraged students to look at a number of Indian gurus. Allegiance to any single guru, however, was considered unhelpful as it would limit a student's understanding of yoga. This approach to yoga was developed within mainstream British culture; it promoted yoga from within the increasingly middle-class British adult education tradition.

The integration of yoga as an adult education subject within the LEA system provided a bureaucratic structure in which classes could be advertised, organised and taught on a low-cost basis. This allowed an affordable way for classes to expand as well as provide

88. Interview with Vi Neale-Smith (17 September 2004).
89. For example, Wilfred Clark writes: 'On October 31 he [Wilfred Clark] attended an enthusiastic meeting in Swansea and arising out of this. Invitations are pending to Newport Mon., where Philip Jones is doing fine work and Cardiff where there is no class as yet.' *Yoga* 6 (Winter 1970/71), p. 3: Also, 'Philip Jones is doing excellent work in Newport and his influence promises much extension work – Cardiff and other places; there is certainly much scope in this highly populated industrial area.' *Yoga* 7 (Spring 1971), p. 3.

yoga with indirect approval from the government. It enabled those with simple curiosity to try the subject in a trusted venue. LEAs influenced the shape yoga took in Britain by encouraging yoga teachers to have a qualification and requiring that yoga conformed to the overtly secular expectations of government-funded adult education in Britain. Subjects taught within the LEA structure were regulated by the principals of the institutes who were answerable to the elected officials of the local authority. Thus, there was an accountability that prevented the subjects from diverging too much from what society found generally acceptable. Conversely, the acceptance of yoga in these institutions conferred a legitimacy and may have encouraged some to pursue the subject who may not have shown an interest as an autodidact. Adult education had been established for the purpose of expanding personal and educational horizons; yoga became popularised in Britain as a continuation of these goals.

Chapter Three

Charismatic Gurus in Adult Education

As early as 1965, Birmingham City Council was concerned about the proper qualifications for yoga practitioners, with 'hundreds' having enrolled for yoga in adult education venues. Apparently, there had been an attempt at 'methodological investigation' of yoga but this had proved 'an irritating business'. *The Times* described how one popular Birmingham yoga teacher had keep-fit qualifications but had learned yoga from books; another teacher was a woman of Indian origin who 'appeared to know quite a lot', but had not 'graduated from a yoga academy'. The article went on to ask, 'If there were yoga graduates, would they, on the whole, be quite the sort of people one really wants?'[1]

In the 1960s the British adult education system was faced with a demand for yoga teaching, but without any established means of assessing the quality or qualifications of a yoga teacher. The guru–*śiṣya* ('teacher–disciple') relationship is often considered essential: is transmission of an authentic yoga tradition possible without such an immediate relationship? In this chapter I will argue that an important contribution in the popularisation of yoga as a global phenomenon has been the institutionalisation of charisma in a way that diverges from a direct guru–*śiṣya* interaction. In many ways, this model of yoga teaching and teacher-training certification developed in response to the needs of the British adult education context. This can be exemplified by examining how a woman named Sunita Cabral (1932–1970) gained the trust of the authorities at the Birmingham Athletic Institute where she taught from 1963 to 1970; her relationship with the local authority teaching bureaucracy will be compared to that of B.K.S. Iyengar (1918–2015), who was accorded special recognition by the Inner London Education

---

1. 'Birmingham Tries to Size Up All This Yoga: Should Prana Force Teaching Come out of Rates?', *The Times*, 23 February 1965, p. 7, col C.

Authority (ILEA) in certifying appropriate 'yoga gurus' for British adult education.

According to those who knew them, both Cabral and Iyengar had an exceptional ability to deliver an almost immediate experiential understanding of something understood as 'yoga', although their methods were somewhat different. According to Max Weber's theories, this type of authority could be termed 'charismatic' (Weber 1947: 328). Weber characterised charismatic authority as the motivating force for change in society, an inherently unstable, potentially revolutionary force which is 'foreign to everyday routine structures' (Weber 1947: 363). For any lasting organisation to be created from charismatic authority, Weber argues, charismatic authority must be 'radically changed', and he termed this process the 'routinisation' of charisma (Weber 1947: 364).

Regarding yoga in Britain, Iyengar and Sunita show two different trajectories in integrating their charismatic authority into the adult education bureaucracy. Although resident in India, Iyengar created a significant bureaucratic framework whereby his understanding of asana could be transmitted in his personal absence. Initially, he corresponded with his students in London answering their questions and commenting on photographs. Then, with the involvement of Peter McIntosh, chief inspector of physical education at the ILEA, he established a structure for training teachers within the LEA system. Iyengar effectively routinised his charisma so that a recognisable teaching of yoga could continue in his absence, including after his death. Highly popular during her lifetime, Yogini Sunita's approach was personal and she never developed – nor intended to develop – a bureaucratic framework for transferring her knowledge. Before her death in 1970, Sunita trained a group of 20 teachers in Pranayama Yoga, and, while this group has continued teaching Pranayama Yoga and training new teachers, no new charismatic authority has revived the popularity or visibility that Sunita herself achieved. With limited social structures to transmit her knowledge, Sunita's tradition has faded as a social movement while Iyengar's charisma has become a globalised institution. In 2004, Iyengar was one of the US *Time* magazine's 100 most influential people in the world and 'Iyengar Yoga' entered the *Oxford English Dictionary*.

'Prana Force on Rates': Yogini Sunita in Birmingham

The majority of those doing yoga in Birmingham in the early 1960s were inspired by Yogini Sunita. She dedicated herself to the popularisation of yoga, largely in north Birmingham, between her 1959 arrival in Britain and her death in 1970. Sunita was raised in Bandra, a wealthy Catholic suburb of Bombay. She was born with the name Bernadette Bocarro, reflecting her Portuguese ancestry, and her family were devout Catholics. English was spoken at home and the family considered itself to be of Brahmin caste (Robins 1961).[2] The young Bernadette excelled at playing piano and thought she might have a career as a pianist. But at sixteen she rejected an arranged marriage with a business associate of her father and felt the only alternative was to enter a convent, joining a Franciscan order of nuns near Bandra and becoming Sister Teresa (Robins 1961).[3]

She explained to a newspaper reporter in 1961 that, at first, she idealised religious renunciation. However, when she refused to continue writing to her mother to ask for gifts of antique furniture for the convent (her family ran an antique shop in Bombay), her life in the convent changed. Suddenly unpopular, the sparse food and 'rigorous discipline' began to affect her health (Robins 1961). She claimed that her time at the convent was 'deeply unhappy' suffering from typhoid fever, lockjaw and undergoing 'several operations'. According to her own report, Bernadette fortuitously found the outer gate of the convent unlocked during evening prayers, walked out of the convent and returned to her parents' home. She described her family as being 'horrified' that she had left the convent, but they allowed her to remain hidden at home (Robins 1961).

Having left the convent, her 'only comfort', she claimed, was to be found in solitary walks by the seashore. On one such walk, she encountered a man with 'wonderful eyes'. Her description allowed her father to identify him as the well-known yogi Narainswami, who was believed to have 'cured leprosy, tuberculosis and many other diseases' (Robins 1961). On a second meeting, he offered to teach her yoga. Through the practice of what Narainswami called

2. This newspaper clipping is in the possession of Kenneth Cabral. The article represents the most complete biography available, and was written soon after her arrival in Britain.

3. Yogini Sunita's birth name and her birthday are confirmed by her death certificate: Bernadette Cabral, OBDX 771214, Entry No. 193, registered 17 April 1970 in the County Borough of Walsall.

Pranayama Yoga, Bernadette's confidence and peace of mind was restored.[4] There is no outside source to confirm this period of Bocarro's life.[5] She did not leave any detailed descriptions of the teachings Narainswami gave her and it is possible that she did not know anything of Narainswami's yoga tradition. Her son Kenneth made it clear that the nature of a teacher's traditional authority in Indian culture would have made these types of question unnecessary for the student.[6] Yet by the time Bernadette reached Britain in late 1959, she felt confident offering both Pranayama Yoga and Japanese massage to others.[7] Recordings of her voice imply a calm authority and confidence in giving instructions (Cabral 2002).

Some time after she absconded from the convent, the Bocarros arranged a marriage to Roydon Cabral, another Catholic Indian of Portuguese ancestry, who worked as a printer for *The Times of India*. Bernadette accepted this marriage and had two children in India, Kenneth and Mignonne. She took employment as a secretary for the Italian Embassy in Bombay and also claimed to have taught yoga in schools while living in India (Cabral 1965: 51). In the 1950s, the Cabrals saw the situation for anglicised Indians becoming precarious and felt their children would receive a better education abroad; the family emigrated to England where some of Roydon Cabral's family had already relocated.[8] Around December 1959, Roydon Cabral found work as a printer in the north Birmingham area and the family settled into a home in Walsall, an industrial town north-west of Birmingham. The children, fair in complexion and native English

4. Personal Interview with Kenneth Cabral (13 July 2007).

5. A photograph of Narainswami appeared in the third edition of her book (Cabral 1971 [2002]: 17) and the fourth edition (Cabral 2012: 17). In the first edition, Cabral mentions Narainswami but there is no photograph (Cabral 1965: 51). I have not seen the second edition.

6. Personal interview with Kenneth Cabral (13 July 2007).

7. Sunita wrote that her training in Japanese massage was from the Oriental School of Massage 'organised by Dr R. Thal Wa Ka, the famous Japanese Masseur. His Training Schools for massage existed in Japan and India' (Cabral 1965: 65).

8. On the subject of Indians in London: 'First ashore were the Anglo-Indians (used here in the sense that it is now used in India, that is, people of mixed English–Indian parentage, not in the sense of Britons born in India), refugees from a country in which they believed that, with the departure of the British, the breadth of their opportunity would rapidly shrink.' 'To the surprise of many Westerners who regard India as a heathen county, Christians make up a large section of London's Indian community. They are perhaps the easiest to identify because they have Western Christian names . . . followed by a Portuguese or Spanish surname' (Davies 1966: 268-9).

speakers, integrated into the local school without any experience of racism.[9] Bernadette initially attempted to return to a career as a pianist, and also taught yoga to a few friends. These yoga students encouraged others to try, and Bernadette found that her knowledge of yoga was in more demand than her skill on the piano.[10]

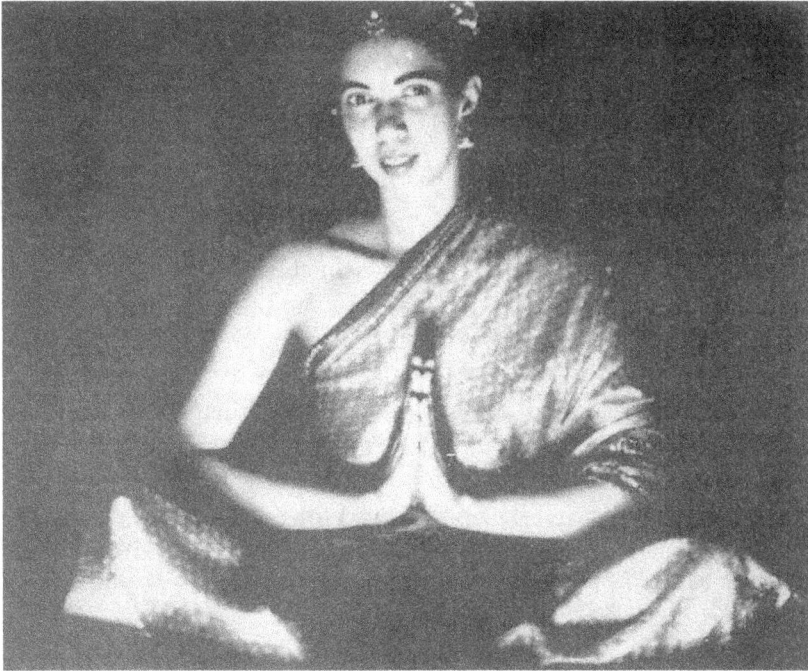

Fig. 3.1 Yogini Sunita, c. 1965. Photograph courtesy of Kenneth Cabral and the Lotus and the Rose Publishers.

By mid-1961, Bernadette Cabral, a Westernised Indian, had transformed into 'Yogini Sunita', a sari-clad Indian yoga teacher – and a living promotion for Pranayama Yoga. Her dress and manner aroused curiosity from onlookers and helped to encourage interest in yoga. An interviewer for BBC Radio 4 *Woman's Hour* described meeting Cabral in September 1961:

> I met Yogi Sunita at a smart West End hotel. She was wearing a flame-coloured sari, sandals and long silver earrings with her dark hair

9. Personal interview with Kenneth Cabral (13 July 2007).

10. *Sunday Mercury* article and personal interview with Kenneth Cabral (13 July 2007).

swept back in a chignon. She was young and attractive and as she took off her sandals and sat cross-legged on the floor. I wondered how she had become interested in yoga.[11]

Customarily dressed in a sari, Sunita usually squatted or sat on the floor for her media interviews, which increased her intrigue.[12] Having got her audiences' attention with her unusual appearance, Sunita impressed her listeners with a calm authority and skill in guiding them into an experience of relaxation.[13]

Her oldest child, Kenneth, recalled his mother's hectic schedule during his childhood. Sunita taught yoga on most weekday evenings and ran the massage clinic all day on Saturday. On Sundays the children often attended mass with their father before returning home to a lunch Sunita had prepared.[14] In August 1961, Bernadette Cabral registered a business in the name of 'Yogi Sunita Clinic' in central Birmingham. In 1964 she used the name 'Sunita Cabral' to register 'The Yoga Relaxation Centre for Great Britain' and 'The Training School of Oriental Massage' as businesses both at the same address in Sutton Coldfield, a predominantly middle-class suburb of north Birmingham.[15] In 1963, her youngest child, Yasmin, was born in what Sunita claimed was a twenty-minute labour; she also claimed to have been up and working only one hour later. She normally needed only three or four hours of sleep daily, it would seem.[16] While one can remain sceptical about these claims, Sunita

11. Unbilled extra on *Woman's Hour* No. 26 (27 September 1961, 14.00–15.00). Yogi Sunita interviewed by Christopher Young Venning, British Broadcasting Corporation Written Archives Centre (BBC WAC). It appears that, at first, she went by Yogi Sunita and later Yogini Sunita.

12. 'Talk on Relaxing in Yogi Style', *Derby Evening Telegraph*, 19 April 1963. Collection of Kenneth Cabral.

13. '. . . just before Christmas she spoke first to the Vegetarian Society . . . and then to the members of the Baha'i World Faith . . . The Yentonians listed carefully to the little lady in the beautiful sari then at her bidding relaxed and benefited thereby.' 'Yogi Sunita Visits Rotarians', *Sutton Coldfield News*, 12 January 1967. See also 'Art of Relaxing', *Derby Evening Telegraph*, 3 May 1963; 'Talk on Relaxing in Yogi Style', *Derby Evening Telegraph*, 19 April 1963.

14. According to her son, Sunita did not attend mass in Britain but never lost a deep conviction about the existence of God. After mass, the children went to the Co-op social club with their father before returning home for lunch. Personal interview with Kenneth Cabral (13 July 2007).

15. Business Registration Certificates numbers 1168078, 1168077 and 1038244, in the possession of Kenneth Cabral.

16. 'Yasmin Looks at the Western World', *Derby Evening Telegraph*(?). Unlabelled newspaper clipping in the collection of Kenneth Cabral. Kenneth Cabral detailed

was undoubtedly very busy.[17] This, combined with a presence that inspired calm and relaxation in her audience, was a striking and attractive combination to many.

When Sunita was interviewed for BBC *Woman's Hour*, the interviewer commented that 'I had always thought of yoga as mind over body, you know, the practice of physical exercises to achieve complete control of the body.'[18] However, the interviewer went on to explain that 'Yogi Sunita teaches only relaxation of the *mind*' and has made a record of the relaxing formula. While the *Woman's Hour* transcript did not record Sunita's words, it is likely that she repeated her 'slip second' on the radio. This is a mental exercise, which takes a minute and a half at most to perform, in which all those people and situations that require personal attention and involvement are brought to mind. Then one tries to let all of these attachments and worries go – just for one second. According to Sunita, this practice will relax the mind and allow one to engage with all the demands of life more effectively. Sunita claimed that one 'slipped second' was equivalent to eight hours of 'perfect sleep'. Sunita advocated that her students practise this exercise thrice daily, upon waking, between noon and 2 pm, and before sleep at night. She also maintained that hearing the teacher's voice was necessary for beginners to learn this method and made recordings for this purpose.[19]

Much of Sunita's charisma was experienced through how she inspired students to 'slip a second' and experience 'deep relaxation.' In her book, she explained several times how the experience of peace 'CANNOT BE TAUGHT' (Cabral 1971 [2002]: 51; author's emphasis). Nonetheless, her calm and authoritative voice delivered instructions which many experienced as leading to relaxation (Cabral 2002 [196?]). Through personal example, she attempted to show the efficacy of the techniques she taught. She claimed that the primary qualification to teach Pranayama Yoga was not technical expertise.

Sunita's term-time responsibilities and travel on public transport which he estimated meant that she rose no later than 5.30 am and did not retire until after midnight. Personal interview (13 July 2007).

17. During 1963, Sunita 'beat the panel' in the popular BBC television programme *What's My Line?* in which the panel attempted to guess the profession of a guest. BBC Television diploma certifying that, on the night of Sunday 10 March 1963, Sunita Cabral 'Beat the Panel' in 'What's My Line?' at the BBC Television Theatre, London W12. Certificate in the possession of Kenneth Cabral.

18. Unbilled extra on *Woman's Hour*, 27 September 1961, BBC WAC.

19. Ibid. and Cabral (1965).

Rather, she explained, '**Above all, there must never be a furrow on the forehead,** THAT IS THE NECESSARY QUALIFICATION' (Cabral (1971 [2002]: 8; author's emphasis) – a comment that highlights the personal example of relaxation and detachment in the midst of a busy life which Sunita attempted to model for her students. Sunita's personal charisma was noted by the principal of the Birmingham Athletic Institute (BAI): 'She had a rare gift of making every student feel they were the only person who mattered to her.'[20] This was all the more significant when considering the number of students in adult education classes; the BAI reported in 1965 that Sunita had taught over 780 students in the academic year.

In autumn 1963, Sunita began yoga classes in the Women's Section of the BAI. In its 1963–64 annual report, the principal reported that 131 students were attending the 'experimental' yoga classes, going on to remark that:

> [The yoga classes] have proved most popular. Many older women find great value from the carefully prepared exercises and the great stress on relaxation both of the body and the mind. Under the right supervision, I think these classes can be very valuable . . .[21]

From this it is clear that the yoga classes were somewhat different from the Institute's other activities, which included traditional sports, gymnastics, judo and courses on 'beauty culture' for ladies. The principal of the women's section of the BAI noted Sunita's 'great ability in the art as both teacher and performer' and consistent reports by the students of the benefits of the concentration and relaxation exercises.[22]

Many students were enthusiastic in their praise of Sunita and her Pranayama Yoga techniques. Testimonials printed in the first edition of Sunita's book *Pranayama Yoga* included:

> Lack of good sleep made life unbearable. Taking drugs did not solve anything . . . And today, I enjoy all the things I have wanted from life.

> It took me three months to achieve the elusive slip-second, but it gives me tremendous energy to cope . . . I have learnt to be more tolerant.

20. Birmingham Athletic Institute Annual Report 1969–1970, p. 2, in Birmingham Central Library Archives.

21. Birmingham Athletic Institute Annual Report 1963–1964, p. 4, in Birmingham Central Library Archives.

22. Birmingham Athletic Institute Annual Report 1969–1970, p. 2, in Birmingham Central Library Archives.

> When I mastered the slip-second, I learnt to rise above seemingly impossible situations.

> Suffering acute attacks of migraine for twenty years, a friend . . . suggested I go along and take a course . . . I am quite over the migraine now . . . it was really Sunita and the amazing calmness that really did the trick . . . (Cabral 1965).

Sunita's students found that her personality and methods helped them cope with their lives more effectively. The large student numbers Sunita attracted at the BAI also testify to her appeal, as does the fact that attendances dropped significantly after her death, as noted by the principal of the BAI Women's Section.[23]

Pranayama Yoga, as presented by Sunita, was a non-religious activity. In India, she wrote, 'Pranayama Yoga is by far the most popular form [of yoga], widely practised, and accepted by recognised organisations, because there is NO form of religion attached to its teachings' (Cabral (1971 [2002]: 57). One of her students, a clergyman, described Sunita's response when he broached the subject of God with her:

> *Do you believe that there is a God?* She said, 'I come from God, and I will return to God one day.'

> *Do you ever ask God for anything?* She said, 'Never, I only thank Him for everything.' By this time, I was most interested.

> *When ill, or there is trouble in your family, surely you ask for Divine help?* She then answered, 'I trust God all the way. God knows what He is about. My children live this way too.'

> I thought she had gone very quiet, she is usually full of beans. Then she told me that at public lectures many people asked her similar questions and she would tactfully divert the conversation as she felt that religion was a very personal matter. Very wise I thought. There was another question, I wondered whether she would mind? . . . *whether she ever prayed for any length of time?* 'Never, I offer my whole life and all it contains as a prayer.' She excused herself politely and was out of the room. Remarkable, I thought, don't you? (Cabral 1965: 9).

Thus, Sunita did not have to adapt her tradition away from a more explicit religiosity when she began teaching in Britain. Her understanding of Pranayama Yoga was that religion was private, while

23. Birmingham Athletic Institute Annual Report 1969–1970, p. 1, in Birmingham Central Library Archives.

Yoga in Britain

the techniques of relaxation were a subject of public teaching. This vicar's comments imply that Sunita avoided the subject of religion in public forums and thus separated her relaxation techniques from religious questions in the mind of her students.[24]

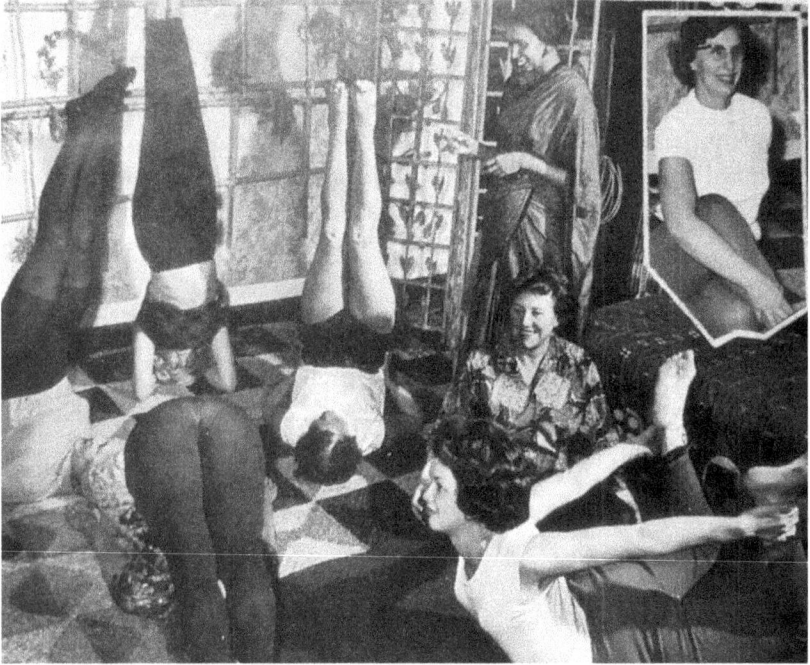

Fig. 3.2 Yogini Sunita teaching at the Yoga Relaxation Centre, c. 1965. Photograph courtesy of Ken Cabral and the Lotus and the Rose Publishers.

Sunita trained her first group of about twenty Pranayama Yoga teachers at Pendrell Hall, a residential adult education centre in rural Staffordshire.[25] She did not intend her teacher-training course

24. Personal interview with Kenneth Cabral (13 July 2007).
25. Pendrell Hall was donated by the Gatskill family to Staffordshire County Council for use as an adult education centre in 1955 but opened for classes only in 1961. Although few records relating to the hall's first seasons remain, it is likely that the Pendrell Hall warden had much autonomy in determining his school's schedule. Weekend courses were run in spring–summer 1964 on subjects such as 'Heraldry', 'Machines in our Society' and 'The Buildings of Staffordshire'. There is a record that 'Mrs Cabral' ran a one-day course for women entitled 'Further Steps in Yoga' on 24 September 1964 from 10.30–3.30. Pendrell Hall 'Prospectus Spring–Summer 1964, William Salt Library, Stafford, WSL pbox C/6.

to provide an automatic qualification for her students to teach yoga in adult education:

> Assuming a student takes the Teachers' Course, and a Yogi is confident that some of the students will be able to teach, it may well be that the Education Authorities do not select a single one from this group to teach for them. In this case a teacher will teach privately . . . on average, one in every thousand is chosen to work for Education (Cabral 1971 [2002]: 57).

She expected adult education officials to choose Pranayama Yoga teachers from among those that had the personal charisma to transmit the tradition of Pranayama Yoga in that context. She wrote that:

> Pranayama Yoga always remains a tradition. The education authorities respect this at all times. A dedication, such as this one, remains a 'pure vocation.' The technical qualification required is a thorough knowledge of psychology, the nervous system, the causes of tension in all its forms in mind and body . . . and in all three hundred exercises involved in Mind Control – Body Relaxation – Breathing and Physical Exercises. The degree of such a Yogi lies in the completion of all these requirements, but . . . the gift and ability to impart such a subject can never be decreed by letters. The recognition lies entirely with human beings who seek the study of the Art of Relaxation, which is the 'key' to health and calmness (Cabral 1971 [2002]: 57).

This method of integrating yoga within adult education was highly dependent on potential teachers' personal charisma. Yogini Sunita's means of transmitting her knowledge ensured the continuation of the tradition of Pranayama Yoga, but not its popularity. There are still Pranayama Yoga teachers practising in Britain, some of whom never met Sunita but were taught by those who had. However, the numbers are small and they have not sought to increase visibility or align themselves with the larger yoga organisations, such as the British Wheel of Yoga.[26]

In April 1970, at the age of 38, Yogini Sunita was fatally hit by a car as she crossed a road.[27] The BAI principal noted that after her death Sunita's newly trained students carried on well and classes continued to be popular.[28] However, Sunita neither organ-

26. Personal interview with Kenneth Cabral (13 July 2007).

27. General Register Office, Certificate of Death for Bernadette Cabral, OBDX 771214, County Borough of Walsall, 17 April 1970, Entry No. 193.

28. 'Despite the death last year of Mrs Cabral who introduced Yoga into the Institute, the classes have continued and flourished under the leadership of teachers

ised nor standardised her teaching in a way that made national popularisation possible.[29] Her emphasis had been on a personal transmission from student to teacher, and she made sure that each potential teacher understood the principles of relaxation: passing Sunita's teacher-training was not a matter of competency in physical exercises or memorisation of technical information.[30] While Pranayama Yoga has continued under teachers trained by Sunita, these teachers have not attracted the same numbers. Sunita taught that Pranayama Yoga was a way of life, of doing one thing at a time, in the present moment, without anxiety. The primary qualification to teach this 'way of life' was approval from the teacher that this understanding was embodied by the student in daily life as well as the yoga class. Although Pranayama Yoga continues to be transmitted in Britain in this manner, it has never been institutionalised and, therefore, remains less visible than other forms of yoga.

B.K.S. Iyengar in Britain

Although based in Pune, India, B.K.S. Iyengar made annual trips to Britain between 1960 and 1974. Instead of focusing on relaxation, Iyengar attempted to make his students completely absorbed in the physical performance of postures and then relax completely at the end of a physically challenging class. Iyengar began to routinise his charisma by standardising the teaching of technical points for asana and pranayama and corresponding with his students during his absence. This put large aspects of Iyengar's teaching into a legal-rational framework that was transmissible without his personal guidance or reliance on personal charisma. Yet the experience that Iyengar wanted to transmit through his asana instructions relied on the ability of yoga teachers trained in his system to apply their own personal charisma within the legal-rational structures. Iyengar also hoped to transmit more than simply physical instructions; however, some individuals understood this more clearly than others. By 1969, Iyengar's yoga had also become accepted within the framework of adult education evening classes. The way Iyengar was able to

---

originally trained by Mrs Cabral.' BAI Annual Report 1970–1971, p. 2. Birmingham Central Library Archives.

   29. Kenneth Cabral believes that his mother had been approached for a television programme prior to her death. Personal interview (17 July 2007).

   30. Personal interview with Kenneth Cabral (17 July 2007).

integrate his distance-teaching with the structure of the LEA system allowed his approach to be widely popularised and less reliant on the charisma of individual yoga teachers.

Born during the 1918 influenza epidemic, Bellur Krishnamachar Sundararaja (B.K.S.) Iyengar was a sickly child of a poor Brahmin family. One of his older sisters was married to Tirumalai Krishnamacharya (1888–1989), who lectured in Indian philosophy (Yoga, Sāṃkhya and Mīmāṃsā) and also taught asana and pranayama, under the sponsorship of the Maharaja of Mysore.[31] At the age of sixteen he was invited by Krishnamacharya to stay with his sister and learn yoga. In the beginning Iyengar recalls that he 'had no genuine interest in yoga' and that, when he was given exercises, the 'pain of the body was unbearable' (Iyengar n.d.).

Krishnamacharya had traditional authority over Iyengar as his brother-in-law and benefactor, but he also had considerable personal charisma. In one account, Iyengar reflects that it could have been his fear of Krishnamacharya's anger that kept him practising yoga. Krishnamacharya trained Iyengar, who was living in his home, to obey his commandments unquestioningly. On his seventieth birthday, Iyengar recalled that:

> My Guru is a man of unpredictable knowledge with unpredictable moods. It was not easy to read his mind. If he said one thing at one time, he used to contradict the same at other time. We were made to accept and obey him without questioning. If I sit in the ordinary cross legs with the left leg first, he would say, take the right first. If the right is placed first, he would say, take the left first. If I stand, he would say 'is that the way to stand?' If I change, he would say 'who asked you to change?' . . . Life became perplexing to me. Difference in age set fear in my heart and his presence was like a frightful nightmare (Iyengar 1988a).

Several times Krishnamacharya demanded yoga postures of Iyengar in public demonstrations which Iyengar was able to perform only by injuring himself (Iyengar 1988a: 8–10). Krishnamacharya's instruction to Iyengar was never limited to asanas: he pushed his student into the zeal and self-discipline that allowed him to dedicate his life to excellence in the 'art' of yoga. Despite his harsh

31. The Maharaja of Mysore's sponsorship of yoga and physical culture has a long tradition. For further context on Krishnamacharya and his influence, see Desikachar (1998), Desikachar (2005), Goldberg (2016: 208–48), Singleton and Fraser (2014), Singleton (2010: 175) and Sjoman (1999).

treatment, Iyengar considered himself very fortunate to have been favoured by Krishnamacharya. As with Yogini Sunita, instruction in yoga was not about religious dogma or specific beliefs; rather, it was an approach to life.

Although Iyengar has claimed that personal instruction from Krishnamacharya in yoga asana was limited to these three intense days only, he practised regularly in the yoga shala with the other students (Iyengar n.d.: 2–3). In October 1935 Iyengar reported that he was judged to have given the best performance of all of Krishnamacharya's students in all three grades of 'elementary, intermediate and advanced courses' of yoga asana (Iyengar n.d.: 3). These might be earlier versions of the sequences that have become Ashtanga Vinyasa Yoga as taught by another of Krishnamacharya's students, Pattabhi Jois. At the age of nineteen, Iyengar was sent by Krishnamacharya to the north Indian city of Pune (then Poona) to teach yoga under a six-month contract. When this expired, Iyengar remained in the city practising asana for many hours a day and looking for students.

Iyengar recalled that, when he arrived, 'yoga was not a popular subject. The economic condition kept people away from Indian thought and heritage' (Iyengar 1988a: 13). He later reflected that fear of Krishnamacharya's temper kept him dedicated to earning a living through teaching yoga. He later reflected:

> I was [more] afraid of my Guruji's moods than to be called a madcap. The freedom had come to me by chance which I did not like to lose at any cost. If I go back, I have to join my Guruji only. That means to live in the web of constant fear (Iyengar 1988a: 16).

He was particularly successful in his attempts to popularise yoga when he took on patients of medical professionals. In 1945 he began teaching the daughter of a rich and influential nationalist, a girl severely affected by polio, with positive results. Having had his success verified by respected Pune doctors, Iyengar made more contacts and gained referrals within Pune's Indian elite (Iyengar 1988a: 36–41).

Having been taught yoga asana by Krishnamacharya as a means of recovering physical health, Iyengar concentrated on the perfection of this aspect of yoga. To some extent, Iyengar's intense focus on this aspect of the yoga tradition can be seen as a novel choice. However, as far as Iyengar was concerned he was simply working with what his guru had taught him. Reflecting on the transmission of knowledge and charisma through the yoga traditions, Iyengar has commented:

> I consider my Guru, and my Guru's guru as father of Yoga who sowed the seed to think and analyse the practical side for further develop-ment in this art . . . coming from the seed, whether it is myself or a col-league, we might change techniques like the branches of the tree, but we all belong to that one tree alone. With this traditional background I carry the message of Yoga when opportunities are thrown (Iyengar 1988a: 14–15).

Iyengar's education apart from Krishnamacharya is all autodi-dactic, consisting of a survey of books on yoga asana in his first years in Pune during the late 1930s, with reference to traditional texts and visiting yogis' lectures as he found appropriate. Iyengar believes he has always taught traditionally because he has not been educated in any other method. His primary education was observa-tion in his own asana practice. He reflected:

> In order to enjoy freedom, I thought I should practise more and strug-gle to learn English as I was not well familiar with it. I began picking up some books on Yoga to read, to get the basic ideas of Yoga. I saw lots of books on Yoga, but they did not interest me at all. I watched a lot of asanas from books. Shirsasana of one person was different to the other. I thought that the practitioners must be presenting according to their whims and fancies. Doubts and confusions led me to do all types of their presentations to find out by trials and errors, for uncovering the wrongs to discover the right ways. I began imitating the poses according to the illustrations which never never gave me any satisfac-tion of right feeling. I never read or looked at books on Yoga again. The moment trials and errors stopped daunting and taunting, my journey truly began in Yoga (Iyengar 1988a: 16).

Although this was a type of autodidacticism, Iyengar continued to work with the model his guru had taught, testing his experience against the tradition as he understood it.

In 1954, Iyengar arrived in Britain for the first time on the invi-tation of the violin virtuoso Yehudi Menuhin (1916–1999). A child prodigy, Menuhin sought in yoga a way of bringing release to his bodily tension and improving his performances (Magidoff 1973: 216–22). He had begun taking lessons from Iyengar while touring India in 1952 at the personal invitation of Prime Minister Nehru. Famously, Nehru made a friendly challenge to Menuhin and the

Yoga in Britain

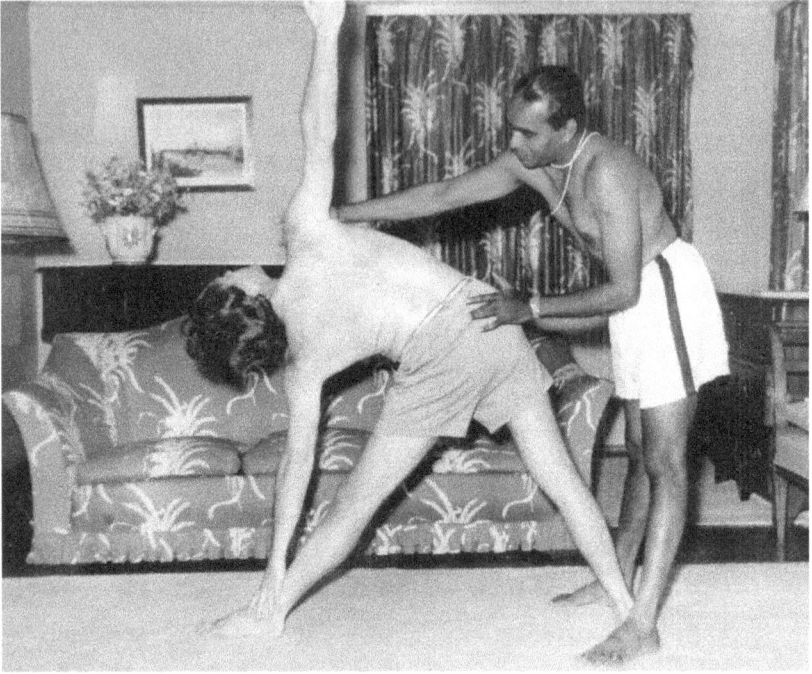

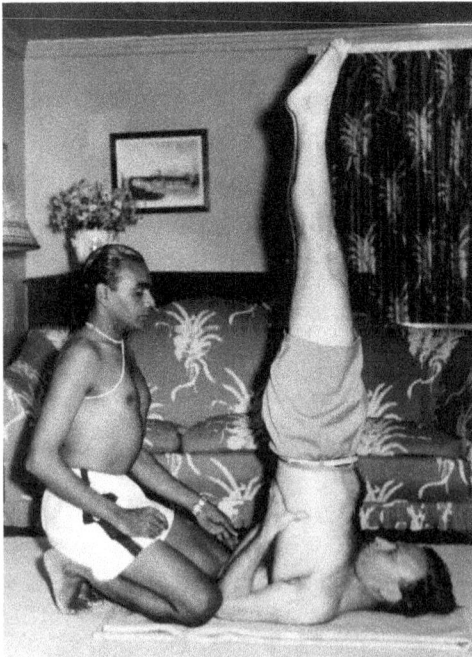

Figs. 3.3 and 3.4 B.K.S. Iyengar teaching Yehudi Menuhin. Photographs used with kind permission of Iyengar Yoga Maida Vale and the Menuhin Center Saanen.

two were found in headstand as the butler came in to announce dinner. When this story reached the press, 'gurus began to queue up wherever [Menuhin] went, each recommended by some prominent patron' (Magidoff 1973: 256–7). A student of B.K.S. Iyengar was part of Menuhin's welcoming party and convinced Iyengar to get on the train to visit Menuhin in Bombay. According to Menuhin, he warned Iyengar that he only had five minutes for him; however, Iyengar guided the violinist into a deep sleep from which he awoke not five minutes but an hour later. Impressed, Menuhin enthusiastically requested Iyengar to teach him during that visit (Menuhin 1996: 259).

This began a regular teaching relationship between the two men. Menuhin brought Iyengar to Europe in 1954 and the United States in 1956.[32] Then, between 1960 and 1975, Iyengar travelled to London to teach Menuhin every summer and was usually resident for at least a month (Menuhin 1996: 259). The New York-born Menuhin was an influential figure in British society, not only for his outstanding musical ability but also for his philanthropic and humanitarian interests.[33] Menuhin's second wife was the British ballerina Diana Gould, and from 1950–84 the couple made their family home in Highgate (Menuhin 1996: 436). It was through Menuhin's annual requests (from 1960) to be taught by Iyengar in London that the latter found his first British students.

Among Menuhin's circle of friends in London was the Angadi family. Patricia Angadi (née Fell-Clark) (1914–2001) was born into an 'affluent and conservative haute bourgeoisie' family in Hampstead.[34] She had met her Indian husband, Ayana Angadi, at a Ram Gopal Kathakali dance performance in London which received good reviews during its pre-war 1939 tour.[35] Ayana Angadi was

32. Iyengar did not return to the United States until 1973 – after his yoga teaching had been established in the LEA in Britain.

33. Menuhin was given an honorary knighthood in 1965 which he could fully accept when he became a British citizen in 1985; he was further honoured by the British government with a Lordship in 1993 (Lister 1999).

34. 'Obituary: Patricia Angadi', *The Independent* (London), 7 July 2001, p. 7.

35. 'Aldwych Theatre: Hindu Dances', *The Times*, 26 July 1939, p. 12, col. C. In Wilfred Clark's unreferenced pamphlet on the history of yoga in Britain, he reports that Ram Gopal taught yoga during this visit. Ram Gopal is better known for Kathakali dance, a physical discipline with some similarities to yoga. A Sri Ram Gopal was also listed as 'patron' on the early *Bulletins* of the Wheel of British Yoga, June 1967–September 1969.

a tanpura player and Trotskyite intellectual who saw himself as a 'cultural ambassador between East and West'.[36] When Patricia was elected head of Hampstead Arts Council in 1953, the couple was well placed among Britain's cultural elite to introduce their passion for Indian music to Britain.[37]

In 1956 they founded the Asian Music Circle to promote performances of Indian music in Britain, with Yehudi Menuhin the nominal president.[38] Menuhin turned to this group to find additional work for his yoga teacher, who had much free time on his hands during his London visits. In 1960, the second time Menuhin had brought Iyengar to London as his personal teacher, Iyengar gave a private demonstration to the Asian Music Circle and a public demonstration in Highgate; that year three people attended private classes at the house of the Angadis in Finchley, north London.[39] Iyengar's impromptu demonstration at a pre-Wimbledon party attracted press coverage as did the demonstrations he gave at public venues such as the Everyman's Theatre in Hampstead.[40] Despite the press coverage and the high-profile students, in the early 1960s Iyengar only had a dozen or so regular students. The morning class consisted of musicians, including the well-known pianist Clifford

36. 'B.B.C. Programmes for the Weekend', *The Times*, 6 September 1958, p. 4, col. F. Ayana Angadi played tanpura on the Third Programme with Ustad Vilayat Khan on sitar and Nikhil Ghosh on tabla.

37. 'Obituary: Patricia Angadi'. 'Garden Parties: Asian Music Circle', Court and Social, *The Times*, 7 July 1962, p. 10, col. C. 'Dance Recital: Asian Music Circle', Court and Social, *The Times*, 1 June 1963, p. 10, col. B. Also Patricia Angadi, 'Iyengar Yoga in the UK', *EuroYoga 93*, in the archives of the Iyengar Yoga Institute, Maida Vale, London.

38. 'Asian Music Circle has provided Londoners with such top artists as Pandit Ravi Shankar, Indrani Rehman, Ustad Ali Akbar Khan, Ustad Vilayat Khan, Shanta Rao and Shinchi Yuize, the famous Koto player from Japan. The circle has staged performances of visiting Asian artists and Mr Angadi hopes to enlarge the scope of the . . . friends . . . the Countess Harewood, Miss Beryl Grey and Mr Benjamin Britten who are the vice presidents devote considerable time in doing something for the Asian Music Circle. In England alone there are 13 major branches and they all enjoy full support of the Art Council of Great Britain.' 'Yoga Exponent BKS Iyengar to Tour England', *Poona Herald*, 1964: newspaper clippings in the collections at RIMYI, Pune.

39. Personal interview with Angela Marris (30 June 2005).

40. *Daily Mail*, 13 June 1960: newspaper clippings in the collections at RIMYI, Pune. *Daily Mail*, 16 June 1961: clipping in the archives of the Iyengar Yoga Institute, Maida Vale. 'Working for Health', *Hampstead and Highgate Express and Hampstead Garden Suburb and Golders Green News*, 7 July 1961, p. 4.

Curzon and famous cellist Jacqueline du Pré, with six attending the evening class.[41]

The small size of these early classes allowed for an intense personal interaction between Iyengar and his keen students. Diana Clifton corresponded regularly with Iyengar during the 1960s and '70s – as did several others among these first students – exchanging news of their families as well as receiving Iyengar's advice on yoga. In 1962, she sent a series of photographs to Iyengar; in reply he wrote:

> I went through all the pictures and remarked in the back. In the whole you have made a good progress. For your husband standing postures and twistings are good . . . Hope members of the yoga class are fine.[42]

This personal feedback was very important for many of Iyengar's early students and they could ask Iyengar directly for advice about how to deal with particular problems.[43] Initially, Clifton led the small group in a weekly meeting to practise their yoga after Iyengar had returned to India (Maimaris 2006: 6–11). She was chosen as group leader because she had no health problems and had already been practising yoga from Indra Devi's *Forever Young, Forever Healthy* (1955).[44] Slowly, friends and acquaintances became interested and Iyengar authorised the group to teach in pairs from 1962.[45] In addition to this correspondence, Iyengar returned to Britain for a month

41. *Daily Mail*, 16 June 1961: clipping in the archives of the Iyengar Yoga Institute, Maida Vale. 'Working for Health', *Hampstead and Highgate Express and Hampstead Garden Suburb and Golders Green News*, 7 July 1961, p. 4. Personal interview with Angela Marris (30 June 2005).

42. Letter from B.K.S. Iyengar to Diana Clifton, 13 February 1962, in the archives of the Iyengar Yoga Institute, Maida Vale.

43. While correspondence may have been kept by those involved, at least some of it has been destroyed at Iyengar's request. Letter from Angela Marris to Lorna Walker, 12 January 2001, in the archives of the Maida Vale Institute: 'When we moved to this flat we were very short of storage space and so we asked Mr Iyengar what we should do with all his letters etc. He told us to destroy all the letters and to give everything else to Silva Metha. We did both . . .'

44. See Devi (1955) and also Devi (1965). Indra Devi (1899–2002) (born Eiženija Pētersone) was taught yoga by B.K.S. Iyengar's teacher Krishnamacharya. She taught yoga in southern California from 1947 and her student, Elizabeth Arden, incorporated yoga into health spas in the USA. She also taught the actors Jennifer Jones, Greta Garbo, Gloria Swanson, Ramón Novarro, Linda Christian and Robert Ryan (see Stasulane forthcoming). From 1984 she lived and taught yoga in Argentina. For more on her legacy, see Goldberg (2015) and Goldberg (2016: 338–63).

45. Diana Clifton, 'The Beginning of Iyengar Yoga in London in 1961', manuscript in the Iyengar Yoga Institute, Maida Vale.

every year over the next fifteen years; in this way a closely knit net-work of students was established.

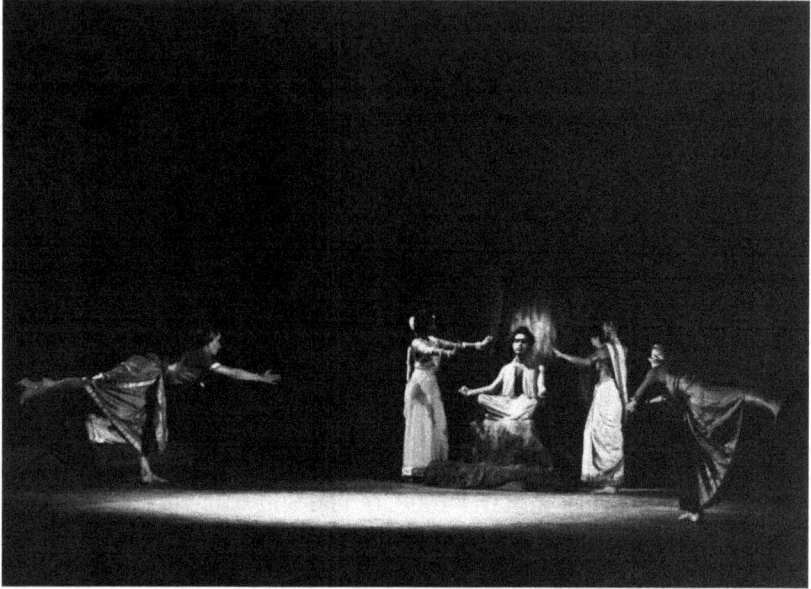

Fig. 3.5 Photograph of a performance of 'The Temptation of Buddha' organised by the Asian Music Circle in London during 1966 and 1967. Diana Clifton is on the left. Reproduced with permission of the Iyengar Yoga Association (UK) Archives, courtesy of John Bradford.

Iyengar and the Inner London Education Authority (ILEA)

In 1969, it was decided that only teachers approved by Iyengar could teach yoga in the Inner London Education Authority (ILEA). The process that led to this decision began in 1967, when a yoga class had been allowed to run on an 'experimental basis' at the Clapton Adult Education Institute. Even before this initial class opened, the ILEA had decided that yoga could be an appropriate subject as 'a means of keeping fit'.[46] Before allowing the class to begin at Clapton, the committee contacted the Birmingham City Council and discovered that 'despite initial adverse press comment and some opposition by Members, the Birmingham Education Committee established the

46. ILEA Further and Higher Education Sub-committee Papers, January–February 1967, ILEA/CL/PRE/16/09, London Metropolitan Archive.

[yoga] classes with continued success.'[47] Therefore, the committee recommended a trial yoga class. The author of the report also noted that the Chief Inspector of Physical Education for the ILEA, Peter McIntosh, was 'keen to assess the value of such a class'.[48]

Peter McIntosh (1915–2000) shaped how yoga was understood and practised in Britain. Something of a visionary, McIntosh's influence on sport and physical culture in Britain extended much further than the ILEA position (which he held from 1959–74). McIntosh wrote the first substantial historical and sociological studies of sport in Britain and argued passionately that physical education developed the cultural, economic and political interests of society (McIntosh 1969 [1957], 1972 [1952]). But he was also an enthusiastic advocate of sport for 'its own sake' and firmly championed the importance of physical culture, linking it with classical Greek ideals. Having read classics at Lincoln College, Oxford, McIntosh had acquired a deep appreciation of Grecian physical culture (McIntosh 1968: 114; Fisher 2000).

Previously, as Deputy Director of Physical Education at Birmingham University from 1946 to 1959, McIntosh designed the first physical education university degree courses in Britain and helped set the culture of physical education in Birmingham which allowed Yogini Sunita's classes to thrive. After leaving Birmingham, McIntosh became more involved with the politics of contemporary sport in Britain as a 'key figure in the formation of the Sports Council', serving on its committee between 1966 and 1974.[49] Among other activities, McIntosh drafted a paper delivered at the 1960 Rome Olympics that catalysed the formation of the International Council of Sport, Science and Physical Education.

McIntosh took a personal interest in introducing the new subject of yoga to the physical education curriculum in London. While excited about the potential of yoga, his influence on ILEA officials led to a focus on identifying a suitably qualified teacher:

> Owing to the growing demand for classes there is a tendency for well-meaning enthusiasts – some perhaps not so well-meaning – to push themselves forward as teachers. Inspectors of physical education

47. Ibid. The City of Birmingham Further Education Committee Minutes, June 1963–1970, BCC/BH 21/1/1/1-7, Archives Department, Birmingham Central Library, has no record of any discussion about yoga in the Birmingham LEA.
48. Ibid.
49. Ibid. and Huggins (2001).

do not have the experience in this particular subject necessary to
ensure good standards of teaching and work.[50]

A September 1968 report to the ILEA identified the newly
founded Wheel of British Yoga as a possible authority for certifying
quality Hatha Yoga instruction and suggested that it be investigated
further.[51] However, ILEA documents make no further mention of
the Wheel. As the Wheel was arguing that yoga was misplaced
as a physical education subject, it is likely McIntosh doubted the
Wheel's syllabus would guarantee high standards within a physical
education department.[52]

McIntosh found the assurances he sought about 'competent
and reliable' instructions on asana and pranayama through B.K.S.
Iyengar. Reportedly, at a social event, McIntosh had a casual conversation about yoga with Yehudi Menuhin's sister, Hephzibah
Hauser, who felt she had benefited from Iyengar's teaching.[53] This
led to McIntosh spending some time investigating and discussing yoga as a subject with Iyengar. Beatrice Harthan recalled that
Iyengar often stayed with Lady Coleraine while he was teaching
Menuhin in London; she further recalled that:

> Lady Coleraine, who was in our practice group, arranged for Peter
> McIntosh and the late Lord Noel Baker [*sic*], Nobel prize winner and
> president of UNESCO's International Council on Sport and Physical
> Recreation, to watch Mr Iyengar teach during his summer visit to
> England . . .[54]

McIntosh reported that he discussed with Iyengar 'the difficulties
in the way of ensuring that those who offer themselves as teachers

50. ILEA Further and Higher Education Sub-committee Papers, October–
December 1969, Report No. 11, presented 3 December 1969, ILEA/CL/PRE/16/24,
London Metropolitan Archive.

51. ILEA Further and Higher Education Sub-committee Papers, May/June 1968,
Report 2.9.68 by the Education Officer, ILEA/CL/PRE/16/17, London Metropolitan Archive.

52. According to ILEA files, during 1968 and 1969 'investigations have been
made into the teaching of yoga in London and elsewhere. The Senior Inspector of
Physical Education has visited a number of classes'. ILEA Further and Higher Education Sub-committee Papers, October–December 1969, Report 25.11.69 by Education Officer, ILEA/CL/PRE/16/24, London Metropolitan Archive.

53. Personal interview with Angela Marris (30 June 2005).

54. Beatrice Harthan, 'The Beginning of the Iyengar Movement in England',
Iyengar Yoga Institute, Maida Vale.

Demonstration

of

YOGA ASANAS

by

B. K. S. IYENGAR

Yoga teacher of Yehudi Menuhin
and
Author of " Light on Yoga "
(published by Allen & Unwin 75/-)

at
COMMONWEALTH INSTITUTE,
KENSINGTON HIGH STREET, W.8.

THURSDAY, 30th JUNE 1966, at 7.30 p.m.
(Doors open 7.0 p.m.)

Tickets 7/6
(reserved but un-numbered)

may be had at the door or in advance from Miss A. H.
Marris, Secretary - Asian Music Circle. 18, Glencairn Road,
Streatham, S.W.16 or Commonwealth Institute.

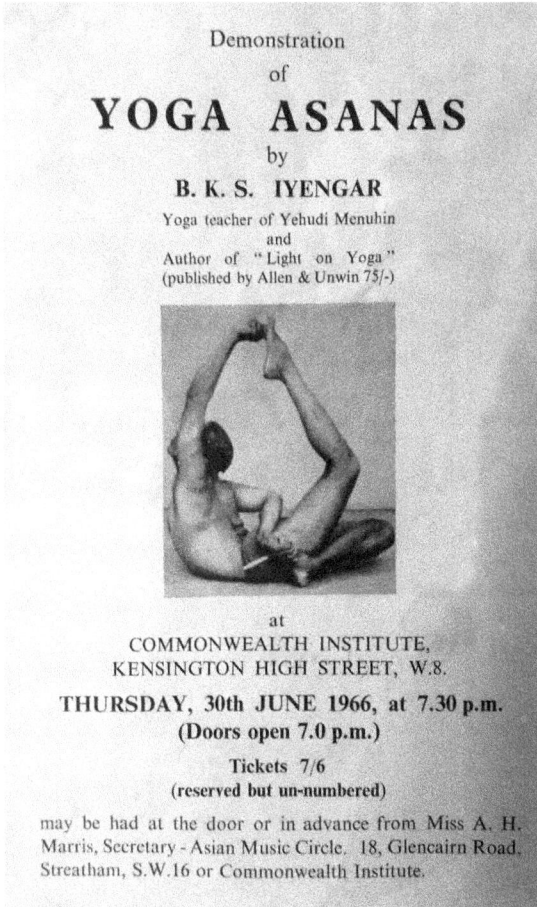

Fig. 3.6 Flyer for a 1966 demonstration by B.K.S. Iyengar in London to promote the publication of *Light on Yoga*. Photograph courtesy of John Yorke.

at Hatha Yoga are competent and reliable'.[55] McIntosh and his colleagues were also impressed by Iyengar's *Light on Yoga*, which the ILEA report considered 'probably the most reliable English text on the subject [of Hatha Yoga]'.[56] It was due to Iyengar's standing as a 'master of Hatha Yoga' (i.e. an expert authority) that Peter McIntosh agreed to let yoga enter the ILEA adult education system. The idea of a qualified 'master' ensures some level of competence but does not have quantifiable standards like those required in passing biomedical examinations. When Peter McIntosh approved 'gurus

55. ILEA Further and Higher Education Sub-committee Papers, October–December 1969, Report No. 11, presented 3 December 1969, ILEA/CL/PRE/16/24, London Metropolitan Archive.
56. Ibid.

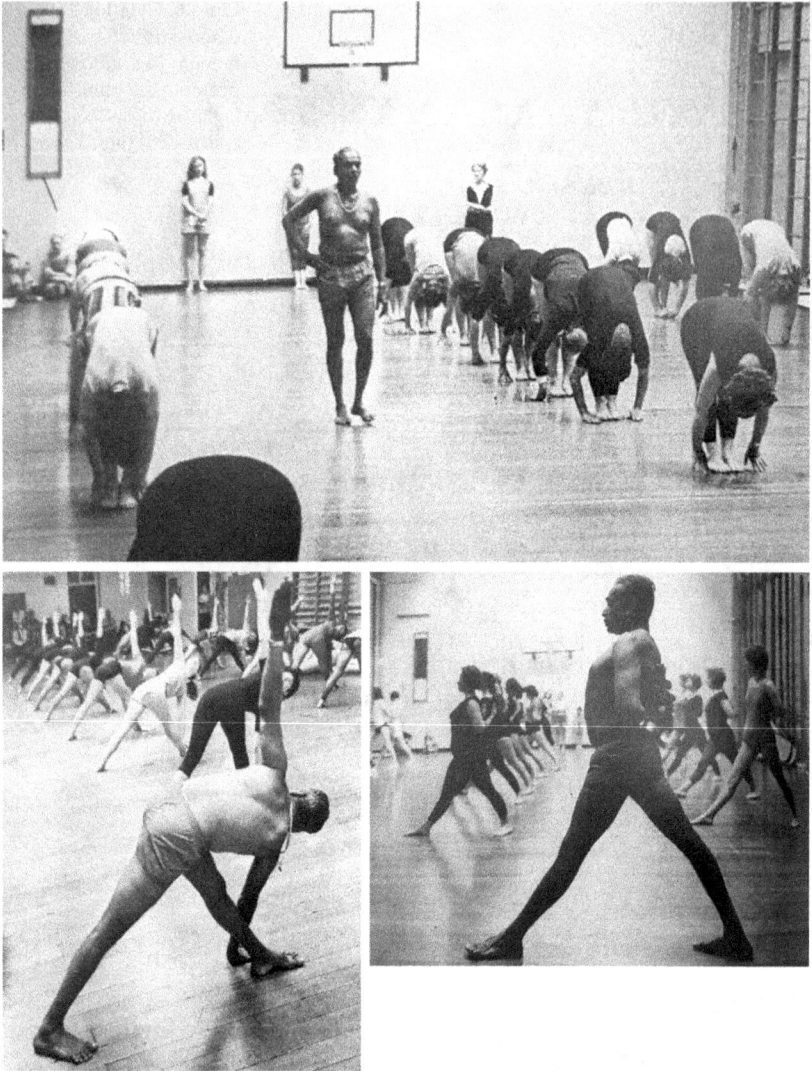

Figs. 3.7–3.9 B.K.S. Iyengar teaching prospective yoga teachers at an ILEA gym in 1971. Source: 'Iyengar Teaches', *Yoga & Health* 1/7 (1971): 22–29.

trained by Mr B.K.S. Iyengar, the author of "Light on Yoga", a recognised authoritative book on this subject', he gave Iyengar-trained teachers a bureaucratic authority as well as an expertise-based authority within the ILEA.[57]

In Iyengar, McIntosh found a quality of instruction in asana and pranayama which he felt could be approved. Yoga was to be taught only 'provided that instruction is confined to "asanas" and "pranayamas" (postures and breathing disciplines) and does not extend to the philosophy of Yoga as a whole'. All yoga tutors were subject to 'prior approval by the Senior Inspector of Physical Education'.[58] In practice, McIntosh approved the yoga teachers that were put forward by Iyengar's appointed trainer in London, Silva Mehta (1926–1994), who was giving a weekly yoga teacher-training class at the ILEA Physical Education College in Paddington from 1971–79. This was a compromise which recognised the traditional-charismatic nature of Iyengar's authority and it was combined with the bureaucratic authority of an ILEA-approved training course.

Silva Mehta was born in Czechoslovakia but attended university at Oxford. During 1957, while living in India, Mrs Mehta began studying with B.K.S. Iyengar twice a week to help with a painful back condition she later described as a 'fractured spine'. She recalled that her two young children, Shyam and Mira, 'came with me to class and made an attempt at some of the postures, but often they played quietly instead'.[59] She returned to England in 1960 with her children, continuing her yoga practice by meeting with the groups organised by the Asian Music Circle. Thus, Silva Mehta was one of the more 'senior' of Iyengar's students and an appropriate choice to lead these classes, which were attended by yoga teachers and aspiring yoga teachers. For the first few years there were no standardised syllabuses of postures or contraindications for specific medical conditions. However, within a few years Iyengar did develop three 'grades' of progressively difficult asana for the ILEA classes.[60]

57. Ibid.

58. ILEA Further and Higher Education Sub-committee Papers, October–December 1969, ILEA Education Committee, Report 25.11.69 by Education Officer, presented to the ILEA, 3 December 1969 (11), ILEA/CL/PRE/16/24, London Metropolitan Archive.

59. Silva Mehta, 'The Story of a Dream', *Dipika: The Journal of the Iyengar Yoga Institute* 16 (1987), p. 25.

60. Recorded in an undated letter from B.K.S. Iyengar to Diana Clifton specifically discussing ILEA classes. Held in the archives of the Iyengar Yoga Institute, Maida Vale.

By 1979 approximately 200 yoga teachers had been trained on this course.[61]

The classes are remembered by participants as being 'tough' and 'highly charged'. John Claxton, an Iyengar teacher in the ILEA from 1974 to 1983, remembered Iyengar's approach as being:

> A strange experience because – he taught in a way that was very un-English really ... He wasn't afraid to express his anger. He wasn't afraid to show real disapproval of what was going on – and to humiliate the teachers for not teaching the practice properly ... He demanded a very high standard of practice and got it.[62]

Much of the instruction focused on details of how to work in the basic postures. One pupil's notes taken from a May 1974 class taught by Iyengar in London consist entirely of anatomical instructions. For example, notes for the yoga posture *Virabhadrasana* I (Warrior I) include 'Turn at the kidneys. Inner arms straight. Raise arms stretching from coccyx.'[63] A large part of the class was practical, with a focus on teaching and demonstrating asana in front of students in mirror image. Iyengar would approve would-be yoga teachers on his annual visits. According to some reports, Silva Mehta sometimes decided when the students were ready to teach in Iyengar's absence.[64]

In response to criticisms that he only taught physical postures, Iyengar described his approach as a pragmatic expedient: 'Better life can be taught without using religious words. Meditation is of two types, active and passive. I took the active side of meditation by making students totally absorbed in the poses.'[65] A student quoted Iyengar teaching during one of his London visits:

61. Silva Mehta, 'A Brief History of Iyengar Yoga in England and the South East England Iyengar Yoga Institute', 19 March 1983. Archives of the Iyengar Yoga Institute, Maida Vale.

62. Personal interview with John Claxton (5 December 2004).

63. Ailsa Herremans, 'Notes Taken at Classes Held by Mr Iyengar in London in May 1974 and in Poona in January 1975', typewritten manuscript in the archives of the Iyengar Yoga Institute, Maida Vale.

64. Sally Finesilver, letter to Lorna Walker, 26 November 1999 in response to a request for memories of 'Iyengar's early days in the UK'. Held in the archives of the Iyengar Yoga Institute, Maida Vale. Personal interview with John Claxton (5 December 2004).

65. Julie Dale, 'B.K.S. Iyengar: An Introduction by One of His Students', manuscript in the library of the Ramamani Iyengar Memorial Yoga Institute in Pune, India.

The end of discipline is the beginning of freedom. Only a disciplined person is a free person. So-called 'freedom' is only a license to act and do as we like. Yoga is to train and discipline the worries and anxieties of men and women.[66]

Through disciplining bodies Iyengar hoped to discipline his students' minds (Iyengar 1993a: 46).[67] Iyengar attempted to give his students control over both their minds and bodies by demanding precision in asana. The continuation of this part of Iyengar's yoga tradition relied on the ability of other yoga teachers to create this experience within the framework of the legal-rational structure of Iyengar's certification system.

Some of Iyengar's approved yoga teachers were able to embody yoga with their own personal charisma. A particularly influential teacher under the Iyengar system was Penelope (Penny) Nield-Smith (1922–1989), who inspired many students to train as Iyengar teachers through her classes all over London (see also Busia 2007: xviii–xxii; Tobias 2007: 285–91).[68] Students recalled that when Penny 'exalted us to stand and concentrate on the way our feet were planted on the ground, she was fond of remarking how man is in a hurry to explore outer space, but is not yet sufficiently aware of what his own feet are doing on earth'. This comment speaks to her personal dedication to global environmental and social causes. Her students remember that she was passionate about environmentalism, the writings of Krishnamurti and African culture, among other causes.[69] Former students Sophy Hoare and Mary Stewart recalled that 'she seemed to involve us in these causes in the very manner in which she told us to drop our shoulders away from our ears or stretch our little toes'. In particular, she used the same words and phrases in every class, often with implicit 'double meanings' – one simple meaning in the class and a greater meaning if applied outside the class.[70] In this way Nield-Smith created an environment in

66. Anonymous, 'The Sutras of Iyengar', p. 11, typewritten manuscript in the archives of the Iyengar Yoga Institute, Maida Vale.

67. Here Iyengar is referring to Patañjali's widely circulating definition of yoga.

68. Kofi Busia was an important populariser of Iyengar yoga in London and Oxford in the 1970s and '80s and Maxine Tobias became an influential Iyengar teacher in London in the 1980s and '90s.

69. Interviews with Sophy Hoare (5 January 2005), Lorna Walker (31 June 2005) and John and Ros Claxton (5 December 2004).

70. S. Hoare and M. Stewart, 'Obituary: Penny Nield-Smith', *The Independent*, 26 July 1989. Personal interviews with Sophy Hoare (5 January 2005), Lorna Walker (31

her classes where attention to the physical body during the asana practice could be transformed into attention to personal and global entelechy. She was a particular example of a yoga teacher under Iyengar who generated her own personal charisma and inspired others to continue within the increasingly legal-rational authority of Iyengar Yoga in London.

Iyengar Yoga in Manchester

In Manchester also Iyengar found students who organised to propagate his teaching. Iyengar first came to Manchester in 1968 at the invitation of two women who were already teaching yoga in the LEA evening classes. The more senior of the two, Pen Reed, had been teaching yoga in the South Manchester Withington Further Education Centre from 1965 having taken lessons in yoga in Birmingham from an Indian, probably Sunita Cabral.[71] The second woman, Jeanne Maslen, came to yoga after Reed demonstrated yoga asana at the end of a keep-fit class in the mid-1960s (Maslen 1997). After seeing a demonstration by Iyengar on television, the two yoga teachers arranged for Iyengar to give a public demonstration on 4 July 1968 at Spurley Hey High School in Gorton, Manchester.

Over five hundred tickets were sold for the event. The two women arranged for some of their regular students to join them for a demonstration in front of friends and family before Iyengar began As one student recalls:

> Jeanne was performing a graceful Virabhadrasana III to the gentle strains of Brahms, balancing on one leg ... when, to her horror, she looked down and saw a brown face with a thunderous expression looking up at her. In front of the 500 people he berated them soundly for desecrating his art, then proceeded to give a demonstration of postures with such purity and clarity that the audience was spellbound and Pen and Jeanne complained not at all about their rough treatment, and only asked to be taught themselves.[72]

June 2005) and John and Ros Claxton (5 December 2004). See also *BKS Iyengar Yoga Teachers' Association News Magazine*, Winter 1989, pp. 17–18.

71. *The Manchester and District Institute of Iyengar Yoga* 1 (March 1972), Manchester Archives and Local Studies, Manchester Central Library.

72. M. Greer, 'The Gentle Octopus', *Manchester and District Institute of Iyengar Yoga* 17 (1988), pp. 26–8.

According to Maslen and Reed, Manchester's Withington Further Education Centre, which sponsored the demonstration, was subsequently inundated with demand for yoga classes. Maslen remembers queues that went 'out the door through the front gardens and round the corner' for the classes (Maslen 1997).

To meet the demand for teachers, the two women quickly set up a teacher-training programme in the Withington and Trafford areas.[73] According to the Manchester and District Iyengar Yoga Institute newsletter:

> The decision of Manchester Education Committee to endorse a course for yoga teachers at Withington, emphasized the need for a specific standard of excellence. With these thoughts in their minds, a number of teachers attended meetings of other groups and looked at their methods. They came back more, rather than less convinced that Iyengar's method with its precision and profound understanding of the body and its needs should be the guiding principle. More decisions followed. The need for a formalized system of training teachers (the present syllabus for our training course is included in this journal) and the need for an information source for the many hundreds of students. All these things led ultimately to the forming of the Manchester and District Institute of Yoga . . .[74]

This 'Institute' had no official premises but was a network of teachers qualified in the Iyengar system in the Manchester area. The Manchester yoga teacher-training programme started in 1971–72 and was open to those who had taken yoga classes under a 'recognised teacher' for at least two years. The course lasted thirty-four weeks, with four contact hours per week and an emphasis on physiology and anatomy. The purpose of this focus was to 'safeguard against physical injury which can be incurred if the complicated posture exercises are taught by a person uninstructed in this direction'. The successful passing of a written and practical assessment in front of yoga instructors and 'educational experts' would result in a diploma 'recognised by the Manchester Education Committee'.[75] While Iyengar did not personally select teachers as in London, he was consulted on the syllabus, which further facilitated the growth of a bureaucratic means of transmitting his understanding of yoga.

73. *The Manchester and District Institute of Yoga Bulletin* 1 (March 1972), p. 6, Manchester Archives and Local Studies, Manchester Central Library.
74. Ibid., p. 1.
75. Ibid., p. 6.

Unfortunately, there was no discussion of this course or its assessment in the Manchester Further Education Committee minutes. Unlike London, Manchester had no sub-committee with an interest in physical education; unlike Birmingham, Manchester had no institution dedicated to promoting access and excellence in sport and physical education. Physical culture offerings at Manchester evening classes during the 1960s and '70s were more limited than in either Birmingham or London.[76] Further Education sub-committees regularly discussed their difficulty in addressing the further educational needs of the Manchester community.[77] It is possible that yoga classes were not closely examined because they subsidised other further-education courses.[78] However, it was in Manchester that courses on 'Iyengar Yoga' further developed their content of asana syllabuses and anatomy basics which increased the legal-rational authority of the adult education environment.

Further Developments of Iyengar Yoga

As the 1970s progressed, Iyengar teachers in Britain in both London and Manchester began to work together to create a national assessment body that issued certificates. In June 1978, the B.K.S. Iyengar Teachers' Association explained to the ILEA that:

> In view however of the great increase in the demand for teachers over the past few years, and in order to safeguard potential students, Mr

76. Manchester Further Education Committee Minutes 1960–70; Manchester Evening Institute Prospectuses Boxes MSC 378 and MSC 370/E and the archives of the Manchester College of Adult Education, Manchester Archives and Local Studies, Manchester Central Library.

77. Manchester Further Education Committee Minutes 1968–69, vol. 34A, 2530. In the east area of Manchester, due to 'reduced expenditure imposed by the council in November 1967' and 'to avert possible serious overspending on the estimates', the principal reported that 'some classes had been closed and others combined. Initially 108 out of 450 had been affected but after review only 45 classes now finally closed with 19 others combined.' Manchester Archives and Local Studies, Manchester Central Library.

78. The Committee clearly considered that it had more important issues to discuss. For example, In 1968, students at the Manchester College of Commerce staged a 'sit-in' due to inadequate accommodation, staffing and book stock at the Manchester College of Commerce. The Education Committee considered that hiring two extra library staff might address the immediate crisis. Manchester Further Education Sub-committee Minutes for 1968–69, vol. 34A, 1595. Manchester Archives and Local Studies, Manchester Central Library.

Iyengar recently decided to issue Certificates to those of his pupils he considered qualified to teach.

Certificates in different grades have been issued. Most people hold the Elementary Certificates which authorise them to teach a number of basic postures and preparatory pranayama. This is perfectly safe for ordinary adult education classes. Some people hold Intermediate Certificates, and a very few Advanced Certificates. We consider, however, that teaching of intermediate and advanced work is outside the scope of ordinary adult education classes.[79]

Elementary and intermediate certificates were assessed in Britain, while advanced certificates were issued by Iyengar personally.[80] From 1978, formal assessments of all Iyengar-trained teachers were made by a professional organisation of Iyengar teachers, the newly founded B.K.S. Iyengar Teachers' Association. At the end of a training period, potential yoga teachers would be assessed by a panel of qualified yoga teachers whom they did not know personally. This system replaced successful completion of a course and the informal approval of the course tutor. This formal issuing of certificates was partially undertaken to ensure that teachers using Iyengar's name would have accountability for at least a certain standard of training.

In addition to teaching in Britain, Iyengar increasingly made trips to North America, Europe and southern Africa, first visiting the latter in 1968 after a South African yoga practitioner attended his London classes. White South Africans travelled to Mauritius for his classes because the Indian government would not allow Iyengar to travel to apartheid South Africa.[81] Iyengar returned to Africa, teaching in Malawi and Kenya in 1971 and Swaziland in 1972, 1973 and 1976.[82] He made his second visit to the United States in 1973 and subsequently gained a larger following of teachers (Vernon 2007: 5). Iyengar's international networks were facilitated by the legal-rational structure developed in London and Manchester.

79. *B.K.S. Iyengar Teachers' Association Newsletter,* June 1978, p. 1. In the archives of the Iyengar Yoga Institute, Maida Vale.

80. Assessments for Teaching Certificates November 1979 and March 1980 in the archives of the Iyengar Yoga Institute, Maida Vale.

81. Iyengar's travels are well documented in the press cutting volumes at the Ramamani Iyengar Memorial Yoga Institute, Pune, India.

82. Newspaper clipping files held at the RIMYI Archives, Pune, India.

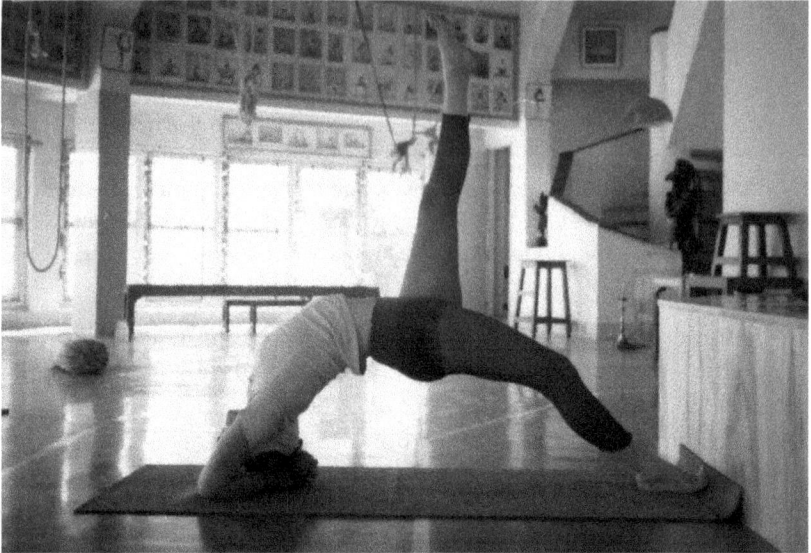

Fig. 3.10 Diana Clifton in Pune, 1977. Reproduced with permission of the Iyengar Yoga Association (UK) Archives, courtesy of John Bradford.

Iyengar's international students funded the opening of a yoga centre in Pune, which became the centre of the international Iyengar network. It opened in 1976, and students worldwide began travelling to Pune for a month or more of intensive daily lessons with Iyengar, his daughter Geeta and son Prashant. This ensured that students felt a personal relationship with Iyengar as a teacher and that teaching was controlled and standardised at this one source. Many of the committed teachers would travel regularly to Pune. However, a new generation of British-based teachers was emerging who did not necessarily have a personal experience of Iyengar.[83] Furthermore, the extensive bureaucratic structures that Iyengar developed ran with minimal personal involvement from him. For example, in 2006, there were 85 newly qualified 'Introductory Level Iyengar Yoga Teachers'.[84] Many of these would have become 'Iyengar Yoga

83. For example, a British person currently wishing to study at the Ramamani Iyengar Memorial Yoga Institute (RIMYI) in Pune, would first have to commit to eight years of study with an Iyengar-certified teacher in their own country. Training to become an introductory-level Iyengar teacher in Britain, on the other hand, could be completed with six years of study with British Iyengar-certified teachers. Hence many new teachers gain qualification without having had any personal contact with Iyengar or his children.

84. *Iyengar Yoga News* 10 (Spring 2007), p. 44.

Teachers' without having travelled to Pune or met Iyengar personally. To become an Introductory Iyengar Yoga Teacher in Britain
currently requires a minimum of six years' practice with Iyengar
teachers and to pass a standard assessment; eight years of practice
are a prerequisite for applying for classes with Iyengar's children
in Pune. Other countries with a lower density of qualified practitioners have less rigorous requirements, particularly for access to
classes at RIMYI in Pune.[85] Iyengar developed a successful method
of routinising his charisma and ensuring the continuation of his
yoga tradition.

Conclusion

Both Iyengar and Sunita presented yoga to the British public as a
non-religious activity that could provide physical and psychological benefits. In contrast to the Wheel, they both concentrated on a
single interpretation of yoga rather than a broad survey of different
approaches. Both had considerable personal charisma, attracting
students with what was perceived as unique insight into essentially
a new cultural practice for Britons. Sunita's classes were popularised
by word of mouth, local newspaper reports and the institutional
framework of the Birmingham Athletic Institute. While this initially
popularised yoga in Birmingham, by relying on traditional transmission of the tradition from one charismatic teacher to another,
Sunita did not institutionalise her charisma.

Pranayama Yoga's lack of institutionalisation can be partially
attributed to Sunita's early death, but there was also a fundamental difference in the method of transmission between Sunita and
Iyengar. Sunita's approach was essentially a traditional transmission of charismatic authority; those students with a deep understanding of her tradition would in turn transmit Pranayama Yoga
to others. The permission to teach others Pranayama Yoga would
be given at the discretion of the established teacher, based on how
well the students understood the system rather than any formal,
bureaucratic method. Her teacher-training course was not designed
to automatically qualify students for adult education classes. For
this, Sunita recognised that few would have the charismatic quality

85. From the guidelines of the Iyengar Yoga Association (UK), published on
https://iyengaryoga.org.uk/iyengar-yoga/pune-institute, accessed 29 August
2017.

required to inspire educational authorities' trust. In her book on Pranayama Yoga, Sunita wrote that 'on average, one [yoga teacher] in every thousand is chosen to work for Education' (Cabral 1971 [2002]: 57). After her death, some students did continue to teach Pranayama Yoga within the Birmingham-area adult education system. However, as Sunita anticipated, most of her teachers would work privately. As the memory of Sunita's personal charisma has faded, this has become increasingly the case. While Sunita's Pranayama Yoga continues to be taught in Britain, none of the teachers she trained have had the charisma to further popularise this yoga tradition into a visible social movement.

In contrast, Iyengar managed to incorporate a legal-rational structure for transmitting important aspects of his yoga tradition. This allowed for entry of significant numbers of recognised, 'qualified' teachers into the adult educational system in Britain. Adult education courses for yoga teacher-training were approved first in London (1969), then in Manchester (1972). Local authorities felt assured of a standard of competence and excellence in the performance of asana, an aspect of yoga that was felt to be appropriate in this context. This successfully popularised Iyengar's tradition of yoga beyond the sphere of his personal influence or reliance on his own personal charisma. Although, the routinisation of Iyengar's charismatic yoga teaching into institutional bureaucracy has created an internationally recognised form of yoga, yoga is less defined by the teacher–pupil (traditional guru–śiṣya) relationships than it is by the institutionalised system. Although yoga now has the benefit of more worldwide availability, the contemporary experience of yoga in Britain is not defined by a relationship with a charismatic personality.

Chapter Four

Middle-Class Women Join Evening Classes

Yoga classes were often in physical education departments in adult education facilities during the 1960s and '70s, in ostensibly gender-neutral categories. However, by most estimates, 70–90 per cent of the students in classes were women.[1] Women began practising yoga for a variety of reasons, but improving their own feelings of physical health and mental well-being was a primary concern. Although yoga classes often focused on participants' subjective somatic experiences, women reported that its effects in terms of better emotional and physical well-being motivated their attendance. Women often reported that they attended a yoga class because it improved their ability to perform social duties and responsibilities at home and work. It was felt by many women that improving their health and emotional equilibrium, two attributes often attributed to yoga classes, better enabled them to care for themselves, their husbands and their children.

The politics of health have long been intimately related to national welfare and ideas of citizenship (Porter 1994). Dorothy Porter attributes the concept of 'health as a right of citizenship' to eighteenth-century French and American revolutionary ideals (D. Porter 2000: 204). Furthermore, public health and modern sanitary reform has been on the British government's agenda since at least the 1830s.[2] Following other states, notably Prussia, in the early twentieth century Britain began encouraging its population to be fit and healthy for the possibility of military action (Hennock 1987). As Ina Zweiniger-Bargielowska has shown, during the interwar period

1. Interviews with Ros Claxton (5 December 2004), Sophy Hoare (5 January 2004) and Lorna Walker (31 June 2005). Hoare also emphasised that she was struck at the 'very varied mix of people attending' in terms of social and age-range mix compared to the dance classes she had been attending previously. It is interesting that these same ratios characterised what Philip Deslippe calls 'early American yoga' which was much less physical in its practice; see Deslippe (2018).
2. For an overview see Szreter (2005: 23–45) and Hamlin (1994: 132–64).

physical culture and public health became associated with eugenic notions of national interest as well as the focus of both private and governmental health campaigns (Zweiniger-Bargielowska 2006, 2007).[3] From its inception, the goal of public health included a need for public education about the causes of disease and its prevention (D. Porter 2000: 203–7).

There has often been a class element associated with both ability and willingness to act on public health recommendations. For example, Simon Szreter has argued that the educated and relatively wealthy middle classes of Britain's South were able to enact community sanitary reforms with greater efficacy than in the North (Szreter 2005: 352–3). More relevant to the case of British yoga practitioners, Avner Offer has shown that, in the second half of the twentieth century, middle- and upper-class women were more successful at maintaining ideal body-mass than women of other classes (Offer 2001, 2006). The participation of middle-class women in yoga classes can be understood as part of a long British tradition of improving health and educational standards. An important element of yoga's appeal in post-war Britain was the way it supported a national agenda of individual responsibility for health and well-being. This was a social message that middle-class women were particularly interested in heeding and well positioned to act on.

Women in Adult Education in Post-war Britain

Courses offered at evening institutes were often highly gendered and women were becoming an increasingly significant component of the adult-education population. During the 1950s Women's Institutes and Townswomen's Guilds grew rapidly in number, as did women's membership and participation in co-educational bodies. While the 1960 Workers' Educational Association (WEA) welcomed this development 'unreservedly', it also noted that:

> so far the influx of women has consisted mainly of those from a comparatively favourable social and educational background. There is still a lack of women recruits from lower income groups and who left school at the age of fourteen or fifteen . . . recruitment difficulties are obvious: the growing practice of married women going out to work,

3. Singleton (2007a) has shown how these eugenic ideals influenced the development of yoga in early-twentieth-century India.

the low age of marriage and child bearing, and also perhaps lingering traditional self mistrust . . . (WEA Working Party 1960: 31).

Although in 1960 49% of female attendees for adult education did not work outside the home, the WEA report did note increasing numbers of women working outside the home for reasons of personal fulfilment as much as economic necessity. Middle-class women did not generally need to work out of economic necessity in the 1950s; those that did work were often looking for more connection to the world outside the home and the personal autonomy derived from earning one's own money. For many middle-class women, freedom and autonomy were psychological and ideological aspirations not economic ones (see Wilson 1980; Ingham 1981; Akhtar and Humphries 2001). The more economically disadvantaged who had to support a family simply did not have the leisure time for either yoga or other non-vocational pursuits.

The revival of feminism in the 1960s was largely pioneered by middle-class women addressing problems originating from their own class. Women had been part of the British workforce before, after and during the world wars; however, for the most part, 'gainfully employed' women were not working from choice but in order to provide food and shelter for themselves and possibly their relations. In previous generations, unmarried women and working-class women worked out of necessity while middle-class women generally only took paid employment when the men were absent in war. Hobsbawm has speculated that

> the very demand to break out of the domestic sphere into the paid labour market had a strong ideological charge among the prosperous, educated middle-class married women which it did not have for others, for its motivations in these milieus were seldom economic (Hobsbawm 1994: 318; Humphries 2000: 85–106).

The resentments of middle-class women burdened with their new duty of managing every aspect of housework and childcare were important as aspirations conflicted with restricted social roles. Ina Zweiniger-Bargielowska (2001: 153) points out that until the Second World War the majority of middle-class households employed domestic help of some kind. Whereas they previously had leisure time to devote to culture and liberal education within the home, now there was only housework. This served as an impetus for second-wave feminists who saw women's status comparing poorly with that of the men. Other classes of women may have experienced similar tensions between personal and family identity but it was the middle-class women who were articulate about their concerns while enjoying relative economic freedom allowing for reflective thought and experimentation in lifestyle. Their sentiments were reinforced by increasing numbers of publications (many by women) address-ing these issues (Sandbrook 2006: 648–64).

Many influential books voiced the discontent and frustration felt women in their failed attempts at having an independent identity; these included Virginia Woolf's *A Room of One's Own* (1929) and the second-wave feminist manifestos of Germaine Greer's *The Female Eunuch* (1970) and Ann Oakley's *Housewife* (1974).[4] The grievances and ambitions of second-wave feminists were echoed in the pages of the British yoga journals, with yoga described as a cure for wom-en's specific problems, such as 'housewife syndrome'.[5] The latter was identified by a yoga teacher who conducted a survey in the 1970s and found many of her students to be housewives suffer-ing from 'monotony and lack of recognition, indeterminate pains and psychosomatic symptoms'. Through the practice of yoga, the teacher concluded that most students suffering from this so-called 'housewife syndrome' found that their lives improved. In fact, she stated that, through yoga, 90 per cent of 'sufferers' regained 'lost vitality' and a woman could 'face her problems without tension'.[6]

Educated, middle-class women's discontent at being confined within the home was noted explicitly by those in the adult-educa-tion community. One participant in a Liverpool initiative to train women as teachers of crafts reported in 1968 that

> the ever-increasing desire of women to do some kind of work outside the home has resulted in many housewives with young families com-ing forward, eager to develop an outside interest and to achieve some degree of status and financial independence (Burgess 1968: 94).

In 1973, another tutor involved in the same programme reported on the reasons given for wishing to join a course to teach crafts in the adult-education system. The largely married female candi-dates would often report in their intake interviews: '"I feel like I am

---

4. For descriptions of other influential ideas and books, see Bruley (1999: 145) and Rowbottom (2001).

5. M.T.M. de Vilar, 'Housewife Syndrome', *Yoga* 27 (Spring 1976), p. 7.

6. Ibid.

becoming a cabbage"; "I cannot stand the four walls"; "I need adult company" etc.' (Hughes 1973: 167). The tutor went on to analyse the situation, remarking that many of these women had educational qualifications that could permit university entry but

> these women, like many others, being conscientious about their role as mother, will not train at the expense of their children's security. . . . [furthermore] The drive is not an economic one . . . employment is not guaranteed, and trainees do not receive any grant (Hughes 1973: 167).

The course only required six hours a week attendance and none of the interviewees were reported to have asked about employment prospects at the time of the interview.

Attending courses on traditionally feminine subjects like crafts, flower arrangement or cooking might have felt less threatening and more respectable than employment outside the home, particularly if there was no financial imperative to leave the house. It is likely that yoga was more gendered in Manchester and the North than in London and the South-east. In an essay on North–South differences in England, Raphael Samuel observed that the North appears to be 'wedded to more patriarchal ways'.[7] Gender distinctions were more institutionalised in Manchester's further education than in London's. Principals of adult-education institutes in Manchester had to negotiate classroom space with the head teachers of the area's schools. During the 1960s and '70s, the East Area Principal complained that gender-segregated secondary schools meant that certain adult-education classes could only be held in certain schools:

> At Lady Barn (a boys' school) there are no cookery classes and dress-making takes place in ordinary classrooms. At Levenshulme and Mosley there are now no classes in woodwork and metalwork . . . I would urge the governors to seek some accommodation where both men and women may have adequate facilities.[8]

7. Samuel (1998a: 161) cites as evidence for this claim the difficulty that the Labour Party has had in promoting all-women shortlists of parliamentary candidates in northern areas. Also McKibbin (1998: 91, 101–5) has argued that between 1918 and 1951, 'Northern' middle classes were identified with non-conformist beliefs and manufacturing interests while the 'Southern' middle classes were generally Anglicans with commercial interests; he concludes that these regional differences were stronger than the commonalities of middle-class culture.

8. Manchester Further Education Sub-Committee Minutes 1970–71, vol. 36A, p. 214, Manchester Central Library Archives.

Also in Manchester, the Withington Further Education Centre listed its mid-1970s yoga course in the Department of Domestic Science, sandwiched between 'cake icing and decoration' (both first year and advanced), 'flower arrangement' and 'ballroom dancing'. Although the course description assured prospective students that 'these courses are equally suitable for men and women of all ages', it is doubtful whether many men would have even bothered to look at the page.[9] During the same year the Mary Ward Centre in London offered its yoga classes under the more gender-neutral Department of Health Education. This may also have been influenced by the agenda of a male teacher at that centre, Alan Babbington, who was committed to the 'philosophical side of yoga' as well as teaching the physical postures.[10]

As a career, yoga teaching in adult education classes offered flexible and part-time hours which particularly suited those who would appreciate some extra money but did not require a full salary. Teaching was traditionally a women's profession and the rates of pay for yoga courses in the LEA compared favourably to other part-time employment open to women during this period. Vi Neale-Smith remembers that, when she started teaching yoga in 1974, the local authority paid her £6 an hour compared to the £3 she made as a part-time medical secretary.[11] More money and fewer hours was an attractive option for married women who had domestic duties and childcare to arrange. Yoga teachers were able to pick and choose classes they wanted at times that suited them – particularly since the family income was not dependent on the work. This flexible and independent employment answered middle-class women's desire for freedom and autonomy more fully than many other available options. Still, teaching for the LEA did not offer a living wage and men who made yoga teaching a profession in Britain took this into account. Ernest Coates and Indra Nath, both males teaching yoga in the 1970s, never relied on it for their primary income[12] – in all likelihood very few did: the majority of teachers would have relied

9. Withington Further Education Centre, *Prospectus Session 1976/77*, pp. 11–12, Manchester Central Library Archives.

10. Mary Ward Centre, *Prospectus 1976/77*, p. 13.

11. Interview with Vi Neale-Smith (17 September 2004).

12. Personal interview with Ernest Coates (19 December 2004) and Indra Nath (18 August 2005).

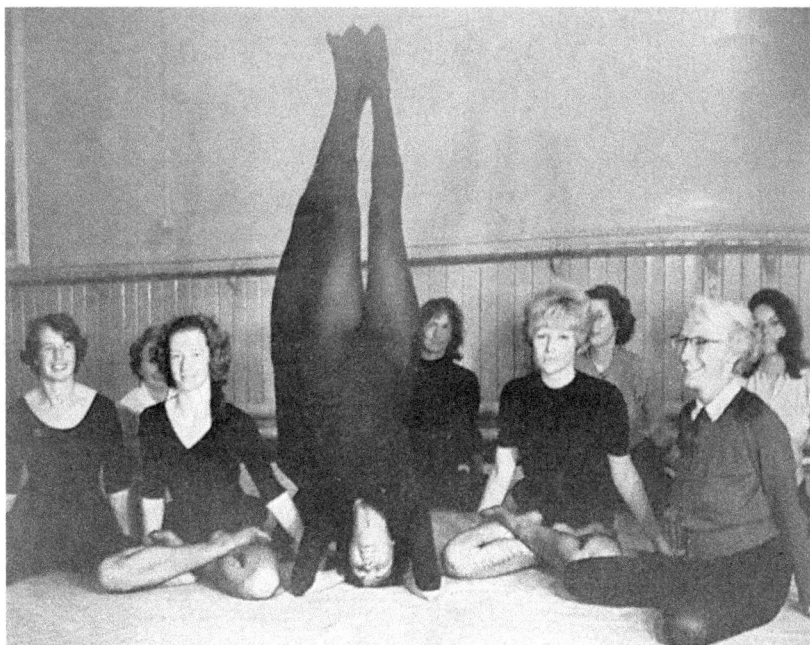

Fig. 4.1 Yogini Sunita's Pranayama Yoga teacher-training class, 1966. Photograph reproduced with permission of Ken Cabral and the Lotus and the Rose Publishers.

on their husbands' financial support, or like Coates and Nath, had reached a point where they had saved enough money to retire.

British yoga teachers numbered less than a thousand during the 1970s and the majority of these were married women.[13] In 1975, one writer in the British Wheel's journal estimated that '99% of Yoga teachers [in Scotland] are housewives with families'.[14] In the Manchester area, a 1972 list of Iyengar teachers includes seventeen names: fifteen 'Mrs', one 'Miss' and one 'Mr'.[15] In 1978 a list of B.K.S. Iyengar certificate holders for Britain includes 214 names, of which 36, or about sixteen per cent, have male first names.[16] During much of the twentieth century, middle age has been a difficult period for women in 'obtaining and retaining well-paid employment' because

13. The British Wheel of Yoga itself claimed 1,500 members and 500 teachers in 1975. *Yoga* 24 (Summer 1975), p. 14.

14. J. Gillespie, 'Scotland', *Yoga* 23 (Spring 1975), p. 23.

15. *Manchester and District Institute of Yoga Bulletin*, p. 1.

16. 'List of B.K.S. Iyengar Yoga Teachers' Certification Holders', October 1978, in the archives of the Iyengar Yoga Institute, Maida Vale.

of a double discrimination of gender and age in many positions (Benson 1997: 80). Many LEAs enforced a retirement age (sixty or sixty-five), but some women continued to teach yoga privately well into their seventies.[17]

In 1982, seventy-two-year-old Clara Buck was offering two private lunchtime yoga classes in London from noon–1 pm for £10 a month.[18] This yoga was at times a meaningful and gainful activity where older women could feel valued. The situation described among those training to be crafts teachers also applied to those attending and teaching yoga classes in the local educational system. It was in meeting women's desire for freedom and autonomy, both mental and financial, that made the adult-education centres an attractive place to spend time. Being state-funded, the activity women were participating in was seen as socially acceptable.

Yoga and Female Physical Culture

Attendance at physical culture courses for reasons of improving health and beauty became part of popular middle-class women's culture during the first half of the twentieth century (Zweiniger-Bargielowska 2005, 2001: 183–97). In this period a woman's physical fitness was sometimes believed to have eugenic implications for the betterment of the national population (Sandow 1919). However, it was generally considered that physical movement appropriate for women's and girls' bodies was different from that which was suitable for men and boys (Fletcher 1984; Hargreaves 1993). In the nineteenth century, middle-class girls might have been taught Henrick Ling's Swedish Gymnastics at school while boys were taught military drills and competitive games such as rugby and cricket (McIntosh 1972 [1952]; McKibbin 1998: 367–71). Ling and his students designed movements to exercise all aspects of the muscular-skeletal system of the body. Employment as a Swedish Gymnastics instructor was a professional career available for women in Britain from the late nineteenth century onwards (Fletcher 1984: 90). Swedish

17. Angela Marris recalled: 'When we started teaching for the ILEA, he [Iyengar] authorised Beatrice [Harthan] to teach but she was already too old – they wouldn't employ her as she was over 60 at the time. And she did go on practising by herself . . .'. Personal interview (30 June 2005).

18. Clara Buck, 'The Choice is Yours', *Overseas* 1982, p. 4. Newspaper clipping in RIMYI archives.

Gymnastics – or 'Drill' – also offered 'remedial exercises' that could correct postural defects that might cause further ill health. Part of its appeal was it required no equipment and could be used to promote public health for schoolchildren (Posse 1908). During the second half of the twentieth century, yoga teaching became a socially acceptable women's profession partially due to this precedent. Singleton (2010: 84–8) has also argued that the global popularity of these exercises for health likely influenced the development of posture-oriented yoga in the modern period.

In the early twentieth century, women interested in physical practices could continue with Ling's system; by the 1920s, they could also join Mary Bagot Stack's Women's League of Health and Beauty, or perhaps participate in Greek Revival dance (Stack 1931; Atkinson 1985; McCrone 1988; Mangan and Walvin 1987). Bagot Stack exercises had many parallels with the forms of yoga as group physical activity that became popular after the war (see also Singleton 2010: 150–2). In her autobiography, Mary Bagot Stack claimed that some of her exercises were based on yoga postures learned while living in India with her husband in 1912 (Stack 1998: 69). Bagot Stack's group movements, often done to classical music, were designed to create health and beauty 'from the inside out'.

During the 1950s, 'Keep Fit' and 'Medau Rhythmic Movement', both of which had been influenced by Ling's system, were attended by large groups of middle-class women. Medau Rhythmic Movement was introduced into Britain in 1931 by the German national Hinrich Medau (1890–1974). Medau had a background in gymnastics and sport and worked with modern dancers as well as Rudolf Bode (1881–1970) and Émile Jaques-Dalcroze (1865–1950). The technique attempted to incorporate a

> variety of rhythm, pace, form, and pattern support and basic training in the technique of movement, which should be effortless, natural, harmonious, skilled and controlled but at the same time retain the unique quality which expresses personality. Instead of teaching exercises, the emphasis was on creating a class to suit the needs of the individuals (Medau Society 2007).

Medau was a popular form of exercise with women and incorporated a variety of aids into its strength and stamina routines, such as Indian wooden clubs.[19] The Medau technique spread through-

19. For Indian clubs in European and American sports, see Alter (2004b).

out the country and was often used in combination with other techniques of women's physical culture. In 1959–60 there were sixteen Medau courses advertised in the London guide to evening classes, *Floodlight,* and in 1971–72 there were eighteen Medau courses compared to thirteen yoga courses on offer. After the 1970s, Medau classes declined in popularity, possibly due to many more physical activities becoming socially acceptable for women.[20]

Also developing during the 1930s was the nascent Keep Fit movement. Eileen Fowler (1906–2000), who would later be associated with the movement, began teaching exercises for fitness and health during the 1930s. During the Second World War, Fowler organised shows and events advocating general fitness as part of the war effort with the Central Council of Physical Recreation. After six years of retirement after her marriage in 1945, Fowler decided to return to teaching physical education in 1951. The Keep Fit Association had its inaugural meeting in 1956, Fowler being a founding member. Keep Fit exercises have been described as a modified version of popular women's gymnastics (Harris 1961).

Fowler popularised 'Keep Fit' by presenting the first BBC radio classes from 1956. It has been estimated that as many as half a million people, mostly women, would rise by 6.45 am to follow along with her radio broadcast. She blamed conditions of prosperity for decreasing levels of fitness from the 1950s onwards and maintained regular radio and occasional television appearances (Anderson 2004). Fowler presented a disco-dance Keep Fit programme on television during the 1970s, providing a more energetic way for women to keep fit at home compared with the Hittleman–Marshall television yoga classes (which will be discussed further in Chapter 6).

The yoga classes on offer in adult education had much in common with Keep Fit and Medau. While quick to declare yoga's difference from Keep Fit, in 1970 the founder of the British Wheel of Yoga, Wilfred Clark, also commented that 'Keep Fit programmes in all Further Education Institutes include quite a large number of Yoga postures'.[21] The 'yoga postures' were perhaps part of the general interlacing of British and Indian physical culture in the early twentieth century. Yoga teachers were often recruited from among Keep

20. Personal correspondence with Lynda Bridges, Administrative Officer, the Medau Society (15 January 2007).

21. W. Clark, 'Teach Yourself Yoga', *Yoga* 6 (Winter 1970/71), p. 10.

Fit instructors. As a woman from the 'North of England' reported in the British Wheel's journal *Yoga*:

> I was originally a teacher-trained Keep Fit leader but after studying and practising Yoga from books I changed over because Yoga is so much better from a health point of view. They [her pupils] all say that they feel marvellous after a class meeting.[22]

Yoga enthusiasts constantly reiterated that yoga could not be reduced to Keep Fit but, nevertheless, yoga, Keep Fit and Medau Rhythmic Movement all appealed to the same population, being presented as an aid to women's health and beauty and taught within the adult-education evening class structure.

All of these physical fitness courses represented safe and interesting places to learn new things and make new friends with similar interests, a social element that was an important part of the appeal of a yoga class for many women. In 1966, the Leicestershire advisor for PE noted in the journal *Adult Education* that there were three types of evening class in his subject: men's activities, women's activities and family activities. In his view the non-threatening expansion of the social network was an important factor for both women and men, reflecting that men's classes were 'often an opportunity to get-together with the "boys" away from the feminine home influence and yet with a clear conscience', while women's 'keep fit' classes were often perceived as 'an opportunity for a good "natter"'' between women (Johnson 1966). This PE educator highlighted a tradition of gendered physical education in Britain: for example, the BAI had separate women's and men's principals from 1937 to 1975.

From the late nineteenth century, certain types of physical exercise had comprised acceptable and attractive activities. During the Second World War, women were encouraged under the sponsorship of Eileen Fowler to 'keep fit' for the war effort, equating their physical health as women 'at home' with national fitness. Bagot Stack's Women's League of Health and Beauty was also active in the war effort to move the nation's women towards 'A1' fitness (Stack 1988: 136–43). Women attended keep-fit classes for a variety of reasons – not least personal enjoyment – but keeping the individual body fit and healthy in the mid-twentieth century was also a goal associated with a greater social and moral good. Certain types of exercise became associated with class distinctions. Middle-class

22. 'Yoga Preferred Over Keep Fit', *Yoga* 4 (Summer 1970), p. 9.

women have a longer tradition of interest in physical exercise, whereas women of other classes have only more recently acquired the leisure and education to devote to physical activity for health and enjoyment.

Yoga and Women's Health and Beauty

As discussed above, in relation to women's physical fitness in Britain, health and beauty have long been related concepts. In the 1970s, the health-and-beauty aspect of yoga was brought to the forefront of media presentations. The glossy magazine *Yoga & Health* and the Richard Hittleman ITV television series both featured toned and beautiful women as models in matching leotards and tights; often the models wore fishnet stockings and a tight-fitting leotard top.[23] Perhaps the female image of yoga on magazine covers originated from a long tradition of women selling things in advertisements, a proven way of attracting the interest of both women and men.

That yoga might be some sort of elixir of youth was part of its particular allure during this period of British history. Fashion followed the growing youth consumer market; designer clothes, such as Mary Quant's short dresses, emphasised and glorified a youthful rather than womanly body.[24] The middle-aged population that made up the bulk of yoga practitioners could not but be affected by the social discrimination against their age, set against the cultural standard of feminine beauty wherein youth was essential (Benson 1997: 82). Youth has long been associated with good health: a young, fit body was also a healthy body, as Mary Bagot Stack consistently emphasised in the Women's League of Health and Beauty (see also Matthews 1987).

A book on yoga written by a British woman in 1969 specifically centres around the popular association between yoga, youth and beauty. With illustrations of middle-aged women assuming yoga postures in the author's garden, Joan Gold promised that through Hatha Yoga exercises:

23. The images of women used to model yoga have tended to change with the ideal body image projected by society; this has become noticeably thinner, especially in comparison to the average body size of women in the general population, since the 1960s (Offer 2001, 2006).

24. For the cult of youth and the influence of Quant on fashion in the context of the 1960s, see Sandbrook (2006: 220).

- You will radiate good health;
- Your eyes will sparkle;
- Your complexion will glow;
- Your step will regain its youthful spring;
- Your arteries will become elasticised and healthy;
- Your system will be regulated and constipation will disappear;
- Your figure will improve, and your body will become supple;
- You will be able to relax (Gold 1969: 3).

Here, traditional tropes of women's beauty are combined with a medicalised language about 'elasticised arteries' and a regulated and unconstipated system. If these promises were not enough to convince the reader, Gold went on to claim that 'yoga will open the door to the secret of eternal youth – it will reverse the ageing forces of nature'. Yoga was presented here as a way for women to achieve both health and beauty 'with a minimum of effort and a great deal of pleasure' (Gold 1969: 3).

Such claims are widespread in 1960s yoga books aimed at women. One 1963 book entitled *Yoga for Women* declares:

> Women can become better-looking through yoga, not only by improving their health but through the development of a more positive interest in life and their own physical and mental problems. Most yoga teachers know cases of women who have astonished everyone, including themselves, by exchanging a drawn and harassed, middle-aged look for a youthful, vital one; by discarding stiffness and tension for suppleness, slimness, serenity and poise (Phelan and Volin 1963: 16).

As Swami Sarasvati, who had a successful television programme on yoga in Australia in the 1970s, claims:

> Breathing, gentle exercise and a little relaxation each day will not only reveal your inner beauty but will also give you a firm body and a healthy mental outlook . . . you will become more energetic, active and younger looking (Would you believe I am forty?) (Sarasvati 1970: i).

Nancy Phelan (1913–2008), Michael Volin (1914–1997) and Swami Sarasvati (born c. 1941) were based in Australia, but their books had a wide circulation in Britain.[25] Having been a model on

---

25. Nancy Phelan was the well-known author of 'numerous bestselling books on yoga, unusual travel memoirs, novels and cookbooks, a delightful account of an

the TV series with Richard Hittleman, British actress Lyn Marshall went on to publish several books based on her yoga practice. They were marketed on the basis of Marshall's reputation as a beautiful woman with a knowledge of how to maintain physical appearance and good health rather than an intimate acquaintance with Indian esoteric religion (Marshall 1975, 1976, 1978, 1982).

A 1970 *Evening Standard* article exemplifies the widespread claims about the 'youth giving' qualities of yoga at that time. A journalist was sent a copy of a booklet that reported: 'those who take hatha-yoga seriously believe that we do not reach maturity at 21 but at 33 and to them the springtime of life is between 55 and 75'. The newspaper's beauty section editor had been attending yoga classes for seven years so her colleague asked her if yoga made her look younger, to which she replied, 'the furrows on my brow look the same as they always have but maybe they would have been worse' – clearly happy to make such claims for yoga without any evidence.[26] Possibly, women felt comfortable making these claims on account of the feeling of 'well-being' regular yoga practise gave them. 'Well-being' was a nebulous idea and could be expressed in a variety of ways. For the more elderly, a manageable activity that increased fitness and mobility was certainly very important. A 'well-being culture' was promoted by a government that encouraged individual responsibility for personal health: personal well-being was understood as a social good, not just an individual indulgence.

In 1982, at the age of seventy-two, Clara Buck, explained to a newspaper reporter how she began her yoga practice:

---

eccentric, sunlit Sydney upbringing and a biography, in 1987, of her cousin, conductor Sir Charles Mackerras' (Christopher Hawtree, 'Nancy Phelan: Obituary', *The Guardian*, 19 February 2008). Michael Volin (Volodchenko), also known as Swami Karmananda, was born in Russia and lived in China during the 1920s and '30s, travelling widely and learning meditation, yoga and Qigong techniques from Buddhist monks. He opened an early yoga centre in Shanghai with Indra Devi in Shanghai before becoming displaced during the Second World War. After the war he relocated to Australia, opening a popular yoga school in Sydney in the 1950s (Daphne Volin, 'Michael Volin (Swami Karmananda)', http://www.agelessyoga.com.au/volinstory.html). Swami Sarasvati became a national figure promoting yoga in Australia from 1968, establishing a yoga retreat centre northwest of Sydney in 1983 (see swami.com.au and 'It's Surreal: The Swami Is Back,' *The Age Online*, 15 September 2003, https://www.theage.com.au/articles/2003/09/14/1063478062266.html).

26. Yvonne Thomas, 'No more rows and wrinkles . . . Ah, Mr Iyengar, You're My Guru', *Evening Standard*, July 22 1970. Newspaper clipping in RIMYI archives.

In 1972 at the age of sixty, I was farming in southeast England. One day a neighbour dropped in and asked me if I would like to go out with her to Hastings, Sussex – our nearest town – where an apprentice Yoga teacher needed 'guinea pigs.' I said I would go anywhere just to get away from the farm for a while, since I worked all hours that God gave me. I was permanently tired and that day more that usual. After one hour of strenuous exercises I felt refreshed and decided to make further investigations. I enrolled in an adult education class and though I had to travel one hour each way, I never missed a lesson. One-and-a-half years later I sold my farm and went to visit Mr BKS Iyengar, in India, who is my Guru. After five years he encouraged me to start teaching, and now, at the age of seventy, I have a profession that makes me feel younger than I felt when I was twenty.[27]

She went on to explain in detail how she had found yoga an aid to graceful ageing. She saw it as her own responsibility to be as fit and healthy as possible, not unnecessarily burdening her children or the public health system:

To keep your body fit and your mind alert is like putting money in the bank for your old age or taking out a life insurance. We tend to forget that family and friends are directly or indirectly subjected to our influence. Growing old in a youthful manner is doing them a favour as well as to ourselves. It is self evident that a healthy person would be more jolly, kindly and affectionate than one who is suffering from various ailments and who would be inclined to be grumpy, moaning and dissatisfied with life. Which way would you prefer to grow old? The choice is yours.[28]

While Clara Buck's level of activity was exceptional for her age, yoga classes offered vitality and interest in life for many women who took up the practice. The perception that yoga was something you could continue learning and teaching well into old age added to its popularity. Middle-class women who were long past the age of childbirth and into retirement described yoga classes as beneficial to their well-being on many levels. For Clara Buck, maintaining health and emotional balance through yoga was a social and moral good that benefited others as well as herself.

The way of thinking about women's health and beauty as presented in these yoga books was in alignment with more mainstream

27. Clara Buck, 'The Choice is Yours', *Overseas* 1982, p. 4. Newspaper clipping in RIMYI archives.
28. Ibid.

ideas in popular culture. For example, *The Vogue Body and Beauty Book* (1978) was illustrated with Richard Avedon's photographs of young, thin models in yoga positions wearing revealing designer clothes, implying that yoga is not only healthy but also glamorous and fashionable. The book's introduction follows the contemporary line that 'Beauty, today, is not a perfect face or a certain look . . . it is glowing health and vitality, it is awareness and action, it is science and technology and of course marvellous looks, a perfect skin, a superb body.' The book provides sensible advice on nutrition, sexual health, and exercises including yoga. Here again, yoga is being presented as an enjoyable method for improving both health and beauty as two desirable and related categories.

The idealised body size had become smaller, and an attainment of this, along with the health benefits purportedly associated with it, was also a motivation to begin yoga (Offer 2001, 2006). A 1972 *Yoga and Health* article describes an Iyengar Yoga class:

> Like most classes in the West, this one is heavily weighted towards the ladies – who also sometimes appear to be heavily weighted. Weight, however, would appear to be removed in direct ratio to attendance at Iyengar classes.[29]

Manchester yoga teacher Penderell Reed reported to a local newspaper in 1972 that she 'took up yoga a dozen years ago in an attempt to lose weight. She succeeded so well that now as a qualified yoga teacher, she can hardly meet the demands for more and more classes.'[30] However, there might have also been an element of self-deselection of the unglamorous women from the yoga classes. One teacher, Sophy Hoare, remembers that, in early classes, 'there were just as many thin people as fat people – [but] in fact I found that fat students didn't last very long in classes because they felt encumbered or self-conscious'.[31]

However, personal reports from the women who continued to practise yoga, for example in local newspapers, established the idea that the activity increased those middle-class ideas of femininity: vitality, beauty and serenity; it was presented as benefiting

29. 'Iyengar Teaches', *Yoga & Health* 7 (1972), p. 23.
30. 'He says goodbye to tension: You don't know whether you're on your head or your heels when you have a guru for a guest', *The Advertiser* (Stockport, Manchester), 27 July 1972, p. 17. Newspaper clipping in RIMYI archives.
31. Personal interview with Sophy Hoare (5 January 2005).

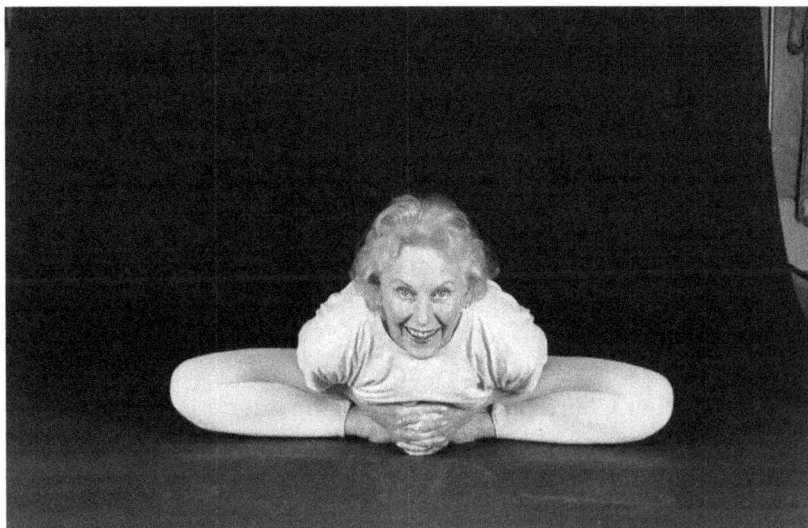

Fig. 4.2 Iyengar teacher Diana Clifton in 1992 in a yoga posture at the age of seventy-three. Images of older women doing yoga, ageing gracefully and in full health, were presented throughout the twentieth century as an inspiration for women. Photograph courtesy of the Iyengar Yoga Association (UK) Archive Committee and John Bradford.

a woman's self-confidence and sense of 'well-being'. A 'Sandwich West housewife', described as 'an advanced student of the centuries-old discipline' and 'turned on' to yoga, explained in the *Windsor Star* in 1976 that yoga leads to 'radiant health of mind and body'.[32] In a medicalised post-war society, these qualities were associated with an individual's moral duty to the state, family and one's self to care for the body. Offer (2001: 92–100, esp. p. 93, Table 2) argues that self-control and fitness disciplines are more accessible to the middle and upper classes: an association between exercise and class is supported by the popularity of yoga among these middle-class British women.

Nonetheless, many women reported attending yoga courses simply to have an activity that made them feel happier and provided social contact with other women. For example, Jeanne Maslen, who was influential in establishing Iyengar Yoga in Manchester, first attended keep-fit classes at her local FE College because 'as a housewife with two small children, I wanted to do something more with

32. Susan Vankuren, 'Yoga: The Ultimate Discipline of Mind, Body', *Windsor Star*, 25 March 1977. Newspaper clipping in RIMYI archives.

my time' (Maslen 1997). Most people in Mrs Maslen's position were restricted by childcare requirements, but at least one Manchester FE college arranged for a nursery to look after children while their mothers attended classes. The courses advertised to these mothers included 'yoga, experimental art, dressmaking, modelling, languages, cookery, embroidery, tailoring, ballroom dancing, piano lessons, wine making, social science, flower arranging, and keep-fit'.[33] British Wheel trustee Vi Neale-Smith remembers attending her first yoga class through another contact in her 'young wives' group'.[34]

Yoga itself was not the only appeal of these classes. According to yoga teacher Claire Buckingham, 'Quite often I felt that . . . they didn't come to class so much to practise yoga. It was their time out to just be still . . . that was part of the attraction to women I think.'[35] Many middle-class women found their lives stressful and appreciated the beneficial effect that the exercise and relaxation of yoga classes had on their 'well-being'. They may not have been able to precisely define it, but such 'well-being' will have included modest improvements in fitness and mood, being in a place of calmness, and access to an extended social network. With the individual's moral duty in mind, as described above, women also perceived yoga as enabling them to better fulfil their duties as wives, employees and, perhaps most importantly, mothers.

Yoga and Childbirth

The late 1960s and the 1970s saw educated women becoming increasingly aware of issues related to their treatment by the medical profession. Initially, discontent concerned experiences during childbirth. A leader in the subsequent 'natural birth movement' of the 1970s described in retrospect the birth of her first child in the early 1960s:

> The day the baby was due I was despatched to hospital by my doctor, although I had no sign of contractions. My blood pressure was up a little and I was told it would be more convenient for the doctor if I

33. 'Whilst Mothers Study . . .', *Gordon Reporter*, 22 September 1967, in newspaper clippings, 'Education Colleges' 158 (Local Studies), Manchester Central Library Archives.
34. Personal interview with Vi Neale-Smith (17 September 2004).
35. Personal interview with Claire Buckingham (14 September 2006).

were to agree to an induction the following morning. Not knowing the pros and cons, I could not weigh them.

Labour was induced at eight in the morning. While I was under general anaesthetic, the membrane holding my waters was broken. I drowsily awoke from the drug half an hour later to find my body in the grip of something like a wrenching tool . . . I asked the nurse to call my husband and my mother, but she gave me pills instead, and my husband and mother were only allowed to stay and hour before being sent home.

I was in labour for fourteen hours under the kind of medication which made me too woolly to deal with myself or anything that was going on. Too weak to stand up for my own rights. I'd forgotten I had any rights. I didn't care how my baby was born. I was put on an intravenous drip to speed up contractions and left alone for most of the labour; shovelled from bed to stretcher to delivery table at the most intense point of discomfort, had a gas mask slapped on my face, and although I summoned all remaining strength to push it away, and was oblivious when my baby was born . . . for reasons never explained to me, I was not permitted to hold my son until hours later, when he was wheeled in to me bathed and cleanly wrapped in his first trappings of so-called civilization. I had to unwrap him like a sterile parcel before I could touch his newborn skin (Brook 1976: 9).

Feelings of isolation, lack of body awareness due to medication, and lack of consultation about intervention strategies comprised just some of the dissatisfactions about the experience of labour which many women were increasingly expressing. They often felt denied of choice about the nature or extent of medical interventions and their own preferences about the process were less important than those of the medical professionals.[36] Educated women were increasingly discussing their experiences, and these feelings of disempowerment and a need for more information and autonomy over their own bodies during the birth process inspired a number of women's self-help organisations.

Labour has been a perennial concern of both doctors and families: in 1907, Mary Bagot Stack's initial training in physical culture at London's Conn Institute focused on a 'scientific system of health-building' designed for all prospective mothers (Stack 1988: 39). In the post-war period, information about the latest advances

36. Interviews with Ros Claxton (5 December 2004) and Sophy Hoare (5 January 2005); see also Brook (1967).

in biomedical treatment and technology was provided by women such as Prunella Briance, who, with an eye on fast-changing medical advances, set up the National Childbirth Trust in 1956 to facilitate access to information on pregnancy, childbirth and parenting. The natural birth movement in Britain primarily aimed to educate women so that they could make informed choices about the medical interventions they wanted during labour.

In 1961, trust in medical expertise was severely undermined when severely deformed children were born to mothers who had been prescribed thalidomide for morning sickness during pregnancy (Lock 1997: 137–8). The idea that doctors might not always know best gained some traction. Anthropological comparisons with other cultures stressed the 'unnaturalness' of giving birth on one's back in stirrups sounded by male 'experts'.[37] The natural birth movement encouraged women to listen to their bodies during the process, and promoted alternative positions to ease the baby out. Many of these overlapped with yoga as taught at the time.[38]

Yoga and natural birth were linked in experience by many of the women staffing the Birth Centre, which had offices in the East West Centre near Old Street (1977) and near Battersea (1980).[39] The East West Centre itself was an early and enthusiastic promoter of macrobiotics and shiatsu and more associated with Japanese culture than yoga. Several women volunteered on phone lines and in an open office for a few hours each week to give advice on the birthing process and related issues and provide speakers on these topics. The Birth Centre also sold a chart of yoga poses for pregnancy.[40] Sophy Hoare remembered that the users of the centre could not be defined by class but were 'women of any class who had had bad – sometimes appalling and traumatic – experience giving birth in hospitals'. However, she reflected, the group running the Birth

37. Particularly influential was Sheila Kitzinger (1967 [1962], 1972).
38. For example the National Childbirth Trust in 1972 produced a series of A5 booklets under the titles of *Breathing during Labour*, *Breathing Control in Labour* and *Keeping Fit for Pregnancy*. Found in National Childbirth Trust, 'Miscellaneous publications not catalogued separately' (1964, British Library). See also Balaskas and Balaskas (1979).
39. Interviews with Ros Claxton (5 December 2004) and Sophy Hoare (5 January 2005).
40. Personal interview with Ros Claxton (5 December 2004). Also influential in this movement were Dick-Read (1960) and Odent (1976 [published in English in 1983]).

Centre was 'probably largely but not entirely made up of educated middle-class women'.[41] Also involved in the early Birth Centre was Janet Balaskas, who was very much influenced by the psychological processing and human potential explorations of the (anti-)psychiatrist R.D. Laing, who wrote a foreword for a book on exercises for childbirth. Balaskas went on to found the Active Birth Centre in North London which incorporates yoga for health in pregnancy (Balaskas and Balaskas 1979).

The Birth Centre group arranged screenings of Frédérick Leboyer's film *Birth without Violence* (1969) and made his book by the same name (1975) available.[42] This work evoked the experience of birth from the child's perspective, encouraging the audience to empathise with the newborn child, in contrast to the conventional medical practitioner's approach to the subject. The book opens:

> 'Do you think babies like being born?'
> 'What do you mean, like being born?'
> 'Exactly what I said. Do you think children are happy to come into this world?'
> 'Happy? But a newborn baby doesn't feel anything. So it is neither happy nor unhappy.'
> 'How do you know that?'
> 'Well, it's obvious. Everyone knows that.'
> . . .
> 'And that makes you think that they don't feel anything either?'
> 'Of course, they don't.'
> 'Then why do they cry so bitterly?' (Leboyer 2002 [1975]: 3).

Birth without Violence poetically championed the newborn and called on parents and physicians to see the child's personhood. Leboyer was highly influential, especially among certain middle-class women's circles; his films and photography added extra emotion to what others only described in words. Body awareness, attention to personal somatic experience and a championing of non-violence all resonated with those practising yoga in Britain during this period.

Leboyer (1918–2017) was a French physician specialised in gynaecology and obstetrics. After undergoing his own psychoanalysis in France, he developed an interest in birthing techniques. He

---

41. Personal interview with Sophy Hoare (5 January 2005).
42. It was reprinted in 1977, 1979, 1991, 1995 and 2002.

travelled to India in 1959 and returned annually for two decades.[43] In 1976, he published *Loving Hands,* a book on baby massage with pictures of an Indian mother. The attention to the newborn infant as a conscious being and the idealisation of India continued in Leboyer's works; this reinforced a connection between the natural birth movement and yoga. In 1978 Leboyer published a book containing inspirational photographs of one of B.K.S. Iyengar's daughters practising yoga late in pregnancy, making his personal association of 'natural birth' with yoga more explicit (Leboyer 1979 [1978]).

In valuing a woman's embodied subjective experience, yoga was a natural complement to the reproductive awareness of the active birth movement. Yoga as practised in Britain was generally done cautiously; the principals of the LEA evening institutes were obliged to provide safe and non-controversial activities for their students. Most classes focused on increasing body awareness through postures and breathing exercises, not on inducing altered states of consciousness or on dramatic contortions. In a more prosaic way, yoga practice increased awareness of the subjective embodied experience and provided techniques to manage stress as well as emotions and physical pain.[44] This was of interest to women in general as well as pregnant women, and also to some men.

One of the few 1970s books explicitly discussing yoga and pregnancy was Wheel member Tony Crisp's *Yoga and Childbirth* (1975 [1976, 1977]).[45] Crisp was concerned with getting the woman's 'body, mind and soul ready for the event of childbirth'. He paid more attention to diet and influencing the unborn child through the mother's emotional and psychological well-being than on asanas, pranayama exercises or anything that might be taken from a Sanskrit text. In fact, the idea of yoga for pregnant women had more to do with 'being' in the body; he advises:

> let any movements or positions occur which suggest themselves to
> you. Let your emotions flow and arise as postures and movements.

43. He travelled to India in 1959 and returned annually for two decades, being deeply influenced by many aspects of Indian culture. 'Tribute to Frederick Leboyer', 2017, https://www.birthlight.com/news/tribute-to-frederick-leboyer

44. For a sensitive positive description of this relationship, see Tourniere (2002), which reflects on her experience with B.K.S. Iyengar in the mid-1970s.

45. Other books include Weller (1978), Berg (1981) and Hoare (1985). Marshall (1975) contains a section for pregnant women, although this is not the focus of the book.

Open to the light, while holding firmly to the earth. Then let the light
penetrate your very being (Crisp 1975: 26).

This is accompanied by suggestions (with photographs) about 'being
a lioness, being a snake, being a baby, being a turtle . . .' (Crisp 1975:
26–36). The idea that a woman's behaviour during pregnancy could
have a profound effect on the unborn child was part of an increasing emphasis in the 1970s on the mother's importance in a child's
psychological development.[46]

As was often noted by those practising yoga during pregnancy,
the physical practice created a sense of freedom and confidence.
This sense of physical liberation for women has parallels with the
cycling trend of a previous generation (Willard 1895; Herlihy 2004).
Yoga provided a technology for experiencing the body as freer and
more autonomous.[47] In valuing a woman's embodied subjective
experience, yoga was a natural complement to the reproductive
awareness of the birth movement. However, until the 1980s there
was little explicit instruction on modifying yoga postures for pre-
or post-natal women; in general women continued with their usual
evening classes as best as they were able, using this increased body
awareness to monitor their body's ability.[48]

Although much of the emotive strength of the challenge against
biomedicine came from birthing experiences, women also found
that yoga addressed chronic complaints that general practitioners could not adequately help with. Kathleen Pepper was drawn
to yoga in the mid-1960s after finding a book called *Yoga and Your
Health* in her local London library. She was suffering from serious
pain and fainting during her menstruation and found relief by
following the instructions in the book.[49] Particularly with chronic
'female complaints' such as menstrual pains, many women found it
difficult to get sympathetic or effective treatment from their (mostly
male) physicians. Even after the feminist-led medical reforms of the
1970s, many women continued to have difficulty with the medical
profession, as explained by Women's Health London in the early
1990s:

46. See the highly influential and popular Spock (1974).
47. For the concept of technology, habits and the body, see Mauss (1979 [1950])
and Martin, Gutman and Hutton (1988).
48. Personal interviews with Ros Claxton (5 December 2004) and Sophy Hoare
(5 January 2005).
49. Personal interview with Kathleen and Roy Pepper (12 July 2005).

> Many women feel distanced from or intimidated by their doctors. They often felt that they are not taken seriously, that they are considered malingerers if they return more than once with the same complaint (Women's Health London 1993).[50]

On account of this experience, many found self-help an important complement to their traditional medical consultation.

Yoga was an important part of women's self-help: 'SELF HELP – yoga, massage, and relaxation techniques, available in many women's centres or adult education institutes can help with high blood pressure, back pain and symptoms of stress' (Women's Health London 1993: 3). Although the limitations of such methods were acknowledged by feminist health groups, activities including yoga had an important impact on women's quality of life. The Women's Health group went on to write:

> Alternative medicine, a change of diet, massage, or yoga may still not make you feel "well" if you are struggling alone to bring up children on social security and living on the tenth floor of a high-rise. However, receiving treatment and/or support for a particular health problem may help you deal with other aspects of your life (Women's Health London 1993: 2).

The self-help attitude that yoga practice fostered in women was as important and supportive as the alleviation of specific physical complaints (Women's Health London 1993: 2). The belief that these same activities made one more slim and attractive was often a secondary albeit appreciated benefit.

Conclusion

Yoga within the LEA structure was able to address the educated woman's desire for freedom and autonomy while simultaneously supporting her traditional obligations to be beautiful, available (for both husband and family) and responsive to her duties towards others. The popularity of yoga among middle-class women can be understood as a continuation of a culture wherein women were responsible for their personal health and the health of their children – directly related to how this population perceived their social responsibilities as wives and mothers. This was especially significant

---

50. For more on the treatment of 'female complaints', see Jones (2001); for physicians' attitudes towards women, see Cook (2005: 273).

as regards the connection between a positive birth experience for the child and yoga in the natural birth movement. Yoga was believed to be capable of creating the 'body beautiful' while simultaneously drawing attention away from physical perfection towards goals of mental stability and general health. Yoga for health and beauty was not simply a selfish endeavour; yoga as an aid to health and relaxation can be understood as a continuation of the wartime message of keeping fit being a national duty – one that many of these women's mothers understood. As citizens and mothers within the British welfare state, women's attempts to improve their health and well-being are more socially useful than a narcissistic quest for lost youth. In brief, women's yoga practice was consistent with their 'traditional' responsibilities yet encouraged, in a socially acceptable way, feelings of freedom and autonomy.

Chapter Five

Yoga in Popular Music and the 'Counter-culture' (the 1960s and '70s)

As this steady base for yoga was growing among the LEA classes, celebrities were beginning to embrace India as a source of musical and personal inspiration. In comparison to some of the high-commitment groups that were brought to media attention, like Swami Prabhupada's International Society for Krishna Consciousness (ISKCON), LEA evening classes would have appeared a very safe way of exploring Indian culture. But widespread coverage of celebrities' interest added glamour and mystery to the idea of yoga and did much to make Eastern spirituality more familiar (Humes 2005: 64; Oliver 2014). The press generally brought scorn or at least scepticism to the stories, which perhaps added a cachet for youth and encouraged them to explore the subject further. Muz Murray's London project *Gandalf's Garden* brought yoga to youth culture by promoting it in association with pop music personalities who would soon become celebrities, including Marc Bolan, David Bowie and DJ John Peel. Exploring yoga and Indian religion became an increasingly common way of looking outside British culture for inspiration, a post-imperial embracing of foreign ideas that had been part of colonial dialogue for several centuries.

India as an Inspiration for Musical Icons

Many British musicians and cultural icons of the 1960s experimented with the image, spirituality and sounds of India. These musicians were often musically inspired by African-American jazz and rhythm and blues music. In deeply racist pre-1960s America, many African-American musicians had turned to non-European cultures for musical and personal inspiration (See Prashad 2000:

38-39; Porter 1998: 95).[1] Indian, African and Arabic cultures all became sources of cultural inspiration; Middle Eastern forms of Islam were a profound influence on jazz musicians in the 1940s and '50s (Porter 1998: 96). An extreme example of this movement is the jazz musician Sun Ra (1914-1993) who attempted to obscure his human origins and claimed to have been sent from Saturn to preach a message of awareness and peace. Although always considered at the edge of avant-gardism, Sun Ra was respected musically, and many major jazz musicians were influenced by his experimental style, including John Coltrane (1926-1967) (Porter 1998: 206).

As early as the 1950s, Muslim bebopper Yusef Lateef is reported to have introduced Coltrane to the Quran, to author Kahlil Gibran and to the writings of Annie Besant's protégé Jiddu Krishnamurti and Paramahansa Yogananda (Porter 1998: 96).[2] Undergoing a withdrawal from heroin in 1957, Coltrane 'communed with God' and experienced a spiritual rebirth that reoriented all his musical output (Cole 1976: 14). According to one biographer, Coltrane heard a beautiful droning sound which became Coltrane's 'Holy Grail':

> ... and the pursuit of it would lead him to the music of India, the Mideast and Africa and to a hypnotic chanting rhythm most easily discernible in compositions such as 'India' from the 1961 *Impressions* and 'Africa' from *Africa/Brass* the same year (Fraim 1996: 35).

In November 1965, Coltrane met sitarist Ravi Shankar (1920-2012). After corresponding with him, he is said to have named his son Ravi as a mark of respect (Fraim 1996: 183). Shankar began touring the classical music venues of Europe and America in 1956, often with the backing of Yehudi Menuhin, an influence that pre-dated by several years the overtly Eastern *Love Supreme* album, which made Coltrane 'Jazzman of the Year' in 1965 (Porter 1998: 262). Coltrane's respect for Indian music, and a spirituality that transcended specific religions, inspired many. One admirer wrote: 'I am not a religious person, but John Coltrane was the only man who I worshipped as a saint or even a god' (Kofsky 1970: 221). Coltrane's sounds have exerted an extensive influence on musicians on both sides of the Atlantic.

---

1. Porter (1998) notes that bebop musicians were likely to turn to mainstream Asian Islam for spiritual orientation; he also notes that some restaurants and venues in the United States would serve a 'Muslim' but not a black man.

2. For more on Yogananda, see Deslippe (2018) and Foxen (2017).

Such personal journeys were not unknown in the British jazz scene too. A well-known 'blue-hot' jazz clarinetist, Cy Laurie, appeared to 'have it all' – a jazz band, a country cottage and townhouse, three cars, and a successful theatrical agency – before he 'mysteriously disappeared without a trace to the consternation of trad jazz fans all over Britain'. In fact, he had 'dropped out' to be with the Maharishi Mahesh Yogi in 1961. Laurie spent several years in India before returning to continue his meditation in an 'isolated farmhouse in England'. By 1969, at the age of forty-two, he was again playing jazz and spreading his spiritual inspiration to the younger generation of musicians.[3] Also inspired by Eastern spirituality, British jazz drummer Glen Sweeney formed an experimental group called the Third Ear Band. Like Coltrane, Sweeney experienced a spiritual rebirth while coming off heroin. By 1969 he felt he was acting as a 'channel' and bringing an 'Eastern sound' to his jazz performances at popular underground venues, such as the UFO club in the basement of 31 Tottenham Court Road in London; he became good friends with Muz Murray at *Gandalf's Garden* (see below).[4]

The Beatles and Indian Musical Inspiration

Perhaps the most significant promoters of Indian spirituality in Britain were the Beatles. The Beatles' celebrity status in 1960s Britain was unprecedented; their lives and interests were avidly followed in the press like 'some all-embracing strip cartoon' (Sandbrook 2006: 201). While the Beatles' chart success only began in 1963, by 1965 their impact on British culture was already so substantial that they were all awarded MBEs. It was also in the spring of 1965 that guitarist George Harrison (1943–2000) discovered what would become a lifelong interest in Indian music. He first saw a sitar on the set of the Beatles' movie *Help!* and immediately had one purchased at Indiacraft, a small import boutique opposite Selfridge's on Oxford

3. 'Cy Laurie: The Vanishing Jazzman', *Gandalf's Garden* 3, pp. 5–6.
4. 'The Third Ear Band', *Gandalf's Garden* 4, pp. 9–11. The UFO club was in operation at Tottenham Court Road from December 1966 to June 1967 and was founded by John Hopkins and Joe Boyd. After a few months at the Roundhouse in Camden, the venture folded completely in October 1967. It retains an important legacy as an early venue for influential bands such as Pink Floyd. See Boyd (2005), Miles (2002) and Green (1988). Also correspondence with Muz Murray (10 July 2017).

Street (Beatles 2000: 196).[5] In October that year, Harrison played a sitar on the single 'Norwegian Wood' (see Macdonald 2005: 162–5).

Help! (1965) has often been dismissed as a 'lightweight' movie. Indeed, at the time of its release director Dick Lester told the press: 'There's not one bit of insight into a social phenomenon of our time' (Robertson 2004: 164). While it might not have been making any self-conscious political statements, viewed historically *Help!* is a significant document of anti-establishment sentiments and Orientalist stereotypes. The plot of the movie is an extended chase wherein members of a Kali cult first attempt to steal the 'sacrificial ring' from Ringo and, when that fails, try to sacrifice Ringo to the goddess. The movie relies on Orientalist stereotypes with white actors playing the part of rather dim-witted Indians. The word 'India' is never used, but Lennon asks at a restaurant, 'Does this Eastern flavour come expensive?' and another character cannot read a label because 'It's written in Eastern.' Equally significant, *Help!* consistently portrays an anti-authority sentiment, with both Scotland Yard and Buckingham Palace found to be incompetent in protecting Ringo either from the Kali cult members or two mad English scientists.

Religion is specifically targeted for anti-establishment sentiments in *Help!*. In the opening scene the leader of the Kali cult, 'Clang', played by Leo McKern, is thwarted in his attempt at human sacrifice (which looks like a Hollywood-style Satanic Mass) and reasons aloud, 'Without the ring there will be no sacrifice. Without the sacrificed there will be no congregation. Without the congregation . . . no more me!' With the last sentence turning into a pathetic whine, the cult leader is no figure of religious inspiration or devotion. Likewise, Ringo himself apparently has a religion, but he is not sure what it is, explaining to the superintendent of Scotland Yard, 'They have to paint me red before they chop me – it's a different religion than ours . . . I think.' In the final scene, religion is shown to be elective with the ring finally falling off Ringo, who puts it on Clang with the line: 'Get sacrificed! I don't subscribe to your religion!' The Beatles portrayed a world in which neither religious institutions or political and governmental authority systems deserved much respect. But *Help!* also portrayed life as a fun, sensual romp where anything was a potential source of amusement.

5. Over the next few years Indiacraft opened several shops.

Amusement for the Beatles became potential sources of musical inspiration. While filming in the Bahamas, it has been reported
that Swami Vishnudevananda (who was beginning to establish
Sivananda Yoga Vedanta Centres in North America at this time)
approached the group and gave each member a signed copy of his
The Complete Illustrated Book of Yoga (1959). Reportedly, none of the
group accorded it any significance at the time, but Harrison later
recalled it when he was becoming interested in Indian spirituality
(Robertson 2004: 160-7; Turner 2006: 135).

While highly influential, George Harrison was not the first musician to look towards India. Dave Davies of the Kinks imitated a sitar
on the single 'See My Friends' (July 1965) which may have been
an immediate inspiration for Harrison to explore Indian sounds. A
friend of Ray Davies, Barry Fantoni, recalled listening to this single with the Beatles, who were subsequently motivated to acquire a
sitar (Clayson 2001: 190-1). The Yardbirds' June 1965 single 'Heart
Full of Soul' also featured a sitar-like sound made with a guitar and
reached number two in the UK charts.

Indian inspiration was also in evidence in classical music: in the
summer of 1966, Yehudi Menuhin and Ravi Shankar preformed a
duet at the Bath Music Festival that formed the basis of the *West
Meets East* collaborative album.[6] There was also crossover from
the classical to popular music scenes. In 1966, Marianne Faithfull
remembers Mick Jagger dancing around to Ravi Shankar and Ali
Akbar Khan during an LSD trip; a sitar, possibly borrowed from
Harrison, appeared in the Rolling Stones' single of the same year,
'Paint it Black' (Faithfull 1995: 124; Newman 2006: 22).

Harrison's interest in the sitar may have also been encouraged by
socialising with Byrds members David Crosby and Roger McGuinn
during the Beatles' 1965 summer tour of the United States. Both
Crosby and McGuinn were known to be enthusiastic about Shankar,
and Crosby had attended Shankar's Los Angeles recording sessions
in the early 1960s (Newman 2006: 17). It is likely that Harrison heard
Shankar's recordings around this period (Macdonald 2005: 165;
Clayson 2001: 192). Indian music was also entering the consciousness of British music aficionados with the lauded appearance of the
carnatic singer M.S. Subbulakshmi (1916-2004) at the Edinburgh

---

6. Ravi Shankar and Yehudi Menuhin, *West Meets East: Historic Shankar/Menuhin
Sessions*. EMI, 1999 [1966].

International Festival in 1963. She subsequently gave performances in London and was recorded by the BBC, before embarking on successful tours of Europe and the United States in the 1960s (Clayson 2001: 191).

Some time in late 1965 or early 1966, Harrison was personally introduced to Ravi Shankar at the house of Asian Music Circle founder Ayana Deva Angadi, who was also facilitating B.K.S. Iyengar's classes in Britain when visiting Yehudi Menuhin. While recording 'Norwegian Wood', Harrison broke a string on his sitar and Angadi was phoned in search of a replacement. His entire family came to Abbey Road Studios to deliver the string and stayed to watch the recording through the glass; Patricia Angadi sketched the performance (Harrison 2002 [1980]: 55; Newman 2006: 23). Harrison remained in contact with the Angadis for several months. The Asian Music Circle found Harrison a local sitar tutor and possibly provided musicians for the track 'Love You To' recorded in April 1966 (Macdonald 2005: 194). Ayana Angadi's son Shankara remembers Harrison and his fiancée Pattie Boyd coming several times a week, staying for dinner, and playing mixes from the recording sessions to the family (Newman 2006: 25). However, Harrison's visits had ceased by late 1966 and he had no further association with the Asian Music Circle, although he continued his friendship with Ravi Shankar.[7]

In September 1966, Harrison and Boyd spent six weeks in India to continue sitar lessons with Shankar. During this visit, Harrison also began to learn yoga postures to enable him to sit and hold the sitar properly and was given books on Indian religion (Newman 2006: 31). Two books significant enough to be mentioned by Harrison's biographers are Swami Vivekananda's *Raja Yoga* (1896) and Paramahansa Yogananda's *Autobiography of a Yogi* (1946) (Shapiro 2002: 80; Greene 2005: 68–71). Paramahansa Yogananda (1893–1952) was very influential in the popularisation of yoga in the United States, having founded the Self-Realization Fellowship in California

7. 'Shankara Angadi: "My father was a difficult character, in some ways. He was chaotic, and never really pulled anything off he set out to do. He probably asked George for money, and that was the end of that relationship. We saw lots of him for six months, but then nothing. When I bumped into him at around the time of the concert for Bangladesh in 1972, he recognised me, and asked someone who I was. When they told him, I heard him say: 'Well, he's not as bad as his father.'"' (Newman 2006: 31).

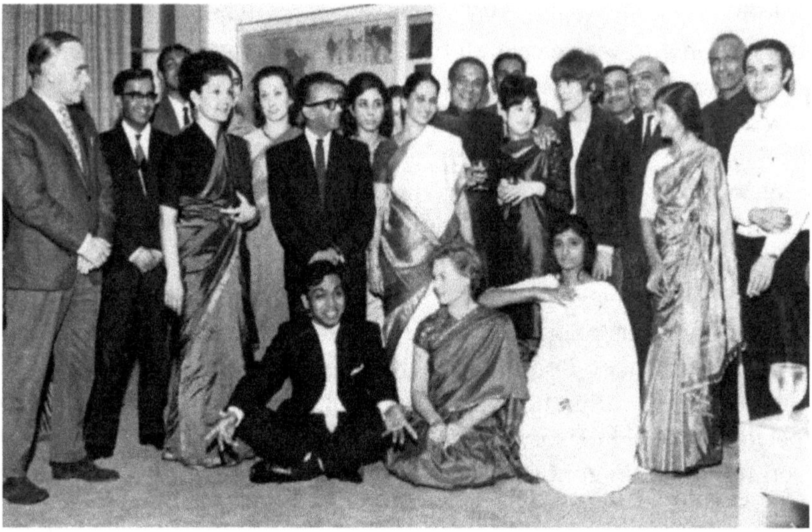

Fig. 5.1 Photograph dating from the mid-1960s showing Diana Clifton in the foreground and George Harrison standing central with members of the Asian Music Circle and a dance group. Reproduced with permission of the Iyengar Yoga Association (UK) Archives, courtesy of John Bradford.

in 1920.[8] However, in Britain, his organisation was less influential, only being established there as a formal charity in 1988, though there were devotees who met in each other's homes and corresponded by post in the 1970s.[9] Yogananda was widely known during the 1960s through his voluminous 'autobiography' which chronicles meetings with a variety of Indian saints and holy men.[10] Harrison never made public statements about Yogananda, yet reportedly carried the book with him, at times reading pages out loud, and he was known to present friends with copies (Giuliano 1989: 115–16).

Yogananda's face and that of other spiritual teachers featuring in *The Autobiography of a Yogi* (namely Paramahansa Yogananda, Śri Yukteswar Giri, Śri Lahiri Mahasaya and Mahavatar Babaji) can be found among the crowd on the cover of the *Sgt Pepper's Lonely Hearts Club Band* LP (1967). As Macdonald suggests, 'when The

8. See Foxen (2017) for more on Yogananda's influence on yoga in the United States.

9. Charity Commission for England and Wales registered charity no. 800412 and Saunders (1972: 175).

10. For authorship of the *Autobiography of a Yogi*, see Deslippe (2018); for style and impact, Foxen (2017: 178–90).

Beatles visually name-checked their cultural icons on the cover of *Sgt Pepper*, they meant to encourage popular curiosity' (quoted in Partridge 2005a: 152). In the estimation of David Reck:

> The acclaim which greeted the *Sgt Pepper* album when it was released on June 1, 1967, was almost universal ... *Sgt Pepper* quickly became one of the canonical icons of 1960's counterculture – joining such works as J.R.R. Tolkien's *The Lord of the Rings,* Hesse's *Siddharta,* the *I Ching,* and the *Tibetan Book of the Dead* and was read for hidden messages, cosmic metaphors and divination of future events (Reck 1985: 108).

Reck also notes that, with the exception of Harrison's 'Within You, Without You' there is very little Indian influence to the music itself. This list of 'counter-cultural icons' is an idealised, Orientalised vision of the 'Eastern' other. Although perceived as new and different, the Beatles were so universally popular that *Sgt Pepper* should not be considered 'counter-cultural'. The album release was a major cultural event, with many radio stations playing the album almost constantly (Macdonald 2005: 249). Popular understanding of Indian religiosity was most often about a more generalised spiritual vision without commitment to any specific tradition, teaching or belief.

In 1966, John Lennon had given a now infamous interview with Maureen Cleave at the London *Evening Standard* in which Lennon claimed that 'we're more popular than Jesus now' (Cleave 2006 [1966]). It caused a furore in the United States but little stir in Britain, perhaps because in post-imperial Britain Lennon's ideas were not so iconoclastic. Lennon's relatively casual approach to comparative religion had already been the focus of public debate in 1963 when the popular BBC television comedy *That Was The Week That Was* aired its 'Consumer Guide to Religion'. This episode compared Judaism, Catholicism, Protestantism, Islam, Communism and Buddhism as if they were washing machines. Hundreds of Britons felt sufficiently moved to send their comments to the BBC; while many were deeply offended, twice as many were complimentary (Sandbrook 2005: 551). In their religious posturing, Lennon and Harrison largely embodied a rejection of institutional Christianity that had already been accepted in British culture (Brown 2001). In this interview, Lennon's comment about Jesus had been immediately preceded by an expression of admiration for Indian culture. Lennon played some Indian classical music to Cleave, apparently given to him by Harrison, and remarked: 'Don't the Indians appear cool to you? Are you listening? This music is thousands of years old; it makes me laugh, the British going over there and telling them what to do. Quite amazing.' In the *Evening Standard* article, Cleave put Lennon's comment in her own context, remarking that Lennon was 'reading extensively about religion' and that 'his mind is closed around whatever he believes at the time, which is likely to change' (Cleave 2006 [1966]).

Part of India's appeal for 1960s pop musicians was musical and creative inspiration. Paul McCartney brought to his bandmates recordings of modern classical composers Luciano Berio, Karlheinz Stockhausen and John Cage (Clayson 2001: 222; Newman 2006: 42–43; Miles 2004: 238). For McCartney, the appeal of Indian music was very practical in terms of songwriting. He said that Indian music was attractive because

> there's nothing greater than not having to bother which a bunch of bloody chords . . . 'what's this? F sharp, H flat minor . . . Oh my God!' Whereas in Indian stuff there's one. And you can go 'Nyahhh' [imitates sitar] for twelve hours if you like . . . (Green 1988: 160).

For professional pop musicians, Indian music was most importantly another way to find inspiration to write something new and better than other bands. India also offered a visual reference in a culture of expanding images.

India and yoga became associated with the 'hippy trail' of adventure, drug use and 'dropping out' of office jobs. Geraldine Beskin, working at the Atlantis Bookshop, did not travel the hippy trail herself, but many of her customers did. Rather than defining the path, Beskin reflected that 'the Beatles widened the road'.[11] She remembered that:

> Fairly early on [there] became an established hippy trail if you like. First, there was a dope route that people took along certain places. But there were also established tea houses where you could leave messages if a friend was coming through in six weeks' time. Places where you could pick people up to travel with safely. And so on and your mate would come back and say 'go here . . .' and people would go off. Sometimes they went alone, sometimes they went together,

11. Personal interview with Geraldine Beskin (12 January 2007). See also Green (1988: 224–33) and Marnham (2005) for an account of travelling from Turkey to Nepal via Iran, Afghanistan and India in 1968.

sometimes they came back in the middle of January wearing a saf-
fron robe saying 'I've got no money, I've got no were to stay' and you
could just crash at someone's place for a while.[12]

The Atlantis Bookshop continued to be a focal point for seekers after information on alternative religiosity. Geraldine Beskin
worked at the Atlantis from 1965 and remembers the clientele of the
period.[13] Like Watkins, the Atlantis served as a meeting place for a
subculture and, from the late 1960s, many of their customers could
also have been considered part of a counter-culture. New bookstores within this milieu and alternative publishers also popped up
in various locations from the mid-1950s onward. Significant among
these were the San Francisco-based City Lights (from 1953), which
published Allen Ginsberg's influential collection *Howl and Other
Poems* (1956), a book that underwent a high-profile obscenity trial
in the United States which greatly increased its popularity. In Britain, Brighton's Unicorn Books was open between 1967 and 1973
and stocked copies of the underground newspaper *Oz* as well as
books popular among the counter-cultural movements of the time.
It closed in the aftermath of an obscenity trial and was replaced by
the cooperative bookstore the Public House Bookshop which maintained the alternative niche locally from 1973 to 1999.[14]

While the Atlantis did not hold meetings itself, it had a notice-
board on which people could post messages for friends that might
drop in as well as open invitations to meeting and events. Beskin
remembers that Yogi Ramacharaka on pranayama and Arthur
Avalon's *The Serpent Power* (1917) sold 'endlessly'. The so-called
dropouts, 'hippies' and young protesters were choosing lifestyles
deliberately different from those of mainstream society. Yoga often
entered these people's lives in a very different way from in the local
education authority (LEA) classes. Beskin remembers yoga practice

12. Ibid.
13. Michael Houghton died in 1962 and his friend and Geraldine's father, Wally
Collins, bought the shop. The Collins family reinvigorated the stock and set the
shop on firmer financial footing, according to Collins's daughter, Geraldine Beskin.
She began working occasionally in the shop after her father died in 1965 and she
completely took over management of it at the age of nineteen in 1971. She sold the
Atlantis Bookshop in 1990 but bought it back in 2002. Personal interview with Geraldine Beskin (12 January 2007).
14. Other major cities in Britain no doubt had bookstores that served as hubs
for local information about alternative ideas of all sorts, particularly from the mid-
1950s to the mid-1980s.

being a popular activity for many of her customers in the late 1960s and '70s:

> Many in this group used yoga as a devotional practice, part of being vegetarian, changing your life, contraception loomed large and tantric sex. Yoga became part of people's devotion practice . . . and was a way of saying that I'm an alternative person.[15]

She also remembered yoga as something people attempting a communal lifestyle might do together as a group activity. The youth culture of the period used yoga in a new way that fitted with their experimental lifestyles and a search for new ways to access the divine. Yoga, in turn, became associated with this group of people.[16]

During the 1960s, the Atlantis Bookshop had a good section on yoga, comprising both new and second-hand books. Additionally, the area around Museum Street held a variety of shops for those interested in esoteric and alternative spirituality. Watkins Bookshop was within a ten-minute walk, and, on the same street as the Atlantis, 'Books From India' ran a business importing specialist books including those on yoga and Indian religions. Both hippies and scholars from America and the Commonwealth would sometimes make a 'pilgrimage' to the British Library, which was then housed in the British Museum, and the bookshops in the area. For those with a broader interest, within a few minutes' walk from the Atlantis Bookshop was the Steiner Bookshop, a Theosophical Society bookshop, and publisher Allen & Unwin's offices. Also with overlapping clientele during the 1960s and '70s was the science fiction specialist Dark They Were and Golden Eyed (c. 1970–80) near Charing Cross, and Compendium Books (c. 1968–2000) in Camden Town which specialised in new and avant-garde political and philosophical literature.[17] From 1969, the Hare Krishna organisation's first London temple was also located near Museum Street on Bury Place (Dwyer and Cole 2007: 31). According to Beskin, 'unsurprisingly' some people involved in this milieu had wide-ranging interests, while others were only interested in a single subject or tradition.

Tolkien's *The Lord of the Rings* had important associations for these travellers:

---

15. Personal interview with Geraldine Beskin (12 January 2007).

16. The Atlantis continued its focus on 'Western' magical traditions such as Wicca, paganism and Crowley-influenced publications and organisations.

17. Personal interview with Geraldine Beskin (12 January 2007).

Everyone set off with a copy of *Lord of the Rings*. Because it was a big thick book. You would split it as well. If you've read the first half and someone came along who hadn't read it yet, you would give them that half. And, you know, pass it around that way.[18]

By using Tolkien's epic to frame their journey through Asia, travellers were understanding their search in the context of a familiar adventure. Many readers have understood the work as an allegorical and archetypal narration of a spiritual quest (Chance 1992; Colebatch 1990; Curry 1997). Chris Tobler, who was very much involved in some of the yogic milieux in the youth culture of the period, remembers spending weekends in bed reading the whole thing. In some ways, the 'hippy trail', with *The Lord of the Rings* as a guide, became an updated *Pilgrim's Progress* for the post-Christian age.

Robert Ellwood has reflected that Tolkien's mythical epic was particularly popular during the 1960s for a number of reasons. One was that mythical and imaginative narrative appeared to teach profound truths that appealed to a neo-romantic sensibility associated with 1960s consciousness expanders and social utopians; it resonated with an anti-establishment world-view, which was supported by identifying 'The System' – an uncaring social system – with the regime of Tolkien's evil fictional empire of Mordor (Ellwood 2002: 132). So many readers identified with Tolkien's stories that social gatherings developed with public readings, dress-up balls and discussion groups focused on the fictional books; there was even a woman in the Mojave Desert in the United States who claimed to have found the actual archaeological ruins of Tolkien's fictional land of Gondor and attracted a small following in the 1970s (Ellwood 2002: 131, 133).

In 1973, the hippy trail to India was already wide enough for the new women's glossy magazine *Cosmopolitan* to offer a feature article on travel to India. It advised that a trip to India was possible for all budgets: 'Package tours cost from around £230 for sixteen days. A really cheap way is overland expeditions from £40 one-way to £90 return' (Leslie 1973: 44). Also, by this point British yoga groups were organising their own tours of India's larger ashrams and holy sites.[19] There was a way of experiencing the magical 'spirituality' of

18. Ibid.
19. For example, 'There is room for just 30 enthusiasts to go on a Yoga tour of India from November 2 for £259. The tour is being organised by Yoga for Health Clubs in association with the magazine "Yoga for Health" and details can be obtained

India on any budget or at any level of adventure. The publications of yoga groups, particularly the glossy magazine *Yoga & Health,* eagerly embraced this celebrity endorsement of yoga. Also in 1973, *Yoga & Health* hailed the group Quintessence as a 'Yoga Rock Band' and gave a celebrity roll call of vegetarians listing Marty Kristian, Pete Murray, Marc Bolan and Cat Stevens, 'among others'.[20]

George Harrison, the Beatles and Transcendental Meditation

In the estimation of music journalist Ian Macdonald, George Harrison was 'arguably more responsible than any other individual for popularising Oriental, and particularly Hindu, thought in the West' (Macdonald 2005: xiii; Spencer 2004: 230–5). Having famously remarked at the end of the Beatles' 1966 US tour, 'Well, that's it. I'm finished. I'm not a Beatle anymore', Harrison increasingly focused on finding the personal contentment that had eluded him (Badman 2000: 244–5). Harrison's first wife, Pattie Boyd, had some contact through friends with the Spiritual Regeneration Movement of the Maharishi Mahesh Yogi (1917–2008). Although the Beatles' association with Transcendental Meditation brought the movement great publicity, the Maharishi had been teaching his meditation technique in Britain since 1960 as part of a mission to spiritually regenerate the world. During his first visit he gave a series of lectures at Caxton Hall and his teachings met with a warm reception from the members of the Study Society (a group associated with the esoteric teacher P.D. Ouspensky[21]) and the School of Economic Science (SES).[22] Both groups had been exploring ways of raising

from Intercapital Travellers Ltd., 9 Old Bond Street, London W1X3TA.' 'Yoga Tour of India', *Yoga: Journal of the British Wheel of Yoga* 16 (Summer 1973), p. 14.

20. *Yoga & Health* 3 (March 1973), p. 29. Quintessence were also reviewed in *Gandalf's Garden* 6, p. 9 and *Yoga & Health* 3 (April 1973), p. 25.

21. Peter D. Ouspensky (1878–1947) was born in Moscow as Pyotr Demianovich Ouspenskii and became a pupil of the Armenian mystic G.I. Gurdjieff (c. 1866–1949) in Moscow between 1915 and 1918. After moving to London in 1921, Ouspensky taught his own understanding of Gurdjieff's teachings and founded the Society for the Study of Normal Man (later known as the Study Society) and subsequently made his home at Lyne Place near Virginia Water, Surrey. For more on Gurdjieff, see Cusack and Sutcliffe (2017).

22. The School of Economic Science (SES) was founded in 1937 by Andrew MacLaren (1884–1975), a Labour MP between 1922 and 1945, who believed that land rather than income should be taxed and encouraged a group of like-minded people to meet and discuss positive social reform. Over time, his son, 'Leon' MacLaren (1910–1994), took over the running of the school and believed that a deeper understanding of human nature was needed in order to enact positive social change.

consciousness and practical meditation and were receptive to the Maharishi's particular meditation technique. In 1961 SES founder Andrew MacLaren organised an open meeting for the Maharishi in the Royal Albert Hall, and that same year the two groups jointly set up the School of Meditation, specifically to teach and study techniques of meditation. However, the School of Meditation distanced itself from the Maharishi while continuing its interest in Advaita Vedānta.[23]

In summer 1967, the Maharishi widely advertised what was to be one of his last public appearances before retiring into silence, like another famous Indian guru, Meher Baba, with a poster campaign on the London Underground (Humes 2005: 77).[24] Lennon, Harrison and McCartney came to hear the Maharishi speak at the Hilton Hotel in London on 24 August 1967 (Lapham 2005: 50). The Maharishi taught that by concentrating on a personally given sound for a half-hour a day, suffering could be replaced by a state of permanent bliss. He taught there was no need for any doctrine and no reason to abandon material and sensual pleasures. The Maharishi, as a contemporary newspaper article explained, 'offers a beautiful soul, without weightlifting or special equipment, without dieting or strenuous training – instant serenity'.[25] It was billed as a natural high that took away any need for drugs.[26] Before the talk, the Beatles were granted a private audience and afterwards decided to join the Maharishi for a ten-day meditation retreat in Bangor, Wales, beginning the next day (Green 1999: 231).

Towards this end, Leon McLaren encouraged the explorations of Plato, Christian religiosity and 'great literature' such as Shakespeare.

23. This was primarily Śāntānanda Saraswatī (d. 1997), the Śaṅkarācārya of Jyotirmaṭh and official successor to the Maharishi's guru, Guru Dev Swāmī Brahmānanda Saraswatī (1870–1953), who held this title, roughly analogous to archbishop of the Anglican Church in England, for the last twelve years of his life.

24. Meher Baba (1894–1969) was born in Pune, India, as Merwan Sheriar Irani and claimed to have been awakened to 'God consciousness' at the age of nineteen. From 1925 to his death, Meher Baba maintained silence, but communicated by pointing to an alphabet board. He travelled to Britain in 1931 and 1936 and gathered a small but loyal British following. He taught that the goal of human life is the conscious realisation of the non-dual nature of God. Pete Townshend (b. 1945), the leader and guitarist of the band The Who, was heavily influenced by Meher Baba from 1967 onwards.

25. 'The Beatles Follow an Old Pilgrim's Road', *The Times*, 14 October 1967, p. 9, col. F.

26. 'The Beatles Get a Thought Each', *The Times*, 28 August 1967, p. 2, col. D.

The Beatles and their wives, as well as Mick Jagger and Marianne Faithfull, joined the Maharishi and 300 others on his Wales retreat. Faithfull remembers the retreat feeling like 'being at school' and described the initiation ceremony in her autobiography:

> We went in separately to meet him. He gave us each a mantra and a few flowers we had brought for him. He giggled a lot and had very cheerful, light vibes which was a relief. It wasn't heavy at all. After we had been given our mantras and flowers, we were terribly sweet and serious about it. Nobody even asked anyone else what he'd said to them (Faithfull 1995: 187–8).

The Beatles received a phone call to inform them that their manager and personal friend, Brian Epstein, had died. The Maharishi, according to Faithfull, told the Beatles that '"Brian Epstein has moved on. He doesn't need you any more and you don't need him. He was like a father to you but now he is gone and I am now your father. I'll look after you all now." I was appalled' (Faithfull 1995: 188).[27]

Initially, the Beatles held onto their new-found meditation, possibly as a way to deal with the loss. Lennon remarked to the press, 'Our meditations have given us the confidence to withstand the shock', and Harrison rationalised, 'There is no such thing as death, only in the physical sense. We know he is okay now. He will return because he was striving for happiness and desired bliss so much.'[28] Six weeks later, on 29 September 1967, Harrison and Lennon appeared with the Maharishi on the well-known broadcaster David Frost's interview show on ITV. The two declared their belief in reincarnation; Harrison affirmed that the goal of life was 'to manifest divinity and become one with the creator' while Lennon affirmed that both Christianity and Transcendental Meditation were the answer.[29] So much attention was generated by this programme that the two were invited back for another interview on 4 October 1967 to discuss their religious interests further with members of the audience (Reck 1985: 108; Macdonald 2005: 274).[30]

---

27. It has been suggested that the Maharishi's reported comment is not so offensive if considered within an Indian, renunciation-focused cultural context.

28. 'Brian Epstein is found dead. News brings the Beatles back to London', *The Times*, 28 August 1967, p. 1, col. F.

29. 'Beatles "believe in rebirth"', *The Times*, 30 September 1967, p. 7, col. E.

30. According to both Reck and Macdonald, Juan Mascaró, author of the Penguin translation of the *Bhagavad Gītā*, was in the audience for the second show and,

In early 1968, the Beatles agreed to visit the Maharishi in Rishi-kesh, India; journalists from many US and British papers were sent to cover the story. According to media reports, the Beatles had expressed a wish to propagate the Maharishi's teaching and they began the six-month training course required at that time to teach the Transcendental Meditation technique. Ringo Starr and his wife left after two weeks; he compared the experience to a holiday camp except 'the food wasn't any good and you had to check out the drain for scorpions before getting into a bathtub' (Laphan 2005: 139). By the end of February, the Beatles had become concerned by a rumour about possible sexual indiscretion on the part of the Maharishi.[31] McCartney returned to London at the end of March telling the awaiting press that he would continue to meditate daily.[32] Harrison and Lennon returned in April. In May, John Lennon said on the US television's *The Tonight Show*, 'We believe in meditation, but not the Maharishi and his scene. But that's a personal mistake we made in public.'[33] In a more enduring form, the Beatles' disillusion with the Maharishi was pseudonymously expressed in the song 'Sexy Sadie', which Lennon told an interviewer that he wrote during the final hours of his stay in Rishikesh (Green 1999: 232). The Maharishi was on tour with the Beach Boys at this time, to a mixed audience recep-tion (Badman 2004: 210–38).

Despite sceptical press coverage and the briefness of the Beatles' association with the Maharishi, the association encouraged thou-sands to investigate the meditation techniques for themselves. In public libraries, books on Transcendental Meditation were put on the same bookshelf as information on Indian philosophy and B.K.S. Iyengar's *Light on Yoga*.[34] Wilfred Clark commented in the *Wheel* news bulletin, 'The only effect of this Beatles business has been

---

in a letter dated 16 November 1967, Mascaró sent Harrison a copy of his earlier book *Lamps of Fire,* an anthology of religious scriptures (Harrison 2002 [1980]: 118).

31. One article implied that Alexis Mardas, the new electronics head for Apple Corps, fed the rumours and scepticism as he did not want to be at the ashram any-way (see Paytress 2004: 303). But other sexual indiscretions on the part of the Maha-rishi are better documented (e.g. Bourque 2010).

32. 'Picture Gallery: Paul McCartney, of the Beatles and his friend Jane Asher', *The Times*, 27 March 1968, p. 2, col. E.

33. Information on the Beatles from Hill and Clayton (2000: 229–44).

34. This is the case in Birmingham and Manchester Central Libraries (personal observation of catalogues and bookshelves during 2005).

increased demands for instruction in meditation.'[35] Despite the public ridicule in the press of the Beatles' escapade with the Maharishi, numbers of initiations into Transcendental Meditation continued to climb until 1975.[36] This press coverage may have stimulated a greater interest in other forms of yoga as well. A 1976 article in *Yoga Today* claimed that 60,000 in Britain were practising meditation and that 'You'll find far more ordinary housewives involved in taking TM classes than jet-setting trendies.'[37] In 1978, a stressed mother of five reported in *She* magazine that she found the experience of Transcendental Meditation 'delightful', although she also reflected that, as her children always interrupted her meditation practice, what she really needed was twenty minutes of silence.[38] Harrison never publicly criticised the Maharishi and, as late as 1992, played a benefit concert for the Maharishi's Natural Law political party in Britain. However, Harrison became more associated in popular understanding with another Indian guru, Swami A.C. Bhaktivedanta Prabhupada (1896–1977), founder of the International Society for Krishna Consciousness (ISKCON).

George Harrison and ISKCON

Although the other Beatles kept a distance from spirituality in future public appearances, George Harrison never went back on his 'ultimate thing', as expressed to David Frost on national television, i.e. 'to manifest divinity and become one with the Creator'.[39] In 1969, a few ISKCON devotees managed to enter the reception area of Apple Corps after Yoko Ono assumed that Harrison had invited them. One of the devotees remembers that Harrison walked straight over to him and said 'Hare Krishna. Where have you been? I've been waiting to meet you' (Greene 2005: 103). Although it felt like a fated encounter to both Harrison and the devotees, several earlier attempts by ISKCON members to get Harrison's attention had failed. These had included sending Harrison an

---

35. Wilfred Clark, British Wheel of Yoga *Bulletin* 25 (November 1967).

36. Worldwide initiations into TM rapidly increased from 1960 to a peak of 292,517 in 1975 alone. However, the numbers of new initiations decreased sharply after this year (Bainbridge 1997: 188–9).

37. 'Meditation: What's in it for me?', *Yoga Today* 2 (May 1976), p. 12.

38. Lee Jancogey, 'Breaches of the Peace', *She*, February 1978, pp. 40–1.

39. 'Beatles "believe in rebirth"', *The Times*, 30 September 1967, p. 7, col. E.

apple pie with the words *Hare Krishna* scrolled across the top in green icing as well as dropping off an inscribed wind-up walking apple and a homemade audition tape of their Vedic chants (for which they received the standard Apple Records' rejection letter) (Giuliano 1989: 101).

Following the encounter, Harrison took a personal interest in the six devotees who had travelled to London from San Francisco in October 1968 to establish Krishna Consciousness in Britain.

Worldwide 'Krishna Consciousness' was the mission of Bengali Swami A.C. Bhaktivedanta Prabhupada. In 1965, at the age of 69, Prabhupada took a boat from India to New York City to spread devotion to God in the form of Krishna in the tradition of Gaudiya Vaishnavism, and the next year ISKCON was founded (see Dwyer and Cole 2007: 28–9). There the poet Allen Ginsberg became interested in his teachings and helped spread support among the popular music and counter-cultural scenes.

Ginsberg was influential on both sides of the Atlantic. Marianne Faithfull recalled an incident with the Rolling Stones during this period:

> in came Allen with a great flourish. He was wearing big, showy Shivaite beads. He went over to Mick, looped them over his neck and asked if he had ever heard of Hari Krishna . . . Then we all went and sat down in a little alcove in the front room. Allen had a harmonium with him and began chanting mantras to Mick, accompanying himself on the harmonium (Faithfull 1995: 191; see also Hopkins 2000).

American devotees quickly moved Prabhupada to the Haight-Ashbury district of San Francisco where he became friendly with some of the area's celebrity and pop music figures. In 1967 a 'Mantra-Rock Dance' at the Avalon Ballroom featured Prabhupada and Ginsberg, as well as the bands the Grateful Dead and Big Brother & The Holding Company (Janis Joplin's band) (International Society for Krishna Consciousness 1982: 48). Through youth culture and popular music Swami Prabhupada had quickly attained his goal of spreading Krishna Consciousness.

Formal initiation into ISKCON involved serious lifestyle changes. Initiates were required to take a Sanskrit name and spend about two hours each day chanting what is known as the *maha-mantra*: 'Hare Krishna, Hare Krishna, Krishna Krishna, Hare Hare, Hare Rama, Hare Rama, Rama Rama, Hare Hare'. Initiates also vow to abstain from all intoxicating substances, including alcohol, tobacco and caffeine, to abstain from all forms of gambling and to eat only vegetarian food (no meat, fish or eggs). Sex was permissible only within marriage and then only for the purpose of procreation. Prabhupada taught that indulgence in these activities is detrimental to spiritual growth and causes anxiety and conflict. Those following Prabhupada believed that their practice would bring awareness of God in the form of Krishna into every moment of their lives. In their desire to spread this Indian version of the 'good news', devotees regularly chanted in public spaces, selling and giving away literature on Krishna Consciousness. This form of union with God through love and devotion is known as Bhakti Yoga.[40]

Although he never became a devotee with all the lifestyle changes that would have been required, Harrison was instrumental in helping ISKCON become established in Britain. By 1969, less than one year after the arrival of six American devotees in London, the 'overground' counter-cultural magazine *Gandalf's Garden* reported that ISKCON 'have made their mission widely known, have set up a commune and temple and have produced a record with the Beatles'.[41] The speed of these developments was largely attributable to Harrison's influence.

Harrison instructed Apple Corps to back the loan for their first British temple. Some of the ISKCON devotees lived for several months in John Lennon's manor home, Tittenhurst Park, and paid their rent by making repairs to the estate. Apple Records released a single of the devotees chanting the Hare Krishna Mantra; with Harrison's endorsement it quickly shot up the charts, reportedly selling 70,000 copies on its first day of release (Giuliano 1989: 104). Harrison's 1970 single 'My Sweet Lord' was also a lasting popular success. The robed and dancing devotees appeared on the popular television show *Top of the Pops* twice in 1970.[42] Harrison also agreed to fund the publication of Prabhupada's translation of part of the *Śrīmad-Bhāgavatam* as *The KRṢNA Book*, a 400-plus-page book with

40. For information on ISKCON, see Rochford (2007); for Britain more specifically, see Dwyer and Cole (2007).

41. 'Krishna Commune', *Gandalf's Garden* 6, p. 25.

42. 'Top of the Pops: programme as broadcast', T12/1,278/1 and R126/270/1 in BBC WAC. The Radha Krishna Temple performed 'Govinda' on 19 March 1970 and 9 April 1970. On the second date, eleven members are noted as being in attendance for filming and on both occasions the song was about four and a half minutes in length.

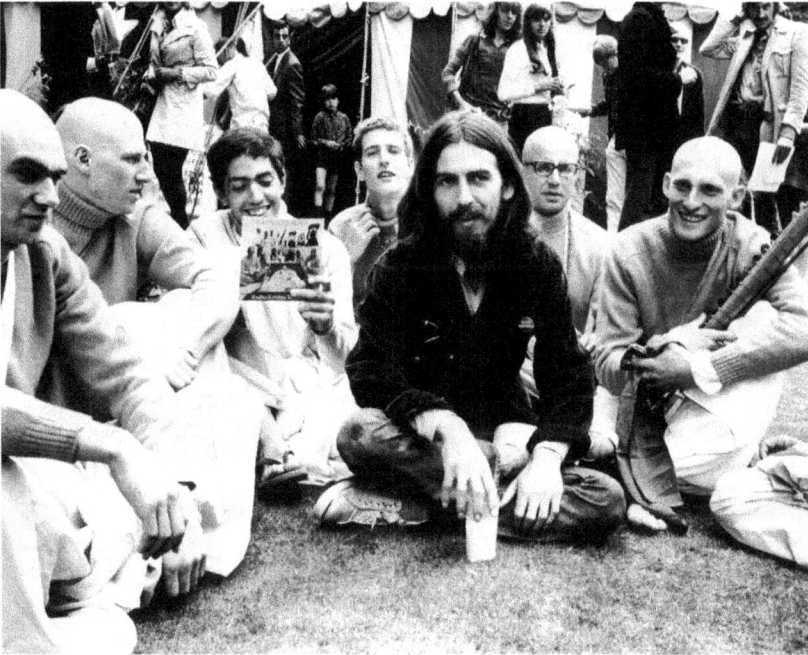

Fig. 5.2 George Harrison with members of ISKCON. Image courtesy of the Bhaktidevanta Book Trust International, Inc. www.Krishna.com. Used with permission.

fifty-four colour pages, at a cost of $19,000 for 5,000 copies. The book details Krishna's childhood and youth, with many anecdotes about the divine life. In presenting the numerous stories, the many aspects of Krishna are described and this is a way of keeping one's mind on God. Devotional reading was an important adjunct to the chanting for which the Hare Krishnas are so famous (Greene 2005: 158–60). ISKCON's efforts in disseminating Krishna Consciousness literature, especially the *Bhagavad Gītā*, in exchange for small donations on the streets of many major cities, also did much to raise awareness of Indian religious paths among the general population. The *Bhagavad Gītā* in its various translations remained closely associated with other forms of yoga, regularly featuring on Wheel of Yoga reading lists. In 1973 ISKCON devotees moved into Bhaktivedanta Manor, a large estate in Letchmore Heath just north of London, a property purchased by Harrison some years earlier.

Harrison established a cultural home for Indian spirituality in popular culture. Many of Harrison's solo albums contain songs based more generally on Krishna and Indian spiritual ideas. The 1971 charity *Concert for Bangladesh* was a high-profile contribution to a raising of consciousness about Indian music and spirituality: Ravi Shankar opened the event and Harrison acted as master of ceremonies for Ringo Starr, Eric Clapton, Leon Russell and Bob Dylan among others. The event drew 40,000 people into its two performances at New York City's Madison Square Garden (Clayson 2001: 308; Greene 2005: 186–94). Harrison's 1973 *Living in the Material World* and 1974 *Dark Horse* tour were also both popular, although they received mixed reviews, particularly with respect to the ex-Beatle's eagerness to moralise and proselytise for Krishna Consciousness (Greene 2005: 183, 213–20). Although many of these ventures were not considered commercial or critical successes, they did ensure extensive publicity for India as spiritual inspiration.

Centre House

Centre House was an influential London-based commune within which yoga was an integral part; it was founded by Christopher Hills (1926–1997) in Kensington, London. The *Aquarian Guide to Occult, Mystical, Religious, Magical London and Around* (1970) listed the commune as simply 'Centre':

> Join in with us and bring your own 'thing' to the Creative Centre. The community at Centre House, 10a Airlie Gardens, London W.8 is a twenty-four-hour a day encounter group, using the growth techniques of meditation, creative conflict, spontaneous music, awareness and sensitivity sessions, creative projects, experiments and discussions. Share their expanding experiences on Thursday evenings at 8.00pm (Strachan 1970: 10).

Centre House also hosted one of England's first macrobiotic cafés (Green 1988). Christopher Hills was deeply interested in promoting human welfare with both science and spirituality. After an early career as a trader in Jamaica, Hills became deeply interested in the revolutionary struggles of the Jamaican and Indian people, forging connections with a variety of influential Indian spiritual and political leaders. Although of an older generation than the hippies, the Centre House commune became a focus for spirituality and exploring human potential. A variety of spiritual teachers came in and out of Centre House during the 1960s while Christopher Hills was writing a book on chakras and the endocrine system, *Nuclear Evolution* (1977

[1968]). In 1970, Hills and his son John were also closely involved in organising a World Conference on Scientific Yoga (WCSY) in New Delhi, India. Hills was also very interested in the potential for alleviating poverty through aquaculture – in particular, developing high-protein algae – and was responsible for bringing spirulina into modern mass production. By 1973, he had moved to the United States where he founded the University of the Trees in Colorado, but the Centre House community continued into the late 1970s.

Closely associated with Centre House was the yoga teacher Malcolm Strutt, who wrote several books on yoga in the 1970s (Strutt (1976a,b, 1977a,b). He was influential among those looking to try yoga during this period and his teaching of asana and pranayama was particularly influenced by B.K.S. Iyengar and inspired by Paramahansa Yogananda (Strutt 1976a: 'Personal Note'). However, his instructions for yoga laid an emphasis on a transformation of consciousness and a reliance on the self as a teacher. He diagrams the effects of the various physical postures of yoga on the 'direction of consciousness' and describes a variety of beliefs and practices found in the alternative milieu of the time as having an underlying unity and contributing to a general uplift of the individual and social consciousness. Evaluating the availability of contemporary teachers originating both from the 'East' and the 'West', he wrote: 'Somewhere in all the new revolution towards evolution you may find this course a stepping stone in your own growth toward fulfilment and enlightenment. Keep looking!' (Strutt 1976a).

Gandalf's Garden

An important figure who bridged the gap between the older Centre House generation and younger generations was Muz Murray (b. 1940). He was born in Nuneaton and, having studied art at Coventry, spent several years travelling around the Mediterranean working on films and taking other odd jobs. Like many of his generation, he was grabbing an opportunity to travel and explore the world. He recalled one day in 1964, aged 23, with £7.10s. to his name, sitting by the sea in Cyprus:

> I just had this very strange feeling like a ghostly hand crept over the back of my head and pressed a sort of etheric brain on top of my brain. And my consciousness appeared to leave the body and just expand right across the ocean, or right across the universe. And I was given information, knowledge that I couldn't get in any other way. Which in

a few minutes changed the whole course of my life. And from then on,
I was on the spiritual path, trying to find out what the hell happened
to me![43]

He claims neither to have taken drugs, read spiritual books nor had
any meditation practice before this experience. Questioning his san-
ity after the experience in Cyprus, he went to the British Library
in Cairo (while working as Art Director for Cairo Television). He
was relieved to find a book on *Cosmic Consciousness* (Bucke 1902),
which satisfied him that he had had a deeply spiritual experience
like many in history before him.[44] After leaving Cairo, Murray had
somewhat more dangerous adventures while hitch-hiking down
the whole length of Africa: long and harrowing journeys, often
without food or money.

Murray considered himself an explorer/adventurer and a poet –
not a hippy. Although in retrospect Murray reflected that he 'looked
like [the] hippies and I had hippy philosophy long before they came
along'.[45] As he travelled down Africa he found his personal preferences changing: he gradually gave up meat, eggs, alcohol and
tobacco. He eventually found himself in South Africa, where he
encountered a Sikh teacher, Maharaj Charan Singh of Radha Soami
Satsang who was initiating people into Shabda Yoga meditation
– provided they had abstained from meat, fish, eggs, alcohol and
tobacco for three months. Finding himself coincidentally meeting these criteria, Murray offered himself for initiation and spent
a week, along with sixteen others, doing meditation practice with
Singh from 1 to 2.30 am every morning while holding down day-
time work in theatre and film. This gave him a desire to go to India
and learn more from the Indian tradition. However, running short
of money for such an extended trip, he instead returned to London,
got a bedsit in Notting Hill Gate, and found a job in television in
order to save money for another adventure.[46]

Back in London, Murray came into contact with many young
people who were ready to 'pour out their problems' to him, seeking spiritual direction but not finding much in an 'underground'

43. Personal Interview with Muz Murray (14 December 2016). See also Muz
Murray's website and publications; at the time of the interview he was writing an
autobiography for publication.
44. Personal Interview with Muz Murray (14 December 2016).
45. Ibid.
46. Ibid.

movement that emphasised sexual freedom, experimentation with drugs and musical self-expression. He got involved with the commune at Centre House and here met Ramamurti Shriram Mishra (later known as Shri Brahmananda Sarasvati [d. 1993]), whom he came to consider a 'guru'. Mishra was an Indian-born biomedical surgeon, who had given up medicine when he found he 'could cure more people with mantra than he could with the scalpel'.[47] Murray also introduced the yoga teacher Malcolm Strutt to the community.

While living at Centre House, Murray attempted, without success, to interest various 'underground' publications in a column on spirituality. Finding little support there, Murray decided to start his own magazine. The first attempt was called *Love Ink*; it folded but he was undeterred. He was inspired by Tolkien's tale of the fight against darkness in *The Lord of the Rings* – and the way elves, humans and hobbits were brought together. Murray claims he wrote to J.R.R. Tolkien to ask permission to call his venture 'Gandalf's Garden' – which was duly given despite the author voicing scepticism about 'hippies'; however, according to Murray, Tolkien did write a letter after reading the first issue to express his appreciation.

After a while, Murray got Malcolm Strutt (his 'straight man') to acquire the lease of an old 'Home and Colonial' shop at the 'rough end' of the King's Road in Chelsea, just opposite The World's End pub. Murray and his friends moved in and cleaned the shop up. He recalls:

> we cleaned that place out, scraping the pigs' fat off the floor and doing a vibration-changing ceremony. [We] made a meeting place in the cellar, and we had upstairs low tables on the floor and cushions. We were selling hippy-made produce and clothes, selling teas and porridge and stuff like that. Very cheap, 6p, at a time. And looking after derelicts on the street who had nowhere to sleep, so we let them sleep in the cellar overnight, and we fed them freely.[48]

From these attempts to give local homeless people and drug addicts spiritual inspiration evolved a programme of talks from various gurus. Murray believes that the physical location of Gandalf's

---

47. Ibid. Mishra wrote *The Textbook of Yoga Psychology* (1972a [1963]) and *Fundamentals of Yoga* (1972b [1959]), and founded the Yoga Society of New York, Inc. in 1958 and the Ananda Ashram in New York in 1964; in 1972, he established the Yoga Society of San Francisco, Inc.

48. Personal Interview with Muz Murray (14 December 2016).

Garden opened up the variety of existing esoteric groups to a new generation of young people:

> all these groups, the druids, the Buddhists, etc., they were all in their own corners. Nobody knew about them and they didn't have young people with them, so I invited all of these, Christians, Buddhists, Hasidim, Chinese, flying-saucer people, every . . . the whole spectrum . . . I gave platforms for all these groups. For the first time, they started getting a lot of young members in their groups.

Spaces like the one generated around Centre Place and Gandalf's Garden were crucial in creating the 'cultic milieu' atmosphere which Colin Campbell (1972) described as a defining feature of spiritual exploration during this period. *Gandalf's Garden* magazine was carried in backpacks of travellers and seekers around the world; people wrote in from all parts of the world and the *Lord of the Rings* spiritual theme spread in 'headshops' and hippy venues throughout Europe. Chris Tobler (who hung out at Gandalf's Garden and later was involved in establishing the first Sivananda Yoga centre in London) remembers Gandalf's Garden as much wilder than Centre House with 'long hair all over the place'. It was a place where you could turn up on a Friday night and be introduced to all sorts of philosophies, ideas, buy underground literature and meet travelling teachers such as Ramamurti Shriram Mishra.[49]

From 1968 to 1971, Muz Murray's Gandalf's Garden project popularised yoga for a younger generation. It had a physical location on King's Road, Chelsea, which was already known for Mary Quant's Bazaar and as the home of many cultural icons of the early 1960s. From this location, from 1968 to 1970 Murray and some dedicated friends produced six irregular issues of a magazine called *Gandalf's Garden*; and the property known as Gandalf's Garden remained open until 1971. Murray attempted to operate outside of the capitalist structure as much as possible, and to a large extent Gandalf's Garden was a counter-cultural gesture. Instead of relying on the capitalist structure of book sales, Murray attempted to spread his ideas by word of mouth and non-capitalist experimentation.

Murray's spiritual vision was inclusive rather than exclusive. He called his experiment an 'overground' movement in contrast to the 'underground' press represented by the *International Times* (1966–1973) and *Oz* magazine (1967–1973) which also were popular among

49. Personal interview with Chris Tobler (12 October 2017).

the London youth culture, particularly as events listings.[50] Yet there was an overlap in readership among Murray's 'overground' and the youth-cultural 'underground'. *Gandalf's Garden's* staff also overlapped with these publications, but this magazine was distinguishable by its spiritual focus. Murray drew on connections with the youth culture more generally to help cover costs. For example, he held benefit concerts in which Marc Bolan/Tyrannosaurus Rex and David Bowie, among others, helped raise funds – musicians who were associated at times with Murray's vision.[51] As much as they might wish to remain outside the system, money was still needed to print the magazine and maintain the premises.

Gandalf's Garden invoked British gardening imagery and Tolkien's *Lord of the Rings* to call for inner spiritual growth with the belief that it could transform the world:

> Between the leaves of GANDALF'S GARDEN a focal point for creators and beautiful people can be attained, and a communication service evolved, whereby all those alone can get to know about each other, can be put in touch and visit each other's creative communes, becoming involved in joint ventures arts and crafts and music-wise.[52]

The magazine was distributed by subscription, street-sellers and specialist bookstores. By its sixth issue, there were stores selling the magazine in the USA, Belgium, Canada, Denmark, Holland, Germany, Norway, Spain and Switzerland, and letters testified to a nationwide distribution in Britain.[53] However, distribution was achieved largely via networks of friends, so only a certain stratum of British society would have been aware of the magazine.

While *Gandalf's Garden* appealed specifically to the late 1960s youth culture, it also overlapped with existing networks of interest in yoga and alternative spirituality. *Gandalf's Garden* enjoyed some circulation among yoga practitioners outside youth culture. In 1969, Wheel of British Yoga founder Wilfred Clark commented on *Gandalf's Garden* in the Wheel's *Bulletin*:

---

50. The *International Times* was also published in 1974, continuously between 1975 and 1982 and again in 1986. Personal correspondence with 'Chis' at http://www.international-times.org.uk, 10 September 2007. The British Library holds the original print run and a few of the later issues.

51. *Gandalf's Garden* 2, p. 10.

52. *Gandalf's Garden* 1, p. 1.

53. *Gandalf's Garden* 6, p. 15.

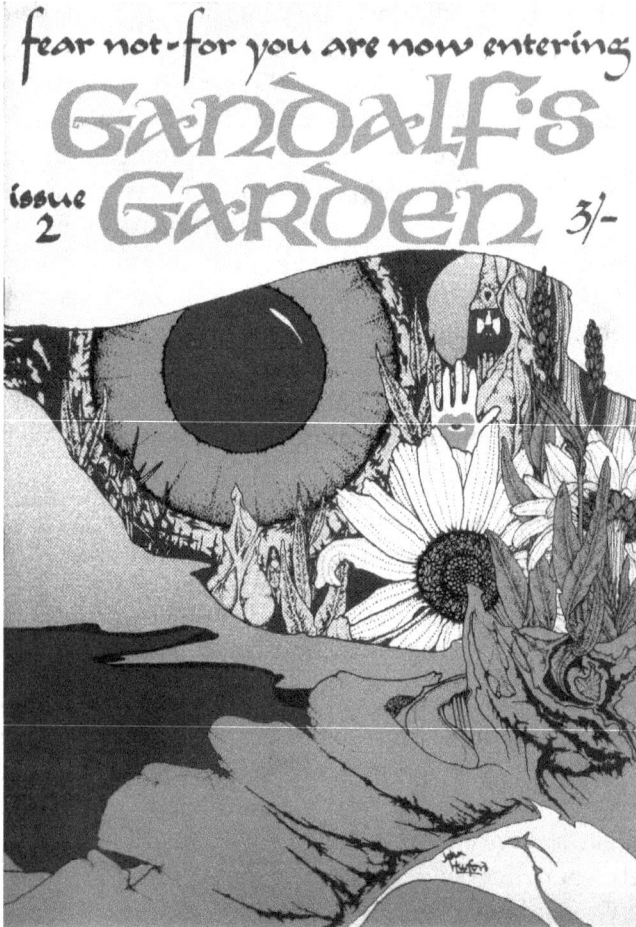

Fig. 5.3 *Gandalf's Garden* Issue 2 cover. Image courtesy of Muz Murray.
Used with permission.

> Should you perchance ever see a jazzy magazine bearing this title
> don't scream; you will find it right up your street. Despite its appear-
> ance (which is definitely aimed to attract youth) it is well planted with
> the Seeds of the Spirit and you shall know it by its fruits. Write to the
> editor Muz Murray . . .[54]

The 'store manager' of Watkins Bookshop wrote a letter to the editor of *Gandalf's Garden*:

54. Wilfred Clark, Wheel of British Yoga *Bulletin* 41 (March 1969).

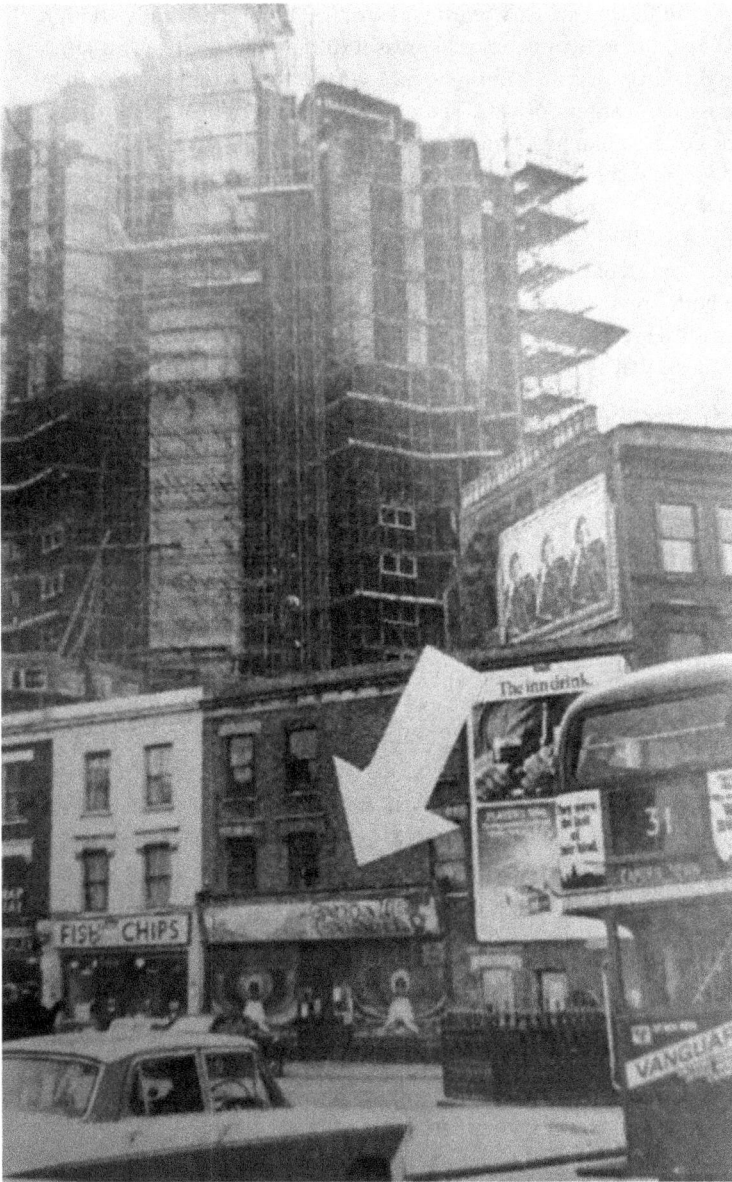

Fig. 5.4 Location of Gandalf's Garden. From *Yoga & Health* 11 (November 1971), p. 15.

> I agree with almost every word you write, although, naturally enough
> perhaps, I would sometimes express it differently . . . one can't jump
> the generation gap . . . the reference was to the pictorial rather than
> the written content of G.G. For pre-McLuhan, pre-Beat and pre-his-
> toric codgers like myself (and there are a lot of us) your lavish (psy-
> chedelically contemporary; or just contemporary?) use of colour and
> above all your imagery are bound to seem a bit bizarre – a marvellous
> melody of ?Beardsley-cum? Bosh-cum? Private Eye-cum all ye faith-
> ful to the call of the Underground (and why not? Nature and History
> are both on your side. The chrysalis is paradigmatic, the Catacombs
> provide a precedent). Well, we shall have to go along with your divine
> madness, that's all.[55]

The 'psychedelic' artwork may have put off some of the older
generation, but the growing British interest in spiritual and esoteric
groups was not specific to those in their twenties. Muz Murray's
project focused on his own generation of 'seekers' yet Gandalf's
Garden could also be understood as a short-lived Watkins Bookshop for a younger generation of seekers. Murray's anti-capitalist
organisation was part of the counter-culture.

Gandalf's Garden was an experiment in both magazine production and as an inclusive open-house shop. Murray relied on vol-
unteers for much of the magazine production and invited those
who were interested in his project to drop in and join whatever was
happening. Friends and interested readers were invited round for
events at the Garden, particularly for yoga classes on Wednesday
and Thursday evenings and Sunday mornings for a mantra-medita-
tion session and cooperative exploration on Friday evenings.[56] The
invitation to the Friday evening gathering makes the inclusive and
spiritual tone of the gatherings clear:

> Soul Gardeners and seekers of the miraculous get together for vibra-
> tion raising, study, discussion, Chinese tea and soul stimulation. Ses-
> sions usually begin with Mantra Meditation (no problem for beginners
> who can just sit and absorb the vibes) to rarefy the atmosphere. (We
> have to close the door during this so please be early). Then follows
> reflections on the *Eternal Why* of our existence from any angel open to
> us, initiated by the Gardeners, or by visiting yogis, occultists, healers,
> mediums, monks, astrologers, writers, researchers or groups, who are
> well into their own thing, who have offered to come along and act as

55. *Gandalf's Garden* 4, p. 32.
56. Typewritten A4 advert stamped in by British Library acquisitions, November 1969, in *Gandalf's Garden* collection.

the catalytic element for discussion. (Prospective catalysts are invited to contact Muz Murray: FLA 6156 or just come along anyway).[57]

This attitude of inclusive openness is also partly why Murray termed the shop and magazine an 'overground' movement. Early issues had columns by the well-known DJ John Peel, who was also celebrated for fostering a similar sense of community on his early broadcasts. Calling his 1967 past-midnight Radio London show *The Perfumed Garden* (perhaps a factor in Murray choice of name for his enterprise), Peel encouraged listeners to write in and join in the musical exploration.[58]

Although Gandalf's Garden itself was drug-free, many of those involved with its message, were interested in experimenting with various forms of 'getting high' and opening their mind to the possibilities of human experience and its meanings. Like many of those coming to adulthood in the mid-late 1960s, Chris Tobler sought experiences with the assistance of drugs such as marijuana and LSD. Tobler's parents were members of the Study Society, did Sufi whirling, and had initiated the entire family into Transcendental Meditation in 1966 when he was a teenager. However, Chris wanted to find his own path and found the scene in Gandalf's Garden more in line with his generation's search than the structures of the Study Society or Centre House.[59] Many others became interested in a variety of mind-changing experiences and lifestyles initially through drugs – experiments that were often accompanied by explorations of yoga and meditation. The consciousness-expanding properties of LSD, its enthusiasts hoped, had the potential to radically transform the world for the better. In the experimental scene of the 1960s, explorations of consciousness linked yoga techniques, meditation and drugs. The Beatles and other popular musicians were known to be experimenting with drugs as well as Eastern spiritualities, as were a number of figures from previous generations such as Aldous Huxley, Allen Ginsberg, William Burroughs, Timothy Leary and R.D. Laing.

57. *Gandalf's Garden* 4, p. 17.
58. *Gandalf's Garden* 2, p. 9. *The Perfumed Garden* went on air in May 1967 and Radio London was taken off the air in August 1967. After this, Peel wrote a column for the *International Times* also entitled 'The Perfumed Garden'.
59. Personal Interview with Chris Tobler (12 October 2017).

Psychedelic drugs were ubiquitous for some populations of young people growing up during this period. As one informant remembers:

> In 1971, aged 14, I had LSD for the first time; nearly all my friends took it too in the early 70s. In 1973 there was a big bust in my school in Sussex; around 200 of the 400 pupils were using cannabis and LSD. Psychedelic experiences led many of us directly into yoga and meditation (and everything 'alternative'). By the time I was 16 I was vegetarian, sleeping on the floor and occasionally experimenting with yoga postures and meditation. Some of my friends became initiated by a guru or ISKCON but many of us just dabbled with all this. We started eating whole foods, went to see all sorts of gurus, including the Dalai Lama, attended free festivals, tried Sufi dancing and all things alternative. Nobody I knew ever went to a yoga class but nearly everyone I knew of my age was experimenting with eastern spirituality, meditation, pranayama, sitting in lotus position, doing headstands etc. I eventually got to India in 1977. One of the reasons for this enthusiasm for India was that there were no road maps in the west for the acid experience (nor, incidentally, were there any guide books for India).

LSD became easily accessible in Britain during the 1960s and was considered enough of a social problem for it to be made illegal in 1966. However, it remained available for those who were interested, at least until the closure of a major manufacturing centre in Wales in 1977 (Roberts 2012). Some who were initially introduced to alternative ideas via drugs eventually looked for other means with which to have transformative spiritual experiences.[60]

From 1969, Yogi Bhajan (1929–2004) was explicitly attempting to appeal to those looking for a natural 'high' having had experiences on drugs with the technique of Kundalini Yoga and the Happy Healthy Holy Order (3HO). Yogi Bhajan (born Harbhajan Singh Puri) combined Sikh doctrine with physical yoga techniques learned from the Delhi-based yoga teacher Dhirendra Brahmachari (1924–1994) and introduced his programme in California from 1969 (Deslippe 2012). Bhajan's Kundalini Yoga was formally introduced to Britain in 1971 when Vikram Singh, formerly Vic Briggs of the band the Animals, established the first London branch and

---

60. For a more comprehensive exploration of the overlap between psychedelics and spiritual experiences, see Partridge (2018) and Clark (2017).

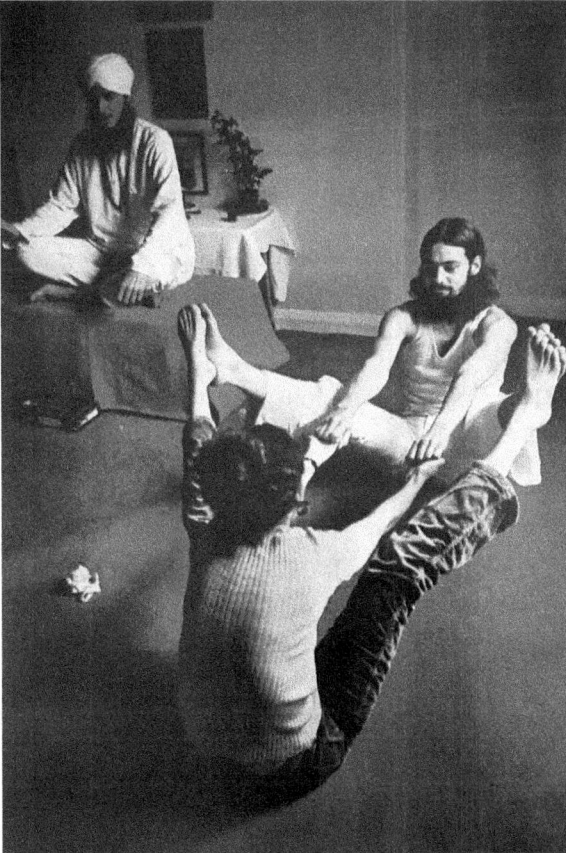

Fig. 5.5 The Happy Healthy Holy Order (3HO). *Yoga & Health* 6 (1971), p. 20.

promoted 'Kundalini Yoga' in the new *Yoga & Health* magazine.[61] *Alternative London* (1972) described the classes thus:

> They say that nearly all their students have been into drugs (though of course everyone is welcome), and that their technique is more rapid than other yogas, providing an immediate 'high' and lasting result … sessions involve straining to one's limits using dynamic exercises and breath control … Classes include some meditation and chanting ('God is me, me is God' repeated vigorously) and finish with that beautiful chorus from the Incredible String Band: 'May the long time sun shine upon you, all love surround you and the pure light within you guide you all the way on' (Saunders 1972: 176).

61. See Deslippe (2012) and Jacobsh (2008) for the history of 3HO/Kundalini yoga as a religious movement as well as the other articles in *Sikh Formations* vol. 8.

This early 3HO centre was meeting the needs of a similar population to the one frequenting Gandalf's Garden in the years between
1968 and 1971, providing a place to meet like-minded people and
experiment with the possibilities of human experience. However,
whereas the 3HO centre was affiliated solely to Yogi Bhajan, Gandalf's Garden encouraged a wide variety of approaches and guest
speakers.

The excitement and transitory nature of the population that
helped spread the message of Gandalf's Garden were also factors in
its rapid degeneration. All those involved in the project were living
in extremely close quarters (Murray remembers from five to fifteen
people all sleeping on the floor in one room) and very strapped for
cash. Much of the money made from selling the magazine often
failed to make its way back to those producing it. After the London
commune folded, Murray spent some time travelling around England and Scotland on his Vespa, trying to help people who had been
inspired by *Gandalf's Garden*. He made it up to Findhorn in Scotland
before returning to Cornwall and ended up leading mantras on the
pyramid at the opening of the 1971 Glastonbury Fayre.[62]

In the 1970s, Murray finally made it to India where he had another
series of adventures seeking out 'every form of yoga available with
many renowned masters of many traditions'.[63] Well known from his
Gandalf's Garden project, he continued to act as a point of contact
for many on a spiritual quest in India. On returning from his three
years of travels, Murray published *Seeking the Master: A Guide to
the Ashrams of India* (1980), a collation of his own personal experience, and reports sent to him by friends, acquaintances and anyone
alerted to his project by word of mouth. This guide summarised
many of the spiritual teachers whom British seekers in the 1970s
might have found during their pilgrimages to India, and it became
the go-to guide to a spiritual journey in India for the 1980s.

The London Sivananda Yoga Centre

Some of those who experienced yoga and meditation at Gandalf's
Garden were inspired to delve deeper into specific yoga traditions.
For example, one of the founders of the first Sivananda Vedanta
Centre in Britain, Barbara Gordon, had initially been introduced to

---

62. Personal Interview with Muz Murray (14 December 2016).
63. Ibid.

yoga at Gandalf's Garden by Doshia Dupré, a student of Dr Mishra.[64] Together with some friends, Gordon was inspired to study yoga at Swami Vishnudevananda's ashram in Val-Morin, Canada, where she met a fellow Englishwoman Judy Tobler (née Stallabrass) who had become interested in yoga while on her breaks in the United States, working as an air hostess for PanAm. Judy remembers her first yoga classes in Los Angeles in 1969. While attending a talk by Swami Satchidananda (who was taught by Swami Sivananda) she experienced a 'light bulb moment'. She became a vegetarian and began regularly attending yoga and meditation with Sivananda teachers in Los Angeles, who suggested that she do the teacher training-course in Val-Morin.

The training programme is remembered as an intense few months. According to Tobler, Swami Vishnudevananda was a strict teacher who insisted on punctuality and criticised a perceived lack of discipline in his students. She recalls:

> ... very much the principles [they] were following [at Val-Morin] were Swami Sivananda's. Often Swami Sivananda's approach was referred to as 'integral yoga'. In other words, he brought together Hatha Yoga, Raja Yoga, Bhakti Yoga, the devotional yoga, and Karma Yoga, the yoga of selfless service. And I would say that Swami Vishnudevananda was very much a specialist in the Hatha Yoga, in the *asanas* and the *pranayama*, the postures and the breathing. But he brought everything else in as well. He was strong on the Karma Yoga, that everyone should help and that kind of a thing. You know, and some meditation and chanting and so on.[65]

Vishnudevananda, in Tobler's recollection was a very passionate character: 'I think he very much wanted to really offer young people something – and the world something.'[66]

The highlight of her time in Canada was a Jubilee festival during which Vishnudevananda invited

> all his brother swamis, particularly ones who had come to the West, to his ashram in Val-Morin. So there was him. There was Swami Venkatesananda, there was Swami Satchidananda, Swami Chidananda.

64. *Yoga & Health* 3 (1971), p. 29. In 1973, Doshia Dupré directed a television programme with Dr R.S. Mishra/Shri Ramamurti (later known as Shri Brahmananda Sarasvati) entitled *Yoga for the Body, Mind and Spirit*, which was produced by Public Access Cable Television (NYC).

65. Personal interview with Judy Tobler (29 September 2017).

66. Ibid.

> He also invited a bunch of what you would call in India wandering
> *bhaktas* or devotees. Men and women who kind of travelled around
> from town to town playing devotional music and chanting and
> going into trances and goodness knows what. And all of this kind of
> descended for a few days on the ashram. And it was the most amazing
> experience . . . It was very colourful and very, very exciting. And very,
> very, very kind of 1960s! I mean, I think every American hippy was on
> the place as well.[67]

Having amassed savings from her well-paid job, Judy was ready
to embrace a radical lifestyle change. She felt an immediate connection with Swami Venkatesananda. She remembers the idea of
opening a Sivananda Yoga Centre in London as arising organically
out of conversations with Barbara in Val-Morin.[68]

They returned to London in December 1970 to the networks of
people dropping in and out of Gandalf's Garden. The two women
searched all over London for an appropriate building to rent for
their yoga centre until, in early 1971, the first Sivananda Vedanta
ashram in Britain opened its doors at 44 Ifield Road in an unassum-
ing terraced house in Earl's Court. Keeping with the youth culture
at the time, from the outset the founders of the centre wanted an
open-door policy. The newly launched *Yoga & Health* magazine
reported:

> There is little to distinguish one Victorian terraced house from the
> next in the road, save for the number over the fanlight and the colour
> of the door; but over the bell push of one particular house is a discrete
> and important little notice. It reads: 'Ring hard, there is always some-
> body in' and it means what it says because it is the home of the new
> English *ashram* of the Sivananda Yoga Society.[69]

As a result of leafleting and word-of-mouth networking, the ashram's yoga classes grew from two students to overflowing capacity
within six weeks.

An early resident in these years, Hector Guthrie, remembers only
about five people living at the centre during the first few years, an
'inner core' of about thirty people associated with the ashram, and
perhaps another thirty 'regulars', with many more people dropping

---

67. Ibid.
68. Ibid.
69. *Yoga & Health* 3 (1971), p. 29. For more general background on Sivananda's
global movements, see Strauss (2002a,b, 2005).

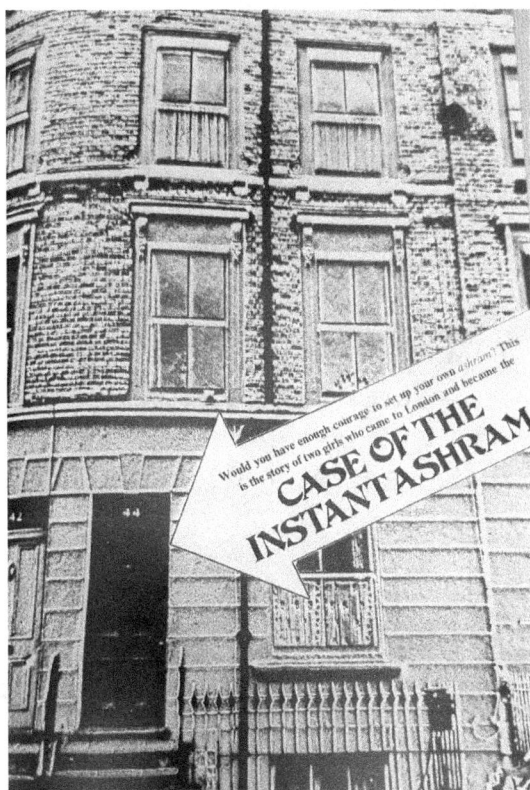

Fig. 5.6 External of the first Sivananda Yoga Centre in London. *Yoga & Health* 3 (1971), p. 27.

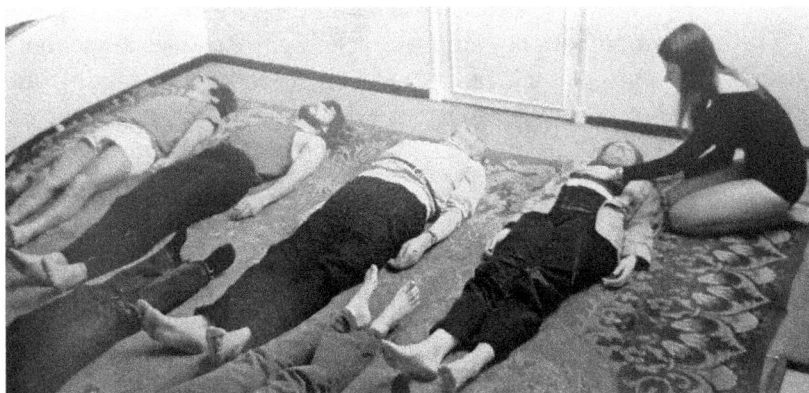

Fig. 5.7 Inside the Sivananda Yoga Centre. *Yoga & Health* 3 (1971), p. 29.

in from time to time.[70] *Yoga & Health* noted the varied population of
people interested in classes at the ashram:

> It is odd that the classes at Ifield Road seem to have attracted as many
> men as women, although their ages may range from fourteen to sixty
> plus, whereas most of the more commercial Yoga classes seem to
> attract far more women than men.[71]

Guthrie remembers that they also ran macrobiotic cooking classes
at the ashram and

> had a real relationship with every other freewheeling spiritual organ-
> isation in London. So, in those days, we were very open, which is
> unlike today . . . we mixed freely with the devotees of this guru and
> that guru.[72]

Swami Venkatesananda was a visitor in the first year, but there was
no resident Swami.

To some extent those attracted to the yoga of the Sivananda
environment may have been reacting against the yoga found in the
adult-education centres, which focused on mastery of physical exercises. Guthrie recalls that:

> I do get the impression from the conversations at the time that peo-
> ple thought that what else that there was around was very stark and
> physical. Goal-orientated. You know, the sort of what we used to call
> the abomination of the Iyengar approach. Which was very, very . . .
> hard-line, and Iyengar at that time really had a strong influence on
> the few teachers around, which meant they were trying to mimic him.
> And it was quite violent, actually. And it did have that reputation at
> the time.[73]

Guthrie remembers beginning to teach yoga classes after about
six months of attendance (he had previously trained in aikido), and
soon thereafter taking on more of a leadership role, directing the
ashram. He recalls the emphasis of the classes at the ashram:

> So it was inhale, arch up and back, exhale down, and inhale, twist
> to the left, and that sort of thing. So there was a lot of emphasis on
> breathing. In doing the *asanas*, the physical thing, again what distin-
> guished us, was: we were telling people do not strain; there is no goal

70. Personal interview with Hector Guthrie (8 October 2009).
71. *Yoga & Health* 3 (1971), p. 30.
72. Personal interview with Hector Guthrie (8 October 2009).
73. Ibid.

here; there is no standard you have to reach. Do it very easily. Sink into the stretch, or sink into whatever it is.

And then it finished with a 10- to 15-minute deep relaxation. And it gave people an experience of relaxation which in many cases they had never experienced before in their lives. And in fact took them to a very deep meditative place. And it was a particular way of doing it, in which we took our time, we dropped our voices. We were soft. We were actually modelling the inner state of relaxation but, more particularly, we were modelling something which, then and now, I think is unknown to many people, which they yearn for, which is we were modelling gentleness and softness and actually kindness towards one's self.[74]

Chris Tobler also moved into the Sivananda Centre when it opened and remembers teaching yoga asana in four or five sequences which began with 'standard exercises' and included shoulder-stands, headstands and spinal twists.[75] The early centre was also a place people enjoyed being around. In Judy's recollection:

There was a lot of hanging out as well. In fact there was a lot of - I really must say there was a lot of fun. I mean, we were very busy being quite spiritual, but we also had a lot of fun. I mean, I can remember, you know, after the yoga classes sitting in the kitchen and just laughing a lot.[76]

The centre grew very quickly and organically at first. This attracted more interest from Vishnudevananda's centre in Val-Morin. By 1972, the Sivananda ashram had moved to another property at 16b Wharfdale Road and the main teaching space to 175 Finborough Road, SW10 and the centre was put under the direction of a resident Swami.[77]

Founder Judy and her soon-to-be husband Chris Tobler left London later in 1971 to follow their teacher Swami Venkatesananda, first to his ashram in Mauritius, then to New Zealand, where Hector

74. Ibid.
75. Personal interview with Chris Tobler (12 October 2017).
76. Personal interview with Judy Tobler (29 September 2017).
77. Personal interview with Hector Guthrie (8 October 2009) and Saunders (1972, n.d.). The first edition of Saunders's *Alternative London* is usually found in card catalogues with a 1970 or a 1971 date; however, the first edition clearly says 'This is the first edition published 12.5.72 by Nicholas Saunders, Alternative London, 65 Edith Grove, London SW10'; there is no date on the second edition, although it is clearly labelled as a second edition. The Sivananda Yoga Centre is not listed in Strachan (1970).

Guthrie later joined them teaching yoga and meditation. They finally settled in Cape Town, South Africa, in 1976, where they continued to live with devotees of the Swami and practise his teachings. The Swami visited South Africa frequently until his death in 1982. This kind of fluid movement around the Commonwealth countries was not uncommon for those involved in looking for alternative ways of being during the 1970s.

Jiddu Krishnamurti and Brockwood Park

Jiddu Krishnamurti (1895–1986) had been identified as the prophesied messiah for the Theosophical Society in 1909.[78] He was adopted by the English suffragette and reproductive health campaigner Annie Besant (1847–1933), who was at that time president of the Theosophical Society, and taken to England for his education.[79] The Theosophical Society believed he was the world teacher for this new age and founded the Order of the Star of the East in anticipation of his mature teachings. Ironically, in attempting to throw off the expectations of his mentors and refuse to be a 'world teacher', he established himself as one. In a 1929 speech in which he dissolved the Order of the Star of the East, he articulated the teachings for which he would become famous:

> Man cannot come to it [truth] through any organization, through any creed, through any dogma, priest or ritual, not through any philosophical knowledge or psychological technique. He has to find it through the mirror of relationship, through the understanding of the contents of his own mind, through observation and not through intellectual analysis or introspective dissection (Krishnamurti 1929).

From the late 1920s, Krishnamurti lived mainly in southern California where he became friends with British expatriate Aldous Huxley (1894–1963); Krishnamurti's first book, *The First and Last Freedom* (1954), was published with an introduction by Huxley. The influence of Krishnamurti on Huxley's world-view is evidenced in *The Perennial Philosophy* (1942) and *Island* (1962).

As an adult, Krishnamurti toured the world as a lecturer attempting to remove the barriers to an experience of 'truth'. In this, he promoted constant awareness, peace and stillness, but also 'an

78. Biographies of Krishnamurti include the authorised one (Lutyens 1990) and a critical personal memoir (Sloss 1991).

79. For Annie Besant, see Taylor (1992); see also Besant's *Introduction to Yoga* (1908).

awareness of self-deception, prejudice and parroted dogmas which can blind us to the wholeness of reality and the oneness of humanity'.[80] Krishnamurti's message was essentially very simple although he phrased it in many different ways: peace, happiness and an improvement of the human condition were to be found through self-exploration, a tranquil mind and the cultivation of love.

Krishnamurti became an integral part of the formation of understandings of yoga in twentieth-century Europe. His teachings were not directly connected to the growing popularity of asana-focused 'modern yoga' although he was very much associated with the same milieu. He lectured in Europe annually from 1961. Mutual connections led to his being taught yoga asana by B.K.S. Iyengar in Gstaad, Switzerland, in the early 1960s, while Iyengar was Yehudi Menuhin's guest. Through Iyengar's introduction, Krishnamurti visited the family of T. Krishnamacharya in Madras in 1965 and became a long-term student of Krishnamacharya's son, T.K.V. Desikachar (1938–2016)[81] for asana and pranayama. During the late 1960s, Krishnamurti was closely associated with the Belgian Gérard Blitz, who founded the vacation company Club Méditerranée in 1950 and in 1973 helped to establish the European Union of Yoga (l'Union Européenne de Yoga) in Zinal, Switzerland (see Desponds 2007). Desikachar's association with Krishnamurti and Blitz greatly increased his visibility in Europe, and to some extent in Britain. Krishnamurti held 'camps' at Brockwood Park, a property purchased on his behalf in Hampshire. From 1969 to 1984 hundreds of people attended annually to hear Krishnamurti speak, many of whom were also interested in other forms of yoga and spirituality. Krishnamurti started an independent residential school there based on his philosophy, as well as a concert series for classical music which continues to promote his legacy into the twenty-first century.

Many teaching yoga in Britain were in some way influenced by Krishnamurti's teachings, which bridged both those popularising yoga within the structure of adult-education classes in the 1960s and the emerging youth culture of the later 1960s. Ken Thompson remembers Krishnamurti's teaching as being very significant within the Wheel of Yoga during the 1970s and '80s, particularly through the influence of Alan Babbington, the founder of the Albion

80. D. Zohar, 'What happened to the boy god?', *Sunday Times* (London), 1980.
81. T.K.V. Desikachar was the fourth child of Tirumalai Krishnamacharya and his wife, Shrimati Namagiriammal, who was the sister of B.K.S. Iyengar.

Yoga movement who taught at Mary Ward adult-education centre in Bloomsbury in the 1970s and early '80s.

Chris Tobler, who was involved in Gandalf's Garden and the Sivananda Yoga Centre, remembers hearing an early 'town hall' talk by Krishnamurti and not feeling particularly inspired: the philosophical message was quite 'hard'. 'He was breaking down, breaking down, breaking down. That was his thing was to get to the core, to get to the essence of whatever issues . . .'.[82] His impression at the time was that Krishnamurti appealed more strongly to an older generation; his parents who were members of the Study Society were very impressed that their son had met Krishnamurti. Not particularly associated with the youth culture of the period, Krishnamurti's ideas appealed to a wide variety of people throughout the twentieth century. Indeed, Krishnamurti had frequent dialogues with a number of very influential public figures and his books remain in print today.

Conclusion

By 1972 there was a huge variety of mystical and spiritual lifestyles on offer that incorporated yoga as part of their teaching. Yoga was both counter-cultural and mainstream. As yoga was popularised, it also diversified. *Alternative London* (1972) lists ten 'Hindu Oriented Groups' and eight 'Hatha Yoga' teaching centres, along with a number of pagan, Sufi, Buddhist and Islamic 'mystical' groups, noting that attendance at these centres is an 'incongruous mixture of old ladies and young freaks' (Saunders 1972: 173). Celebrity example created a popular mystique for Indian spirituality, particularly among the young looking for alternative beliefs and lifestyles to those of their parents. Postcolonial critical theorist Robert J.C. Young recalled the late 1960s London environment of his youth:

> So it was that the first real awareness of India as a country and as a culture came for many of my generation in the later 1960s when India became iconic for the counter-culture, an environment wonderfully satirized years later in Hanif Kureishi's *The Buddha of Suburbia* (1990). India for many of us at that time was fully represented by Indiacraft, a shop bristling with goods from India, which appeared opposite Selfridges on Oxford Street in London, and which became the shrine where everyone went to buy their sticks of incense, beads,

82. Personal interview with Chris Tobler (12 October 2017).

silk scarves, trying in vain to look like one of the Kinks, the Moody
Blues, or George Harrison. Indiacraft shops sprang up all over the
country during those years, and in fact there is one in Little Clarendon
Street in Oxford which still improbably lingers on from those days.
This was when I first read the *Gita*, along with Basham's *The Wonder
That Was India*, and no doubt other equally orientalist texts. I then also
first learnt about and began to see classical Indian dance and listen
to classical Indian music, the result of the fact that a friend of mine
who was learning Indian dance at the now famous Bhavan Centre
in Baron's Court encouraged me to come along to the performances
and concerts. That was the first time I met people from India (Young
2006: 3).[83]

Young's memory of this time reflects an idea of India popularised
by the musical celebrities of the period divorced from any experience of the actual country or its people. While here he dates his
growing awareness of India to the late 1960s, it might more accurately be his impression of the early '70s: the Bharatiya Vidya Bhavan opened in London in 1972. While his reflections are no doubt
greatly influenced by his later understanding of the postcolonial
position (at the time of writing this reflection, he was teaching postcolonial theory at New York University), Young's description of a
young middle-class Londoner's idea of India and Indian spirituality
during the late 1960s/early1970s is likely not too far off the mark for
many of his class and generation.

While other topics in *The New London Spy: An Intimate Guide to the
City's Pleasures*, a 1965 guidebook to London, exhibited a detailed
and rather subtle knowledge,[84] the 'Indian London' section focused
on food and stereotypes of immigrants (Davies 1966: 76). It complained that 'Most Indian restaurants in London aren't strictly
Indian at all but Pakistani, and from one small part of Pakistan
at that.' As for the culture of Indians in London, the guide rather
voyeuristically remarked that:

> Call at the North Star public house in Swiss Cottage any Saturday
> night and you'll see most of North London's au pair community

83. Young (b. 1950) currently teaches postcolonial theory from his position
of Julius Silver Professor of English and Comparative Literature at New York
University.
84. For example, in 'London Churches, Part Two' the guide explained that 'in
Roman Catholic churches, it's the ceremony that matters, not the sermon. In Non-
conformist churches, it's the other way around . . .' and discussed the subtleties of
Christian worship.

[German] with their Indian boyfriends enjoying some typically British
pub life (Davies 1966: 270).

It also noted that there was a great diversity of Indian families in
London, including Muslims, Sikhs, 'Parsees', Jews and Christians;
that most Indians were very family-oriented, did not live in specific ethnic neighbourhoods; and that they found it 'hard to make
friends with the British' (Davies 1966: 269).[85] If this 1965 description was accurate, it might explain why many young middle-class
Britons took their ideas about India from music and popular culture – rather than from direct contact with Indian people – despite
increasing immigration.

Through the Beatles and other celebrities, India became associated with an Orientalist vision of salvation. Cultural icons such as
George Harrison, Terence Stamp and Pete Townshend, as well as
a host of more minor celebrities, found salvation in Indian spirituality. Yoga, as something related to Indian spirituality, became
associated with this popular quest. Of course, Orientalist idealisation and selective borrowing from Indian religion had been the
practice of the Theosophical Society since the late nineteenth century, but mass media distribution and celebrity example created
a new level of idealised India and yoga. With these personalities
attracting national and international media attention, yoga became
more familiar. Meanwhile, the changes in consciousness that yoga's
physical techniques can promote became of interest to young people who were experimenting with drugs and alternative lifestyles.
The involvement of youth and popular culture added another layer
to the already complex perception of yoga and Indian cultural ideas
in Britain.

85. 'Unlike in India, London's Indians have not grouped together on a communal basis and are sprinkled throughout many suburbs – Swiss Cottage, Bayswater
and Kilburn [being] the more popular.'

Chapter Six

Yoga on the Telly

The expansion of the media during this period increased the accessibility of yoga and standardised its presentation. Yoga on television made it possible for viewers to attempt exercises in the privacy of the home without actively seeking out an esoteric printed manual or a teacher. In the 1970s several regular television features exposed what was still a minority interest to a much wider cross-section of the British public. Contemporary estimates suggest that the number of committed British yoga practitioners may have increased from 5,000 to 100,000 between 1967 and 1979. A much wider audience had been exposed to yoga through the mass media during the mid-twentieth century: the 1971–74 *Yoga for Health* television series alone reached an estimated audience of four million and the accompanying book sold over a million copies (see Table 6.1).[1]

The content of yoga television programmes was usually modelled roughly on the format of adult-education classes and emphasised safe stretching, relaxation and fitness with practical benefits for health. While yoga in the adult-education system had implicit governmental approval (at least at the local level), yoga on television offered an implied authority beyond that of a teacher. In Britain, the authority of the British Broadcasting Corporation (BBC) was explicit because of its educative mandate and its historical role as the 'voice of the nation' (Samuel 1998b: 172–93).

Television was a very different medium compared to an interactive adult-education class. McLuhan identified a dichotomy between 'hot' and 'cold' forms of media, a useful intuitive distinction between the different effects that a medium can have on information transmission. For McLuhan, 'hot' media, such as radio and film, are 'high definition', i.e. information-dense and involving little

1. 'Howard Kent: Obituary', *Daily Telegraphy* (London), 21 March 2005, p. 23, from Kent, 'How the Hittleman TV series was born', Lexis-Nexis Professional, http://web.lexis-nexis.com/xchange-international.

Year of estimate	Number of practitioners in Britain
1950	1,000+[a]
1967	5,000[b]
1973	50,000[c]
1975	25,000–80,000[d]
1979	100,000[e]
2000–2002	265,000[f]
2002	450,000–500,000[g]
2004– 2015	2.5 million[h]

Table 6.1 Estimates of numbers of yoga practitioners in Britain

a   From the number of students reported to have voluntarily completed a questionnaire for Desmond Dunne's School of Yogism in London in Desmond (Dunne 1951).

b   Personal estimate of Wilfred Clark in a letter to Ken Thompson, 16 March 1967.

c   Kent, 'How the Hittleman TV series was born', Lexis-Nexis Professional, pp. 20–21, http://web.lexis-nexis.com/xchange-international. The figure is based on an estimate of over 2,000 yoga classes in evening institutes in Britain with an average of twenty-six students per class. Kent also estimates in this article that over four million viewed the *Yoga for Health* television series.

d   Estimate found in the British Wheel's journal *Yoga* 24 (Summer 1975), p. 14. In this article, the British Wheel of Yoga itself claimed 1,500 members and 500 teachers.

e   Personal estimate by Georg Feuerstein, in 'Introduction', *Bulletin of the Yoga Research Centre* 1 (Summer 1979), p. 3.

f   The Kendal Project also looked at how many people were doing yoga in Kendal between 2000 and 2002; extrapolating from that small northern town, they concluded that 0.4% of the population did yoga in any given week, which would equate to about 265,000 (very roughly) doing yoga classes weekly in Britain (Heelas, Woodhead *et al.* 2005; Kendal Project, 'Methods and Findings', 2005, http://www.lancaster.ac.uk/fss/projects/ieppp/kendal/methods.htm).

g   Personal correspondence with the British Wheel of Yoga, 2002.

h   The 2.5 million figure is from a market research firm's estimates as reported in Carter (2004) and also repeated in *Yoga* magazine (2015). The Integrated Household Survey (IHS) undertaken by the Office of National Statistics (ONS) on 'well-being in the UK' in 2010/11 conflates yoga with the category of 'keep-fit' which includes 'aerobics, yoga and dance exercises'. The authors extrapolate that 7.1% of the population of England (nearly 3.8 million) are regularly doing these 'keep-fit' activities, with a similar percentage of the population likely to be participating in such activities in Northern Ireland, Wales and Scotland (Seddon 2012). The ONS's General Household Surveys between 1980 and 1993, which also lumped yoga in with keep-fit (also incorporating Laban, Margaret Morris, Medau, aerobics, and Dalcroze movement-based activities), revealed a fairly constant c. 9% of the total British population from the mid-1980s to 1993, with women up to 17% and men around the 5% mark in these activities (roughly 5 million of the total UK population).

participation in interpretation. In contrast, 'cold' media, such as television and telephone, provide comparatively limited information and leave room in the production of meaning for the audience to 'fill in' (McLuhan 2006 [1964]: 24). According to this model, yoga on television is cold, in contrast to the classroom situation, where teachers will usually interact to ensure at least a minimum of standardisation in the students' understanding. In some cases, such as with B.K.S. Iyengar, the concentration and attention to the details of physical performance demanded by the teacher left very little to the students' imagination. Yoga on television provided visual examples, but it was up to the viewer to interpret the instructions, and only limited interaction was possible to address any problems or misunderstandings. This chapter will argue that the presentation of yoga on television encouraged viewers to imagine their own meaning for the exercises. The extension of yoga instruction to this new medium led to its being understood as a physical exercise with tacit soteriological and spiritual significance.

The First Yoga on Television: Sir Paul Dukes

Sir Paul Dukes gave the first demonstration of yoga exercises on BBC television in 1948.[2] The BBC began experiments in television broadcasting in 1932, but suspended broadcasts between September 1939 and June 1946. BBC Radio's role in informing the British public of wartime developments had created an idea of the BBC as 'the voice of the nation,' an idealisation 'unquestioningly accepted by the "television service"' when it resumed in 1946 (Thumim 2004: 13). Only a single television station was broadcast from Alexandra Palace in London, until the commercial Independent Television Network began operation in 1955. Thus, in these early days especially the BBC had an authoritative role in informing and educating the public, and its programming was assumed to be for public benefit. Although in 1951 only about 5% of British households had

---

2. 'TV Talks "Yoga" 1948–1950, T32/367'. BBC Written Archives Centre, Reading. This file contains the notes: '28th May 1948 – Mr Cecil Madden – Yogi Programme: Sir Paul Dukes and Mrs Verscholyle – 9.15–9.30 pm approximately and 23.9.49, Saturday 1 October 1949 – Yoga for the Middleaged'. However, there is no further information on these first two programmes.

(black and white) television licences, television was quickly becoming more popular and accessible.[3]

The presenter of the BBC's instructional broadcasts on yoga was Sir Paul Dukes (1889–1967), the son of a Congregationalist minister who was knighted for espionage services in Russia during the Bolshevik Revolution, when Dukes most likely passed on information about the 'operational effectiveness and morale of Bolshevik naval forces in the eastern Baltic' (Hughes 2004).[4] From his youth, he showed an interest in unusual forms of spirituality and made contact with Theosophists and a Gurdjieff-like 'Prince Ozay' during his years abroad in Germany and Russia who instructed Dukes in breathing exercises and the 'vibrational' power of the Lord's Prayer when sung properly.[5] After being knighted, Dukes lectured in America where he visited the office of Yogi Ramacharaka in Chicago, to discover that the author likely had no personal knowledge of India (Dukes 1950: 121). Dukes also spent several months at Pierre Bernard's 'Country Club' in Nyack, New York where 'Hatha Yoga' techniques were taught.[6] Here in 1922 he met his first wife the wealthy socialite Margaret Vanderbilt, who was to inherit a million dollars over the next year; the marriage lasted only until 1929.[7] In 1939, Dukes returned to espionage, having been asked by the Foreign Office to investigate the disappearance of a Czechoslovakian industrialist en route from Prague to Switzerland. At this time he published his observations on the Nazi regime, emphasising its similarities to Bolshevikism (Dukes 1940).[8] It is likely that it was during

3. In 1951 there were 14.49 million households in Britain, and 764,000 television licences were issued (Office of National Statistics 2002). Between 1947 and 1957 television ownership rose from less than 1% to 48% of British households (see Gershuny and Fisher 2000: 640).

4. See also 'Mr Paul Dukes Knighted', *The Times* (London), 3 November 1920, p. 13, col. D. Dukes also wrote his memoirs of his espionage days (1938).

5. There has been an assumption that Prince Ozay was in fact the Armenian mystic Gurdjieff (c. 1866–1949). Gurdjieff's 'official' biography takes this identification as a fact (Moore 1991: 341) and it is repeated in Washington (1993: 175-6). However, Taylor (2004) offers a robust argument that Prince Ozay and Gurdjieff were different people.

6. On Pierre Bernard see Love (2010) and Urban (2001).

7. 'Sir Paul Dukes Married', *The Times* (London), 19 October 1922, p. 12, col. E; and 'Vanderbilt Estate: Legacy for Lady Dukes', *The Times* (London), 8 March 1923, p. 10, col. F. In 1959, Dukes married Diana Fitzgerald.

8. In 1947 Dukes also published a book in which he attempted to explain the breakdown of British–Russian Relations in the Second World War.

the late 1940s that Dukes began teaching physical yoga techniques in Britain. His high-profile associations would no doubt have made for a respectable and interesting host for what would have been an unusual public-interest series.

During this period most material was transmitted live – a 'once-only' performance; filmed material was expensive and 'telerecord-ing' on tape only became available in the late 1950s (Thumim 2004: 1). As such, no recordings survive of Sir Paul Duke's four-part series on yoga, which aired at 9 pm on Saturday evenings in April, May and June 1950. However, extant production paperwork provides infor-mation about the programme's intention and reception.[9] Dukes was given a time slot immediately after the 'main Saturday evening fea-ture', a position designed to maximise 'flow viewers' from the pre-vious programme.[10] Janet Thumim (2004: 3–5) has argued that the programme's design was similar to that of a print magazine where short pieces on various subjects were placed together. According to the promotional listing for the show:

> Yoga does not aim to make people live forever, but to keep the temple of the body as a worthy holder of the spirit. Throughout the series of four programmes, Sir Paul will show how the principles of Eastern yoga can be applied to Westerners.[11]

This implies the presence of both spiritual and demystifying ele-ments: yoga apparently had something to do with an undefined 'spirit', but also was suitable for 'Westerners'. The titles empha-sised the practicality of yoga for certain categories of British people: 1. 'What Yoga Is', 2. 'Yoga for the Office Worker', 3. 'Yoga for the Housewife', and 4. 'Yoga for Britain Today'. The authoritative voice of the BBC would have implied to the audience the public benefit of exploring yoga. While some of the audience were interested in an explanation of how yoga related to the 'spirit' and other meta-physical issues, it appears that Dukes mainly focused on physical

9. 'TV Talks "Yoga" 1948–1950, T32/367. BBC Written Archives Centre, Read-ing. This file contains the notes: 'For SE Reynolds 23.9.49, Saturday 1 October 1949 – Yoga for the Middleaged' and '28th May 1948 – Mr Cecil Madden – Yogi Pro-gramme: Sir Paul Dukes and Mrs Verscholyle – 9.15–9.30 pm approximately'.

10. 'View Research Report Week 22', in 'TV Talks "Yoga" 1948–1950, T32/367'. For 'flow viewing', see Williams (2003 [1974]: 94).

11. Yoga (22 April) BBC press schedule in 'TV Talks "Yoga" 1948–1950, T32/367'.

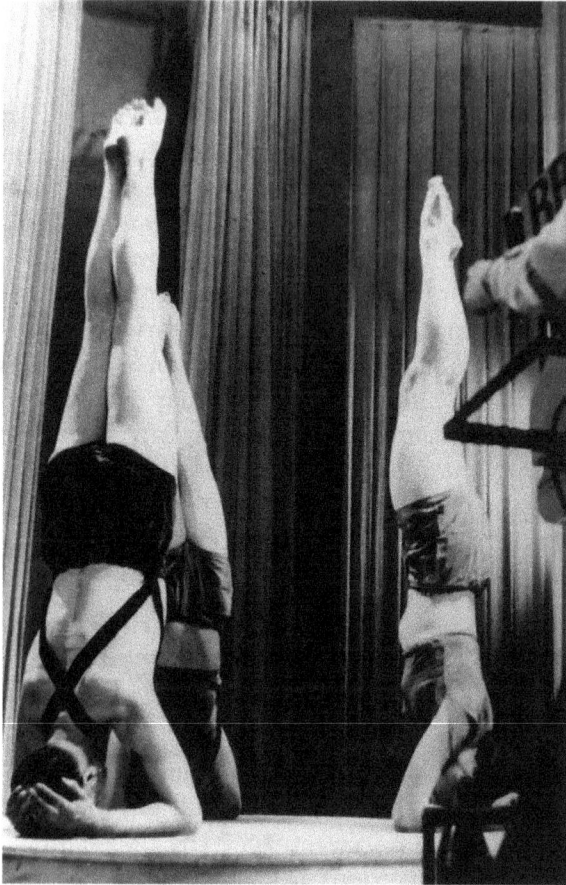

Fig. 6.1 Still from one of Sir Paul Dukes's BBC appearances in 1949. Sir Paul Dukes papers, Box 4, Hoover Institution Archives.

exercises.[12] Shortly after his television appearance, Dukes published his autobiography, *The Unending Quest* (1950), which recounted his personal journey for spiritual fulfilment without specifying yoga techniques.

He was assisted in the television programmes by Russian ballerina Nadine Nicolaeva-Legat and two of her young pupils, 'Beth

12. 'Many letters ask for further and more precise breathing exercises of which very few were demonstrated' and 'Comment on the series as a whole further suggested that a number of viewers gave each demonstration a trial, in the hope that eventually some explanation would be given on the doctrinal aspects of Yoga. Hence there was considerable disappointment that little or no reference was made in the programme to the ideology of the Yoga cult, and many viewers were of the opinion that as, in their own words, "the series consisted mainly of repetitive physical exercises, the whole system could easily have been explained in one demonstration".' 'TV Talks "Yoga" 1948–1950, T32/367.

and Pamela'. He most likely had connections to Nicolaeva-Legat from his time in Petrograd before the Bolshevik Revolution. Nicolaeva-Legat's husband Nicolai Legat (1869–1937) had been Ballet Master and Principal Choreographer at the Imperial Ballet of St Petersburg, before emigrating to England in the 1920s. Legat established high-profile ballet schools in Britain during the 1930s, which his wife continued running after his death.[13] These professional ballerinas' high level of fitness may have been somewhat at odds with a presentation of yoga for the general British public. The programmes received 'about 1,000 letters' the majority of which asked for further instruction and made inquiries about books. One segment of viewers appeared to enjoy the programmes 'if only as a graceful and entreating spectacle'. About a third of the 1950 audience were convinced that 'principles of muscle control, as demonstrated by "Sir Paul," were sound and valuable as the basis for a health-giving cult'. While some viewers had followed the exercises 'with considerable benefit' since the first television demonstration, the total audience numbers declined over the course of the series.[14]

However, this minority interest was not strong enough to deny Dukes's series some of the lowest audience reaction ratings for a 'television talk' programme.[15] The reports noted that, while Dukes appealed to some, 'rather more thought he appeared too self-satisfied and several even accused him of talking down to his audience'.[16] Dukes also upset the BBC production team: Dukes's two references in the first episode to Madame Nicolaeva-Legat's ballet school were perceived as promotional, and putting his arm around her young students' waists did not meet with approval.[17] Both the supposedly inappropriate behaviour and the gratuitous promotion

13. The Legat school during the 1930s was a competitor to the Dame Ninette de Valois's Sadler's Wells Ballet School which moved into the Royal Opera House in 1946 and received a royal charter in 1956.

14. 'Paul Dukes: Analysis of Correspondence Re: Yoga', 'TV Talks "Yoga" 1948–1950, T32/367'.

15. The 'Audience Reaction Index' was an idiosyncratic tool the BBC used to compare audience approval among programmes. For more on BBC audience research, see Thumim (2004: 29–30).

16. 'Paul Dukes: Analysis of Correspondence Re: Yoga', in 'TV Talks "Yoga" 1948–1950, T32/367'.

17. Memo, Norman Collins to H. Tel. T, 4 April 1950, in 'TV Talks "Yoga" 1948–1950, T32/367'. 'In particular if Dukes is supported by young ladies please ensure that he does not put his arms around them when talking as this friendly gesture is liable to be misinterpreted by viewers.'

ran counter to the BBC's public service mission.[18] On the heels of such controversial behaviour, the producer of the series reported in an internal BBC memo that 'after the last of the current series we can afford to give Yoga a good long rest'.[19]

Dukes himself, however, did not give yoga a 'good long rest' but continued to make it a focus of his life. He spent a few years in South Africa just after his BBC appearance. Stella Cherfas, who ran a successful yoga studio in London in the late 1960s and early 1970s, remembers taking her first class yoga class with Dukes in Johannesburg before her son was born around 1951. Previous to her interest in yoga she was athletic and also interested in Grantly Dick-Read's methods of natural childbirth. When she was in her late twenties, out of curiosity she attended a talk on yoga by Dukes, and followed it by attending the class he mentioned during the talk. She came back for more classes:

> ... slowly I got not so much the postures but the whole philosophy of it. As you saw, using every single part, dividing the class into *pranayama* breath, which is so important – it's the first thing you take in and the last thing you relinquish in your life and that's paramount. Moving the body and the glands and the joints. And the total [whole body] – we started as relaxation but it is now visualization.[20]

According to Cherfas, a yoga class should be structured into three main sections: pranayama (breathing exercises), bringing movement and awareness to every part of the body, and closing with a relaxation or visualisation exercise. Now with two young children, Cherfas taught a few classes in Johannesburg in the 1950s. According to Cherfas, Dukes spent some years teaching regularly in South Africa, with Diana Fitzgerald, a dancer who would become his wife

18. Memo from senior producer Mary Adams to series producer S.E. Reynolds: 'These projected programs on Yoga were to be absolutely straight-forward demonstrations with simple explanations from Sir Paul on the theory and practice of Yoga. I was very much disturbed to find that his first program on Saturday did not carry out these instructions. Sir Paul's manner was coy and frequently facetious, and the demonstration became a variety turn ... I feel so strongly on this matter that unless Sir Paul is prepared to revise the presentation entirely, and take the fullest instructions from you, we shall have to consider taking off the last two programmes in the series.' 'TV Talks "Yoga" 1948–1950, T32/367'.

19. Memo from S.E. Reynolds to H. Tel. T, 3 April 1950, in 'TV Talks "Yoga" 1948–1950, T32/367'.

20. Personal Interview with Stella Cherfas (17 January 2013).

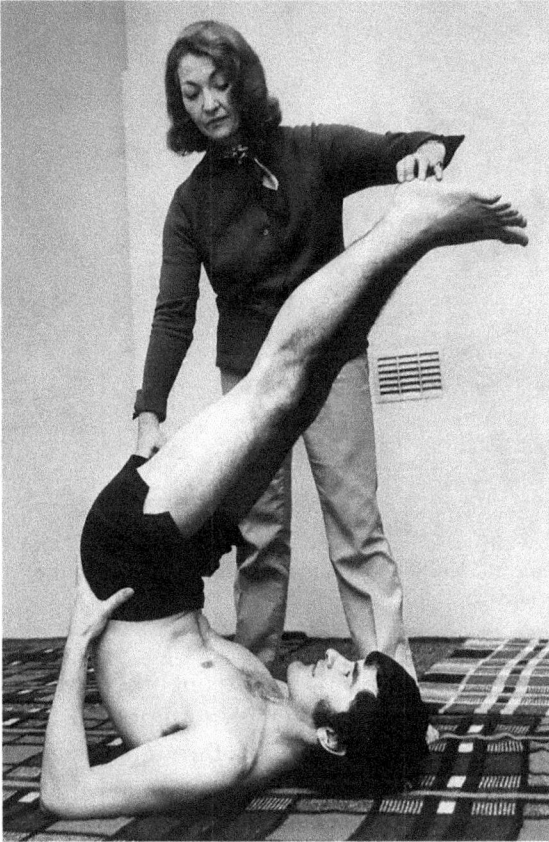

Fig. 6.2 Stella Cherfas teaching cricket player Alan Knott (early 1970s). Image courtesy of Stella Cherfas. Used with permission.

in 1959.[21] Dukes never discussed with Cherfas how he learned yoga, his experiences in Russia or those in Nyack.

As her children grew older, in 1962 Cherfas and her husband decided to emigrate to London. She remembers being at a hair salon in Hampstead where a young man was complaining of anxiety so she invited him for a private yoga class; he was amazed at the effects. Through personal networks, Cherfas began teaching. A student found a property for her studio in Westbourne Grove. A few years later, one of her students helped to secure her a lease to teach out of a more central property in Manchester Square, W1, which she called the 'The Yoga Studio'.[22] This was perhaps the first British

---

21. Personal Interview with John Roycroft (17 January 2013).

22. *Alternative London* (Saunders 1972: 184) described the centre as follows: 'Classes are held every day except Monday – mornings, afternoons and evenings. Lessons last for one hour, and must be booked in advanced at 4 for £3.50. They do

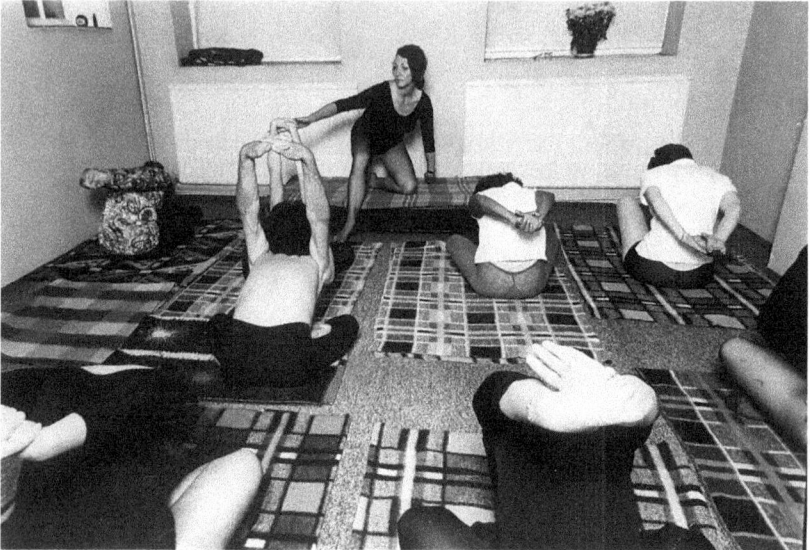

Fig. 6.3 Stella Cherfas teaching at Manchester Square (early 1970s). Image courtesy of Stella Cherfas. Used with permission.

venue to go by the name of 'yoga studio'; it frequently appeared in mainstream media in the 1960s and '70s with a number of those who taught yoga during this period walking through its doors. So, through Cherfas's teaching, Sir Paul Dukes continued to have an influence on the shape of yoga in Britain long after his death in 1967.[23]

Yoga on ITV: Yoga for Health

The next attempt at televising yoga classes was in 1971 – a very 'long rest' indeed, and long after yoga had been established in adult-education classes and music celebrities had gone on their 'Orientalist' journeys.[24] This time it was ITV, who had spotted the success of

not involve meditation or chanting – it's exercise for health and relaxation – though the teachers may come from various ashrams.' Cherfas, when interviewed in 2017, maintained that there were not teachers 'from various ashrams' and that the only teachers were herself and her close associate Jack London.

23. Cherfas left London in the late 1970s, teaching yoga in Vienna before returning to London in the early 1990s. At the time of writing she continues to teach weekly yoga classes in the Covent Garden area.

24. There were occasional references to yoga on BBC and ITV before 1971; for example, Iyengar appeared on BBC television in a special feature, 'Menuhin and

Richard Hittleman's syndicated programme in the United States.[25] Like the BBC's presentation of yoga as public health, Hittleman's form of yoga was a 'sensible program for physical fitness on a national scale' in the United States (Hittleman 1964: 7–9). Hittleman (1927–1991) reported that he had learned yoga from 'his parents' Hindu maintenance man at a getaway called Utopia in the Catskills' (a mountain range in upstate New York) (Mills 1995). However, Hittleman was not far from Pierre Bernard's Nyack Country Club, so it is also possible that he had contact with yoga through members of this group, or other teachers in New York City.[26] Hittleman reported that he founded his own yoga school in Florida in 1957 and produced his first successful half-hour television series in the United States in 1961.

Hittleman's programme hit New York City's television schedules in 1966,[27] aired on weekdays at 9.30 am with an audience that would have largely comprised women at home, perhaps having returned from the school run; it was scheduled opposite a popular exercise programme on a rival channel. The format was clearly positioning yoga as physical fitness for women but it also implied that it might offer something more: its listing promised that Hittleman would demonstrate how one might activate 'the great vital forces of the body and mind which become lazy and dormant if not correctly stimulated'.[28] This formulation is similar to New Thought, a philosophical and spiritual movement that developed out of the work of American Phineas Parkhurst Quimby (1802–1866), which had a significant influence in nineteenth-century USA and on the yoga books of Yogi Ramacharaka (Albanese 2007; Jackson 1975, 1981; Melton

his Guru', being interviewed by David Attenborough in 1966. BBC Written Archive Centre. Dukes's yoga teaching is also recorded in his books (1953, 1960).

25. The importation of the Hittleman series can be seen as part of a long and well-established American influence on British fashions and trends (see McKibbin 1998; Marwick 2000: xviii).

26. I have not found an autobiographical explanation as to why Hittleman practised yoga. Shri Yogendra (born Manibhai Haribhai Desai and also known as 'Mastanami') (1897–1989) taught yoga in Harrison, New York and Long Island around 1920–24. Hittleman's books always focus on a practical, demystified, physical fitness practice and it is likely that Hittleman found he was able to earn a living from the mid-1950s by teaching yoga in this manner.

27. 'Yoga Show Entered in Health Race', *New York Times*, 10 January 1966, p. 45.

28. Ibid. Christian Science grew out of this movement, although it is now considered distinct (see Singleton 2007b: 64–84; Satter 1999; Melton 1992: 15–29).

1992; Satter 1999).[29] New Thought is not a strict belief system, but rather a position of personal exploration in relationship to an interconnected reality. While there is no formal theology that New Thought groups share, they are united in an emphasis on positive thinking, affirmations, meditation and prayer.[30] By 1970, the pilot had been syndicated as a series on over forty television networks in the United States.[31] Hittleman's first book *Be Young With Yoga* was published in the United States in 1962 and his books continued to remain in print until the end of the 1980s.

The idea of making a British series under the same principle as Hittleman's was one of many business possibilities explored by producer Howard Kent (1919–2005) on a 1967 business trip to New York.[32] Kent was familiar with yoga having read works by Mahatma Gandhi some thirty years previously. After a contact suggested producing a Hittleman-type series in Britain, Kent brought back some of Hittleman's 'practice-along-with' records and found that his whole family enjoyed the exercise.[33] It was decided to make the programme from scratch using the new colour technology. Richard Hittleman was not the automatic choice, but unable to find a more suitable instructor they flew Hittleman to England in summer 1970. He brought with him a regular student, an attractive and thin blonde woman named Cheryl. It was decided that a second model, with no previous experience with yoga, was to be chosen in England. As Kent explained, 'It was necessary to demonstrate the progress which can be made by any reasonably fit person . . . everyone can have a shot at this and feel the benefit.'[34] Lyn Marshall was selected, although her background as a model and ballerina hardly qualified her as average.[35]

29. For the identity of Yogi Ramacharaka, see footnote 13 on page 48.

30. For more on New Thought's relationship to the development of a modern yoga, see Singleton (2007b).

31. H. Kent, 'Yoga for Health: A Breakthrough Television Programme', *Yoga & Health* 1 (1971), p. 17.

32. H. Kent, 'Elliseva Sayers: Where are you now?', [unknown journal] 6, pp. 18–19, in Yoga for Health Foundation newspaper clippings collection.

33. Ibid.

34. H. Kent, 'Yoga for Health: A Breakthrough Television Programme', *Yoga & Health* 1 (1971), p. 17.

35. J. Still, 'Obituary: Lyn Marshall', *The Independent* (London), 9 May 1992. Lyn Marshall also ran her own yoga centre off Baker Street in London in the 1970s. See C. Nash, 'Lyn's New Yoga Studio', *Yoga & Health* 2/10 (1972), pp. 24–25, 43.

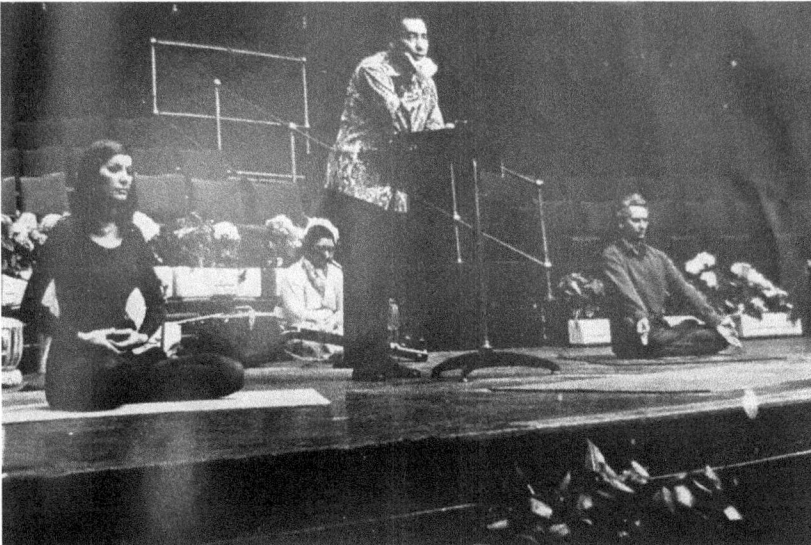

Fig. 6.4 Richard Hittleman's Royal Albert Hall appearance on 8 July 1972. Lyn Marshall is on Hittleman's left and Alan Babbington on the right. *Yoga & Health* 2/8 (October 1972), p. 3.

Yoga for Health ran on ITV between 1971 and 1974 and reached an estimated audience of four million.[36] Television programming in the early 1970s was not continuous and there were often short gaps in the schedule. Initially, *Yoga for Health* was screened for twenty minutes at around 3.45 pm on Wednesday and Friday. Its exact broadcast time varied but it appeared to be part of a 'tea time' programme that included children's cartoons.[37] The initial series would have encouraged 'flow' viewing, primarily by mothers at home. After its original run it was also screened on a number of regional stations. Unfortunately, the original series does not appear to have been preserved but to accompany the series Kent also produced practice books and a glossy magazine entitled *Yoga & Health*. Building on the success of yoga in LEA contexts and celebrity associations with India, the television series *Yoga for Health* offered new visual associations and exposure to yoga in the privacy of one's own home.

36. 'Howard Kent: Obituary', *Daily Telegraph* (London), 21 March 2005, p. 23.
37. British Universities Film & Video Council, TVTimes Project 1955–1985, listings for April and May 1971, http://tvtip.bufvc.ac.uk, accessed 7 May 2007.

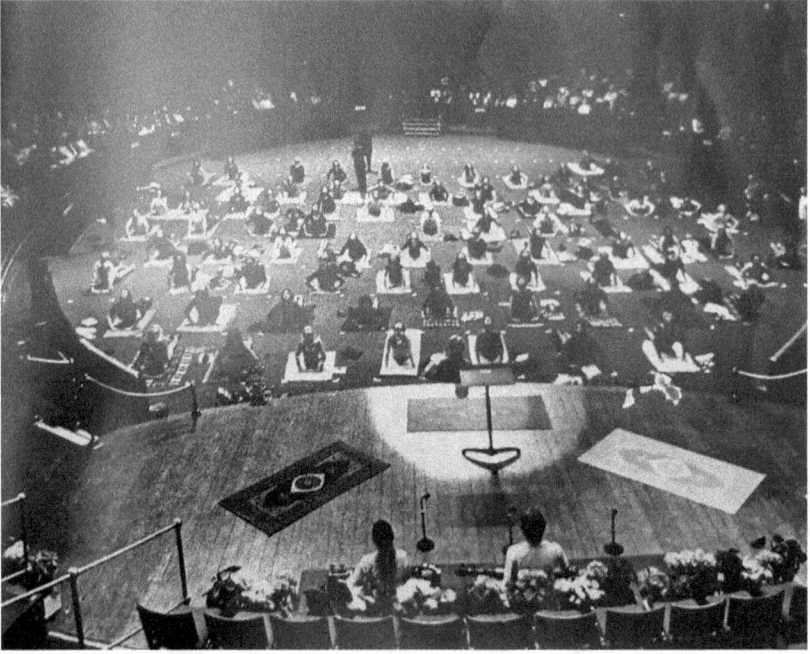

Fig. 6.5 View from the stage at Ronald Hittleman's Royal Albert Hall appearance on 8 July 1972. *Yoga & Health* 2/8 (October 1972), p. 3.

Yoga & Health ran from 1971 to 1975,[38] regularly referring to Hittleman's television series and highlighting minor celebrities practising yoga. In the opening issue, editor Joyce Finch wrote:

> Yoga is for health, relaxation and poise; for anyone to develop the best in themselves in their own particular way. Yoga is a key to prolonged youthfulness and to the power of the mind. It is a way of living and it costs you nothing more than a little time each day. Yoga is not asceticism.[39]

The idea that 'yoga is not asceticism' was a key aspect of Indian spirituality as popularised by the Beatles. Yoga was presented as an activity that did not require renunciation from sensual pleasure,

38. *Yoga & Health* ceased in 1975 and another national magazine, *Yoga Today*, began in 1976. Howard Kent ran the magazine *Yoga for Health* as part of his Yoga For Health Clubs from 1975–77. *Yoga Today* was renamed *Yoga and Health* around 1990. The Library of Congress Catalogue has the national US magazine *Yoga Journal* beginning its run in 1975 and has no serials with 'yoga' in the title before this date.

39. H. Kent, 'Yoga for Health: A Breakthrough Television Programme', *Yoga & Health* 1 (1971), p. 17.

but still promised to effortlessly promote improved self-control and physical fitness. Although Richard Hittleman's exercises featured in nearly every issue, the magazine promoted a wide variety of yoga teachers including J. Krishnamurti, Yogi Bhajan, Ram Dass (Richard Alpert), Sri Chinmoy, Swami Vishnudevananda, B.K.S. Iyengar, etc. Howard Kent and *Yoga & Health* magazine also sponsored (with Inter Capital Travellers) one of the first British yoga holidays to Yugoslavia in 1972, which cost £65 for the 35 participants and was led by yoga teacher Ernest Coates.[40]

The *Yoga for Health* phenomenon successfully repackaged yoga as a public health activity in the commercial sphere and featured many endorsements by minor British celebrities. The *Yoga & Health* magazine offered a monthly step-by-step course of asana with television actress Janet Waldron under the title 'Yoga with Jan'. The actress was reported to have had a 'genuine interest in yoga' because of a 'genuine problem due to a trip abroad'.[41] A US television actress, Celia Kaye, testified in the pages of *Yoga & Health to* how yoga is 'something you can look forward to', having discovered it while working in London.[42] More famous celebrities, such as Miriam Karlin, who appeared in *The Entertainer* (1960) and *A Clockwork Orange* (1971), testified that after two years of yoga classes she had stopped taking pills for sleep and anxiety and her self-confidence and fitness was 'much improved'.[43] Celebrity testimonials were commonly paired with letters from and interviews with 'ordinary' people who reported benefits of yoga in terms of fitness, health, confidence and mental stability. The implication was that if Hittleman's yoga was so successful for these glamorous women, it could work for the ordinary housewife or office worker.

Yoga with Lyn Marshall

The *Yoga for Health* television series with Richard Hittleman ran until September 1975 at which point Hittleman's British model Lyn Marshall (1954–1992) took over with her own ITV series, *Wake Up*

40. 'Yoga Holiday: Special Report', *Yoga & Health* 2/11 (1973), p. 7.
41. *Yoga & Health* 1 (1971), p. 31. The exact problem was never mentioned.
42. *Yoga & Health* 2 (1971), p. 38.
43. 'Interview with Miriam Karlin', *Yoga & Health* 1 (1971), p. 9.

with Yoga, at 11 am on Sundays.[44] In 1976, it moved to 9.30 am the
same day and was renamed *Keep Up with Yoga*, under which banner it continued through 1977.[45] These series were also followed up
with their own books featuring Marshall demonstrating simple and
practical routines of yoga postures: *Wake Up to Yoga* (1975), *Lyn Marshall's Keep Up with Yoga* (1976),.*Lyn Marshall's Yoga for Your Children*
(1978). From 1983, Marshall took her yoga to the BBC with a series
entitled *Everyday Yoga*.[46]

Wearing her signature unicoloured leotard, Marshall focused
on one posture in each episode: in an episode recorded in April
1976 she demonstrated 'the fish movement'; a transcription of her
instructions illustrates the style:

> The fish movement arches the spine upwards to make it more supple.
> At home, if you are ready, we are going to begin by lying into the
> corpse, the total relaxation position. So, slowly, there is no hurry, lie
> back down – legs and feet together. And let's relax by letting the toes
> fall open. And let the hands rest on the backs of the hands and let
> the fingers curl. Now close your eyes. Now, ideally, if you know the
> movement, you keep your eyes closed . . .
>
> All right, let's begin. Bring the legs and the feet together. First
> straighten your elbows and make fists of your hands. Push with the
> elbows, push with the hands. And push up. Don't try to come up as
> far as I am. Just go to your own limit and stay there. And now we
> are going to hold for a count of five. One . . . two . . . three . . . four
> . . . five. You can still hear me. And now, slowly, let your head slide
> back. Don't rush. Just let the back sink down very gently. Now when
> you feel your back on the floor, just relax. Let your feet relax. Let your
> hands relax. Now sit up slowly.[47]

44. Lyn Marshall died at the age of 38 of: 'I a. subarachnoid haemorrhage and
b. ruptured artery aneurysm (stroke) and was certified dead on arrival at the University Hospital Nottingham. Her maiden name was reported as Wallis, occupation
as secretary, wife of Kenneth Michael Marshall, Legal Executive.' GRO Death Certificate for Marshall, Lyn QBDX 803775, Nottingham, Nottinghamshire, November
1992, Vol. 8, 958, entry no. 114.

45. TVTiP database of London TVTimes 1955–1985, digitalised by Bournemouth
University.

46. The series was produced by Peter Ramsden and accompanied by a book
(Marshall 1982). Episodes of the series have been preserved by the British Film and
Television Archive.

47. *Keep Up with Yoga*, episode 1. ITV production 3971, recorded 5 April 1976,
aired 5 September 1977. British Film Institute Archive.

While Marshall explored a variety of asanas on her programme, she always presented the same instructions about relaxing, breathing into the pose, only going to your own limit, holding gently for a count of five, gently relaxing out of the position and finally completely relaxing in the corpse position.

In every episode, Marshall would read letters from her viewers and invite a few of the correspondents onto the show for personal tuition. Those who appeared on screen were very ordinary-looking, emphasising the appeal to the general public. The gentleness of Marshall's approach was also appreciated by many of the television audience. A mother and son appeared on screen for help with a 'standing side bend'. The mother had not practised yoga before seeing the show, and remarked,

> I have always been very anti-exercise in the past. I always felt agonised for days after doing normal exercise. But this is so gentle: I feel if you were eighty you could do this and not suffer any adverse effects. And I feel really marvellous![48]

The teenaged son (perhaps just happy to be on television) eagerly agreed with his middle-aged mother. Simple physical exercises for health, fitness and beauty, with celebrity endorsement, clearly had popular appeal.

Marshall's popularity continued, evidenced by her continual presence on televised yoga programmes until her last programme, *Everyday Yoga*, on the BBC in 1983. In the accompanying book, she described her 'special style of yoga' in more detail:

> ... as you go slowly through each movement, your mind is totally concentrated and absorbed in what you are feeling and doing and whether your mind likes it or not, all other thoughts and preoccupations are simply forced out ... you are completely indulging in yourself and your sensations and feeling wonderful. At the end of the movement, you feel not only physically good and relaxed but mentally at peace as well (Marshall 1982: 11).

This popular approach is more in line with what Heelas and Woodhead (2005) have described as a 'subjective-self' style of spirituality, except that Marshall did not pressure her viewers to do yoga for a spiritual purpose. She wrote that:

---

48. *Keep Up with Yoga*, episode 3. ITV production 3973, recorded 3 May 1976, aired 19 September 1977. British Film Institute Archive.

> My main concern is that as many people as possible simply *use* this
> way of moving their body to improve their lives right now – today!' . . .

> There are many people who after being introduced to Hatha or phys-
> ical yoga, do wish to get involved with the philosophy, but in my
> experience, very many more don't. They simply enjoy what they get
> out of their practice and the benefit they feel in their lives as a result,
> and don't want to take it any further. The choice therefore is yours
> (Marshall 1982: 13; emphasis original).

At the end of the *Everyday Yoga* book, Marshall listed 'common
conditions and ailments helped by yoga' and suggested specific
postures for these problems as well as general routines for twenty,
thirty and forty minutes. However, she made a point of deferring to
biomedical expertise:

> Although it is clear that Yoga improves your health and can be
> extremely therapeutic when used for many conditions, **it must never
> be used as a substitute for medical treatment.** If you are suffering
> from an illness or have a history of serious illness you must check
> with your own doctor before commencing the routine. He knows
> your personal medical history and therefore is qualified to tell you
> whether you can safely undertake these movements (Marshall 1982:
> 19; emphasis original).

By deferring to the doctor, Marshall presented yoga as a self-help
complement to medical treatment which did not undermine but
rather reinforced medical authority. Marshall's yoga was primarily
a means of allowing responsible individuals to better care for their
mental and physical health.

Pebble Mill at One: Yoga on the BBC Television Magazine

The success of Hittleman's ITV programme spurred the BBC to
recommence presentation of yoga. Initially, instruction in yoga
exercises were a regular feature of *Pebble Mill at One*, a Birming-
ham-based lunchtime television talk show,[49] broadcast between
1973 and 1986, which included current affairs, discussions, interviews and guests who demonstrated crafts, dancing and singing.
It was a manifestation of the BBC's continuing charter to educate,
inform and entertain its audience, and it carried the authority of a
light news and general interest magazine. As a lunchtime broadcast,

49. 'Yoga for All', R43/1,650/2, BBC Written Archive Centre.

it too targeted women at home during the day. While yoga on this programme was evidently a response to the success of the Hittleman series, there appears to have been regular, friendly correspondence between Lyn Marshall and both the BBC and the Pebble Mill programme instructors.[50] However, the instructors chosen were Hazel and Frank Wills who lived within commuting distance of Birmingham.[51] While the broadcast footage was not recorded, the BBC did produce a small paperback book to accompany the series entitled *Yoga for All*, which featured the postures and pranayama, but also tried to present yoga as a path to peace and serenity. It appears that yoga was a hit with the 1970s *Pebble Mill at One* audience; *Yoga for All*, a thin paperback volume with a sale price of 65p, exhausted its print run of 17,500 copies between 1973 and 1978.[52]

By using the photographic technique of solarisation, where the dark and light areas of a black-and-white photograph are reversed, *Yoga for All* attempted to bring some youth culture tropes into its visual aesthetic while being aimed at middle-class women. The book intended to:

> cover some of the background common to all forms of Yoga, but deal mainly with two forms – Hatha yoga and Pranayama Yoga. Each chapter contains an introduction to one aspect, with a number of 'asanas' or postures which relate to that aspect. Each posture is fully illustrated with photographs.[53]

Although the silver-toned images were illustrations for asana practice, much of *Yoga for All*'s text covered the need to address the stresses of 'alienation' and 'disharmony between mind and body, between our inner self and the person others see' which was common to both housewives and the youth of the counter-culture (Wills

50. 'I was surprised to hear from Tony that you have been ill (as I thought yogis never were.) I hope you are fully recovered now though, and that I'll see you for a natter next time you are in London.' Lyn to Hazel, 16 January 1973, 'Yoga for All', R43/1,650/2, BBC Written Archive Centre.

51. 'Yoga for All', R43/1,650/2, BBC Written Archive Centre. Mrs Hazel Wills lived in Grinshill, near Shrewsbury.

52. 'Further to my memo of 30th November 1973, will you please arrange to reduce the reprint of Yoga for All from 10,000 to 7,500 copies at 65p. This will make the revised total print order to date 17,500 copies. J. M Hore.' 'Replied 28 November 1978 – John Hore – Yoga for All. Now out of print. No more copy available.' Memo dated 1 February 1974, 'Yoga for All', R43/1,650/2, BBC Written Archive Centre:

53. Memo dated 18 September 1973, 'Yoga for All', R43/1,650/2, BBC Written Archive Centre.

and Wills 1974: 9). Frank Wills, who was a sociologist, was probably responsible for the use of the term 'alienation', against which there are footnotes about its technical use in the discipline of sociology. While the author admits that 'there is nothing new in this . . . but the conditions of modern life, the pace of change, make many people feel left out altogether' (Wills and Wills 1974).[54] Here yoga is being presented as a way to address all sorts of problems related to stress, materialism and emotional imbalance. Rather than being strictly associated with Indian religion, Wills writes, 'hatha yoga is an excellent base' for all religious and spiritual teachings. The back of the book gives contact details for those who want to learn the Maharishi's Transcendental Meditation technique as well as for the Beshara Centre in Gloucestershire, which is described as a ' "school without lessons, life itself being the lesson" based on communal living and Sufi meditation techniques' (Wills and Wills 1974: 63). In this way, the BBC promoted yoga as part of a greater idea of mind–body harmony and as an appropriate public service for a happier, healthier populace. But no specific religious ideology was included in the public service of asana instruction.

It is likely that Hazel and Frank Wills had learned yoga from Dr Gopal Singh Puri (1915–1995) and his wife Kailash (1926–2017), a couple who were both born in the Punjab but settled in Liverpool around 1968 (Nesbitt with Parry 1996: 2).[55] Dr Puri lectured in biological sciences at Liverpool Polytechnic's College of Technology and his wife became a well-known 'agony aunt' offering advice to women in the Punjabi language (Puri and Nesbitt 2013).[56] The couple taught yoga from their large home three times a week, for about twenty years (Puri and Nesbitt 2013: 117). Kailash Puri explained that they began teaching soon after the Beatles had returned from Rishikesh and recalled that 'when they came back, yoga centres and yoga classes mushroomed like anything . . . everyone who knew

54. 'Hazel Wills has a degree in physiology and education and has taught in remedial education for the last seven years. Her husband was a sociologist working for a child guidance clinic.' 'Yoga for All', BBC Written Archive Centre.

55. In a short autobiographical piece in *Wake Up to Yoga*, Lyn Marshall reported that she had studied yoga with an 'Indian doctor' who had been interested in the subject for fifteen years. It is possible that this refers to Dr Puri.

56. Also personal interview with Kailash Puri (25 May 2007). Also a novelist and 'sexologist', she was editor of the Indian women's magazine *Roopvati*, where she wrote on health, beauty, relationships and cookery. She also advised Marks & Spencer about introducing Indian food to their range in the 1970s.

even a little bit would open centres'.[57] Kailash was not clear about where her husband learned yoga: 'I was sixteen when I got married. I had no idea. I had never been to university or college and everything I learnt from my husband.'[58] Her husband encouraged her to teach asana, *śavāsana* and pranayama while he in his spare time gave philosophical lectures and made Ayurvedic (traditional Indian medicine) herbal prescriptions. He saw yoga and relaxation as an extension of his interest in ecology: 'For him a sound ecological balance was inseparable from harmony within the human psyche and between individuals and groups.'[59] He was asked to give talks on yoga and relaxation in Grimsby and Glasgow, and, at first, Kailash accompanied him giving demonstrations on health foods and cooking with vegetables.

The couple were also inspired by a meeting with the Indian High Commissioner to Britain (1969–72), Apa Pant (1912–1992). Pant was the son of Bhawanrao Pant Pratinidhi, the Raja of Aundh, who had done much to popularise the modern practice of *sūrya namaskār* (popularly known as sun salutations) in the first half of the twentieth century. The Puris attended a Day of Yoga and Relaxation that Apa Pant had organised in Crosby in 1971 (Puri and Nesbitt 2013: 116). Kailash remembers Pant remarking that 'This [yoga] is the best and subtlest way of Indianising the British' (Puri and Nesbitt 2013: 116). During his time as High Commissioner, Pant was proactive in promoting yoga through the British Wheel of Yoga and through his diplomatic profile.

Following this inspirational encounter, Kailash remembers the students who came to their home to learn yoga as having comprised a high proportion of middle-class professionals. According to Dr Puri's handbook on yoga, he viewed his work on yoga as 'experimental discourses' which had shown 'great success' (Puri 1974: 1), and promoted the natural benefits of relaxation for mental and physical health. The Puris gave many demonstrations and lectures on yoga in Liverpool and across Britain (Puri 1974: 22). While the Puris were observant Sikhs, they did not present their religious beliefs as part of yoga. In later life, Kailash Puri reflected:

57. Personal interview with Kailash Puri (25 May 2007).
58. Ibid. and Puri and Nesbitt (2013). According to her report, Puri never undertook any project without her husband's encouragement.
59. Personal interview with Kailash Puri (25 May 2007).

> Sikhs will object that here is no place in our religion for yoga. Didn't
> Guru Nanak refute the yogis of his day? Fanatics denounce any Sikh
> who dabbles in yoga, or worse still, teaches it, as Yogi Bhajan (alias
> Harbhajan Singh Yogi, also a Puri) did so conspicuously in America as
> the founder of Sikh Dharma of the Western Hemisphere. To these crit-
> ical coreligionists I say 'Whatever brings true peace of mind is good. I
> am a devout believer in Guru Nanak and the Guru Granth Sahib from
> which I read daily. Through my faith will come my salvation, but my
> faith is not restricted to a narrow path.' Gopal and I both practiced this
> and learned a great deal both from Guru Granth Sahib and from yoga,
> the science of relaxation (Puri and Nesbitt 2013: 117).

Indeed, an appeal to pragmaticism, kindness and moderation was
a hallmark of all of Kailash Puri's interventions in her work as an
author and educator as well as in teaching yoga. The BBC book *Yoga
for All* was dedicated to Dr and Mrs. Puri and was written in the
same spirit of balanced health promotion.

Every Body Knows: Yoga Demystified

In 1975, the BBC broadcast a second series featuring yoga which
highlighted themes of mental and physical health. In ten episodes,
Every Body Knows was transmitted on BBC1 on Thursdays at 11
pm between 13 January and 24 March.[60] It was categorised as 'further education television' and continued the pattern of yoga as a
public health message. However, the late-night time slot targeted
adults only, perhaps in recognition of something more experimental in the programme. The first half examined 'a different approach
to reducing stress and tension': for example, two episodes examined the Alexander Technique; others discussed karate, 'retreats',
meditation techniques, Zen Buddhism and the 'philosophy of the
I Ching'.[61] The second half of each episode comprised 'elementary
yoga classes taken by Arthur Balaskas together with a small group
of pupils'.[62] The weekly yoga sessions offered a continuity between
these different possibilities for increasing mind–body awareness
and reducing stress.

---

60. David McGowan, BBC Written Archives Manager, personal correspondence
(25 January 2007).
    61. 'Programme Content', in 'Everybody knows (keep calm)', 1974–75, Gen
Pubs Edit, BBC Written Archives Centre.
    62. Ibid.

Only the first episode of *Every Body Knows* has been preserved.[63] It opens with the lines:

> Everybody knows that every body experiences tension and stress in their everyday life. This programme is about the roots and causes of stress. And, while some tension is needed, we hope to point out some simple and effective ways of minimising unnecessary tension and stress in our everyday life.[64]

After this introduction, lights fade into an image of a naked baby spotlighted on a stage. A voice-over explains:

> When we enter the world we are at one with our body and our senses. We are direct with our communication of our wants and needs. We are whole beings . . . As we grow up, we appear to lose the simplicity and directness of early childhood. As our mental attitudes harden, our bodies too become less flexible. Our heads, because they carry our brains, for many become the most important part of our bodies . . .[65]

The introductory programme went on to explain how stress causes the body discomfort, anxiety, muscular tension and illness. The narrator compared the human body to a machine and explained that, unfortunately, the 'manufacturers do not provide a handbook'. So the programme offered itself as a kind of handbook, dealing with stress and how to manage the body responsibly, as if it were a machine. The first programme explained: 'Our programmes are a step backward towards expressing that [baby] suppleness of mind and body.' Yoga was a primary means of becoming more youthful and flexible; and the guide to this method of bodily upkeep was yoga instructor Arthur Balaskas (1940–1995).

Balaskas offered a much edgier approach compared to either Hittleman or Marshall. He was introduced to yoga through R.D. Laing (1927–1989), whose critique of psychiatry and championing of individual experience and expression had been a topic of discussion in the media from the early 1960s. Additionally, he was an important figure during this period for those experimenting with consciousness-expanding drugs, especially LSD.[66] As Balaskas's

63. 'Everybody Knows 1: Help Yourself – 13 January 1975', British Film Institute Archive.

64. Ibid.

65. Ibid.

66. For example, Alan Marcuson talks about bringing a girl on a bad LSD trip to Dr Laing's house in order to ride out the trip (in Green 1988: 178–80; see also Clay 1996: 80).

first wife, Mina Semyon, later explained, Laing 'had these people around him with a similar wish to find their own being from a being that got invaded by other authorities, parents and society, teachers, and others'.[67]

Semyon was Laing's patient, but soon her family were also social-ising with the famous psychiatrist (Semyon 2003). Laing introduced yoga to Balaskas and his wife around 1970 when he was beginning to explore Indian spirituality himself. Initially, the group worked through sequences from B.K.S. Iyengar's *Light on Yoga*.[68] In 1971 Laing spent a year in Sri Lanka and India where he studied Bud-dhism and Sanskrit, spending three weeks under Gangotri Baba, a Hindu ascetic, who initiated Laing into his Shakta-Tantra tradi-tion which is associated with Kali worship (Clay 1996: 158). Dur-ing this time, the Balaskases had daily lessons with Iyengar-taught Dona Holleman and attended classes with Iyengar when he was in London. Holleman had originally met Iyengar through J. Krishna-murti and spent much of 1964 and 1969 studying with the former in Pune. During the 1960s, she ran a B.K.S. Iyengar Work Group in the Netherlands until moving to Florence in 1972, at which point her teaching was influenced by another former student of Iyengar, Vanda Scaravelli. Holleman often travelled to London to teach yoga, developing a small, dedicated following of students.[69] Balaskas was soon teaching yoga at Laing's Philadelphia Association in Hamp-stead and remained associated with the psychiatrist for many years. Balaskas shared Laing's interest in the birthing process, including work in active birthing and rebirthing.[70]

As with the other 1970s television series, an accompanying paperback was produced. *Every Body Knows: Yoga Demystified* was twenty-two pages of photographic illustrations of the yoga postures with an initial print run of 20,000 and a cost of just 50–60p. While the marketing notes suggest a general-interest audience of both sexes between the ages of twenty-five and forty, 'promotional opportuni-ties' listed LEA yoga classes and also the women's pages of Sunday papers. The illustrations were attractive and showed some of the simpler postures demonstrated on the programme. The introduc-tion discussed the assumptions behind Balaksas's approach:

67. Personal interview with Mina Semyon (16 August 2006).
68. Ibid.
69. 'Biography', http://www.donaholleman.com, accessed 6 September 2007.
70. Balaskas and Balaskas (1979).

Over the last twenty years, an increasing number of people have found that some combination and interpretation of classical physical yoga postures have helped considerably to reduce some of the stress of life. Despite growing popularity a great deal of mystery still surrounds yoga.

... there is no mystery in this; yoga postures work directly on the physical repository of stress and tension – our muscles and joints. Yoga works systematically on all parts of the body, helping to release tension by stretching and contracting those parts which are most tense – most often the shoulders, neck and hamstrings (Balaskas 1975: 5).

Here, the BBC was again promoting the health-giving properties of yoga exercises and their effect on mental tranquillity. In 1977, Balaskas brought out a 190-page hardback book based on his yoga practice with an introduction by R.D. Laing (Balaskas 1977) – further evidence of a continuing and expanding market for yoga practice during the 1970s.

Balaskas was not only the series' yoga teacher but also its 'principal consultant', presumably influencing the choice of topics explored in the first half of the programme.[71] While the sense of duty implicit in keeping oneself fit and healthy was the same as previous television presentations of yoga, *Every Body Knows* was also influenced by the growing human potential movement concerning psychological development.[72] On the programme it was claimed that through the practice of asana an individual could find 'a new awareness and freedom. And, unlike any other system of exercises, many people find that with practice these exercises can produce a feeling of outer calm and inner stillness.' On *Every Body Knows* the presentation of yoga expanded from relaxation and fitness exercises towards yoga as a tool for personal exploration and dynamic change. However, the message that yoga was a technique for better mental and physical health remained the underlying theme.

Conclusion

Yoga on television can perhaps be best understood as a continuation of the adult-education cultural form. Raymond Williams has

71. 'Programme Content', in 'Everybody knows (keep calm)', 1974–75, Gen Pubs Edit.
72. For more on the human potential movement, see Goldman (2012), Heelas (1996), Kripal (2007) and Puttick (2000).

identified a close correlation between television, national culture and an implicit 'consensus version of public interest' (Williams 2003 [1974]: 34). There were also important authoritative implications: all these programmes encouraged their viewers to follow the instructions of the television presenters, and, as such, the television was accorded an educative authority formerly only embodied in a book or real-life teacher. As part of the *Pebble Mill at One* magazine show, yoga was imbued with a semi-official BBC sanction. These observations suggest that yoga was becoming increasingly accepted in Britain as an activity with assumed public health benefits. Its presence on British television had an important familiarising and popularising effect, reaching millions of Britons in their own homes. With its minor celebrities and attractive personalities, television added a veneer of glamour to the yoga provided in adult-education classes, although it remained much the same kind of yoga: an emphasis on safe, health-giving and relaxing activities for all. The evidence suggests that television presenters remained silent about – and in fact looked to 'demystify' and decouple it from – any religious and spiritual associations, instead promoting the public benefit of greater fitness and relaxation.

Media theorists have argued, and audience studies have confirmed, that readers and viewers will have their own interpretations about any presentation of information (Williams 2003 [1974]: 134; see also Rose 2001). By leaving the ideological content undiscussed, yoga on television left quite a lot of room for the viewer's interpretation and variable engagement. As McLuhan has argued, television's very form encourages an independent, imaginative relationship with the content. With the absence of a real-time teacher, many questions would have remained unanswered and 'errors' uncorrected. Popular enthusiasm to engage with Indian spirituality, encouraged by celebrity endorsement in the 1960s, was bolstered by the portrayal of yoga on British television (see Partridge 2005b; Campbell 1999, 2007). Television broadcasts, like the publicly funded educational contexts, tried to minimize explicit discussion of religious or spiritual ideas related to yoga; plenty of space was left for individual viewers' own interpretations of the meaning of these practices.

Chapter Seven

Yoga as Therapy

Anecdotal reports suggest that physical suffering was a frequent motivation for taking up yoga. Yoga teacher Ernest Coates began yoga in part to deal with stress from work and a resulting duodenal ulcer for which he did not want an operation.[1] Beatrice Harthan came to yoga partially because of a spinal injury. In 1961, she was photographed doing a forward bend in a swimsuit and was quoted as saying:

> I've got a damaged spine ... at the hospital they told me I must just learn to live with it and that I mustn't bend forward. Now I find I can bend any way I like. The pain has lightened and I feel much freer.[2]

A May 1973 *Yoga & Health* article reported that Swami Satyananda cured 'people who have been suffering from drug addiction, depression and many other mental afflictions' with Kriya Yoga.[3] Instead of accepting a surgical supporting belt for spondylolisthesis, another person turned to yoga and claimed that it kept her back 'free from pain'.[4]

The individuals who were interviewed about yoga on BBC Radio 4's *Woman's Hour* in the 1960s attributed improved mental and physical health to their practice. In 1962, Muriel Goodwin in Scotland had developed her own yoga routine from books and reported that yoga has 'helped my rheumatism very much and my husband's hay fever completely cleared up'.[5] In 1964, Neville Braybrook described that 'I myself began [yoga] in the hope that it might help my

1. Personal interview with Ernest Coates (19 December 2004).
2. 'The World of Topsy-turvy People', *Today*, 19 August 1961, press clippings at the RIMYI, Pune.
3. *Yoga & Health*, May 1973, p. 16.
4. *Yoga Biomedical Trust Newsletter* 14 (May 1991), p. 10.
5. 'Yoga for Everybody: Elsie Russell asks Muriel Goodwin about a system she has devised', *Woman's Hour* from Glasgow, 23 November 1962, BBC Written Archive Centre.

lumbago. I now know it can do much more than that.'[6] Several years later, in 1970, Eileen Williams from Leeds recalled how she began taking yoga seriously when she was bed-bound and recovering from major surgery. She reported that it was 'due to those exercises that my recovery was so rapid and complete' and described yoga as 'a science which points the way to leading a good and healthy life'.[7] There was a popular assumption that yoga could either alleviate physical pain or help one manage it better.

By the early 1980s, sociologists had noted a revival of interest in non-orthodox medical treatments. The mood of the period is captured in the introduction to a 1984 edited book on alternative medicine:

> A spectre is haunting scientific medicine: the spectre of alternative approaches to health and healing. A popular resurgence of interest and activity has recently manifested in a wide variety of new and age-old therapeutic modalities which challenge the contemporary form of medicine in advanced Western societies (Salmon 1984: 1).

A renewed popular challenge to the theories and practices of bio-medical doctors began in the mid-1950s as Thomas Szasz and R.D. Laing challenged psychiatric diagnosis and the dehumanising treatment of psychiatric patients.[8] Meanwhile Thomas McKeown argued that improvements to health were more a result of better nutrition and municipal sanitation than improvements in scientific/medical technology (McKeown 1976: 16). By the early 1980s the language of 'holism' and 'holistic health' dominated discussions of alternative medicine (Power 1991).

In the numerous surveys of 'alternative medicine', which began appearing in the post-war period, yoga held an ambiguous place. Brian Inglis (1916–1993), a well-known journalist, historian and television presenter, became a key figure in the popularisation of alternative medicine in Britain. In *Fringe Medicine* (1984), Inglis devoted a chapter to yoga, which he described as 'the best known of the methods' by which 'the individual can train himself to what amounts to a higher level of health' (Inglis 1964: 131). Yoga was

6. 'Standing on My Head: Neville Braybrook, *Woman's Hour*, 24 July 1964, BBC Written Archive Centre.

7. 'Healthy and Happy: Eileen Williams on Yoga', *Woman's Hour*, 10 December 1970, BBC Written Archive Centre.

8. In Szasz (1997 [1970]) although his criticism dates from Szasz (1956); see also Laing (1959).

omitted from the 1978 *Alternative Medicine: A Guide to the Medical Underground* which states in its introduction that yoga would not be covered and neither would colour therapy, Tai chi or the Alexander Technique (Eagle 1978: 8). In Inglis's 1979 book *Natural Medicine,* he positioned yoga as a type of 'auto suggestion' along with hypnotism and biofeedback (Inglis 1979: 189–92).[9] Yoga was also not included in the report of a 1981 Threshold Foundation survey of complementary medicine in Britain (Monro and Fulder 1981: 2).[10] Part of the reason for yoga's omission was that it lacked a system of qualifying practitioners in parallel with more established alternatives such as osteopathy and homeopathy (Squires 1985; Collins 2005). However, by the late 1970s many yoga teachers were leading classes and taking private students with 'remedial' conditions, i.e. specific health problems. Soon British yoga organisations attempted to professionalise in order to gain greater social authority in treating these cases.

Because yoga teachers claimed to have specialised techniques for improved health and well-being, they could have been perceived as infringing on the area of expertise claimed by the medical profession. Medicine and law were often considered the original 'professions' and were the focus of initial theories of professionalisation (Burrage and Torstendhal 1990: 1–23).[11] Two of the major characteristics of medicine as a profession were the relatively high level of knowledge required for practice and income that depends on clients rather than employers (Burrage and Torstendhal 1990: 1–23). The medical profession was among the first to attempt to monopolise their area of professional expertise through a legal framework. However, the 'orthodox/unorthodox interface still remained relatively fluid and undefined by the end of the [nineteenth] century' (Saks 2003: 16; see also Porter and Porter 1989; Porter 2000). Mike Saks has argued that professional self-interest was the primary motivation for the distinctions between orthodox and alternative medicine, rather than objective measures of efficacy and patient benefit (Saks 1986).

9. The association between yoga and hypnotism goes back to the birth of the subject of hypnotism (see Baier 2009).

10. 'Psychotherapy, Personal Development and Self-Help' were omitted from the report but 'most of them are included in our computerized database'.

11. On professionalisation, see also Berlant (1975), Brooks (1986), Burnham (1998) and Kirk (1976).

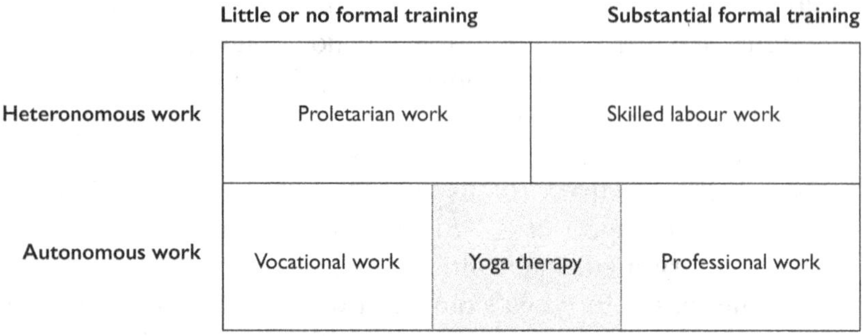

	Little or no formal training		Substantial formal training
Heteronomous work	Proletarian work		Skilled labour work
Autonomous work	Vocational work	Yoga therapy	Professional work

Fig. 7.1 Where yoga therapy fits in 'types of work'. Adapted from Figure 1: 'Four Types of Work' (Beckman 1990: 120).

This chapter will argue that yoga in Britain largely avoided overt conflict with the medical profession by simultaneously profession-alising with educational qualifications and deferring to medical expertise. There are many different ways of defining professional-isation and professions. Figure 7.1, adapted from Svante Beckman, defines professional work as autonomous and requiring substan-tial formal training, whereas vocational work is autonomous but requiring little or no formal training (Beckman 1990). The medical and legal careers are professions because they require both auton-omous client-centred work and a high level of formal schooling. Vocational work could also be called 'lay work' which, Beckman explains: 'though the successful performance of such work may require substantial skills, there are no requirements of formal train-ing' (Beckman 1990: 121). As will be recalled, two of the main pro-moters of yoga in Britain, B.K.S. Iyengar and Sunita Cabral, did not possess any internationally recognised standard of training in yoga, although both had high levels of skill and charisma. However, as yoga entered the adult-education system, local authorities wanted evidence of 'formal training' to verify instructors. In response, Iyengar and the British Wheel developed teacher-training courses to attempt to move yoga teaching from vocational work towards professional work. These distinctions became more important in the context of treating medical problems.

As will be shown, most yoga teachers positioned themselves, socially, higher than vocational professions yet deferred to the professional standing of the medical profession. This prevented direct conflict with medical expertise while claiming a degree of professional legitimacy in treating a variety of medical conditions. Three yoga organisations will be used as case studies in demonstrating this social positioning: the Yoga for Health Foundation, the 'remedial yoga' work of the teachers following B.K.S. Iyengar, and the Yoga Biomedical Trust (YBT). While there were many other yoga organisations in Britain, these were the first to be established that dealt directly with medical conditions, and they took very different approaches. Both groups created policies that helped establish 'yoga therapy' as more than simply vocational work, but with less authority than the medical profession.

Neither the British Wheel of Yoga nor the Friends of Yoga (FRYOG) directly addressed medical conditions within their organisations. Teachers associated with these groups who were interested in working with medical conditions networked with the Yoga for Health Foundation or the Yoga Biomedical Trust (established in 1983). Paul Harvey has been the primary student of T.K.V. Desikachar in Britain, a tradition that also works with therapy and established the Association for Yoga Studies for networking within this tradition in 1981. In the twenty-first century there have been new organisations seeking to integrate yoga as a therapy within the National Health Service, with some success at the local level.

Beckman has also offered a model for looking at professionalisation in terms of authority in which professional authority is positioned between bureaucratic authority and 'expert authority'. As he explains, expert authority is 'goal-based and clings to the presumed performative skills of a person, e.g. expert advice from fiscal consultants to astrologers' (Beckman 1990: 129). In contrast, bureaucratic authority is derived from 'institutionally defined rules and roles relating to goals and contractual tasks' (Beckman 1990: 130). Professional authority, according to Beckman, has an authority on the borderline between being institution-based and person-based and contains elements of both.

The authority of yoga teachers in post-war Britain could be described as bordering between expert and professional authority. The British yoga organisations, with regard to use of yoga for therapeutic purposes, have attempted to establish training with more bureaucratic authority. Yoga therapy organisations have also emphasised their person-based authority as a credential in opposition to medical objectivity; the use of yoga as therapy attends to individual problems and the individual 'patient' is the final judge of

efficacy. However, in the development of yoga institutions that can
'certify' yoga teachers as being qualified to treat medical conditions
there has been an attempt to move towards a more institutional,
bureaucratic authority.

Institution-based	Bureaucratic authority
	Professional authority
	Yoga therapy
Person-based	Expert authority

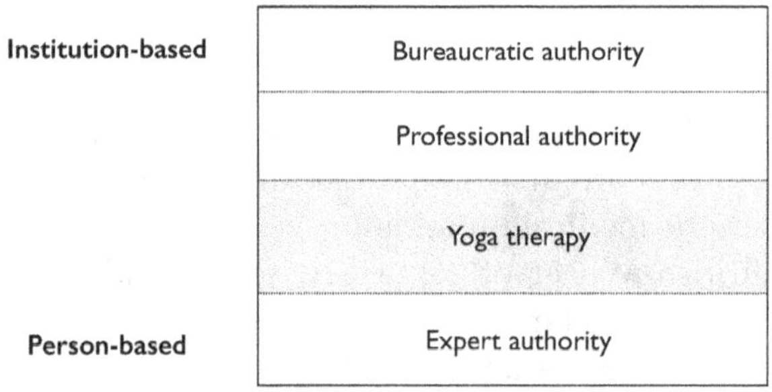

Fig. 7.2 'Types of authority' including yoga therapy. Adapted from Figure 2: 'Four types
of authority' (Beckman 1990: 129).

The Yoga for Health Foundation

The Hittleman television series concentrated on mitigating the
effects of stress, and improving fitness and self-esteem through
yoga exercises. The series producer, Howard Kent, focused increasingly on practical techniques that could benefit everyone, regardless of ability. Kent wanted to promote a kind of yoga that could
'combat the strains of present-day living, combining both mental
and physical fitness' (Kent 1974: 56). However, he also made general claims for yoga's health benefits. In 1974 he asserted of regular
yoga practitioners:

> They will exercise the muscles and create greater flexibility; They
> will massage the internal organs, so that they are properly condi-
> tioned; They will eliminate the strain and tension which is automat-
> ically reflected in the seizing up of muscles and pressure points and,
> thereby, they will provide the first step to mental relaxation, since a
> physically relaxed body cannot be achieved in a state of major mental
> tension (Kent 1974: 8).

Relaxation was a key component of these exercises, and moving
consciously and without tension was prioritised. Kent emphasised
the healing potential of this approach over precision in physical

positions. The exercises themselves varied from merely purposefully moving the eyes to more ambitious back-bends like *ustrasana* (camel pose). The focus was on breathing, and movement within an individual's range of ability and relaxation.

After seeing Hittleman's *Yoga for Health* programme in the 1970s, a Scottish physiotherapist contacted Kent and together they developed yoga-based exercises for those with multiple sclerosis (MS). Initial results showed MS patients experiencing significant benefits.[12] 'Yoga for MS' was designed 'to improve both the morale and the mobility of the sufferer'. Further goals were set to contain the disease and possibly to reverse its progress.[13] Work on yoga for MS continued: in 1984 the British Wheel of Yoga's journal reported on the Bedfordshire venue Ickwell Bury:

> Perhaps one of the most important facilities here is the remedial help given to visitors suffering from multiple sclerosis. I have seen for myself the improvement in individuals who, when I first visited the Bury some years ago, were confined to wheelchairs and are now walking unaided.[14]

Becoming more focused on exploring the potential of yoga for health and healing, Kent extended the Yoga for Health Clubs concept by founding a registered charity, the Yoga for Health Foundation, in 1976 (Kent 1997: 10), which was run by a board of trustees but primarily directed under Kent's leadership. Its registered aims were to:

> Research into the therapeutic benefits to be obtained by the practice of yoga both mentally and physically and the promotion of such benefits by means of training therapists, publishing relevant material and setting up centres for the practice of the principles of therapeutic yoga and by any other means upon which the trustees may decide.[15]

Initially, the Yoga for Health Foundation focused on organising groups of MS patients to meet regularly for yoga classes under a Yoga for Health Clubs instructor.[16] Other groups were set up for people with conditions such as hypertension, arthritis, asthma and

12. Howard Kent, 'Acceptance is the Name of the Game', *Yoga and Life* 1 (October 1977), p. 10, in Yoga for Health Foundation newspaper clippings.

13. Ibid., p. 22.

14. *Spectrum*, Spring 1984, p. 37.

15. Registered Charity No. 271648 statement of aims available on the Charity Commission's website.

16. 'The Yoga for Health Foundation', *Yoga and Life* (Summer 1977), p. 26.

back trouble. There were also groups for those with learning disabilities and for partially sighted children.[17]

Changing attitudes about pain and suffering was an important
aspect of the Yoga for Health Foundation's approach. Tony Perkins
had been an alcoholic for 15 years before he was taken off daily
Valium and asked to do physical yoga exercises daily at the Ley
Clinic in Oxford. Before checking in, he had been bankrupted,
served a prison sentence, and had a twenty-year ban from driving
a car for motoring offences. Perkins attributed his recovery to the
yoga offered at the clinic: 'Yoga taught me to live a contented life
without drink. I began to feel more relaxed and free from tension
than at any time in my life before.'[18] As well as finding a way to
rebuild his own life, Perkins saw yoga as a tool that could help others and began teaching at the Yoga for Health Clubs. He also ran a
yoga class for alcoholics under the framework of Alcoholics Anonymous.[19] In 1977, Perkins claimed a success rate of 25% of yoga-prac-
tising alcoholics becoming alcohol-free, which contrasted with a 1%
rate using medication or psychiatric interventions, although Perkins did not explain precisely how he measured his success.[20]

In 1977, Perkins began nagging Howard Kent to start a residential centre and showed him prospectuses of country mansions for
sale. To this end the former placed a small, boxed advert appealing
for help in this project in the Yoga for Health Clubs magazine *Yoga
and Life*:

HELP
It was an act of faith in yoga
that made recovery from
alcoholism possible.
It is an act of faith which guides
me to open a yoga residential
guest centre.

17. Ibid.

18. 'Remedial Yoga: How Yoga Cured an Alcoholic', *Yoga and Life* (Summer
1977), p. 25.

19. Véronique Altglas (2005a) has suggested that there is an overlap between
twelve-step programmes such as Alcoholics Anonymous and members of other
neo-Hindu (particularly Siddha Yoga) groups in France and Britain. The November
1979 B.K.S. Iyengar Yoga Teachers Association newsletter contains a collection of 'I
resolve . . . just for today' statements, the format taken from Alcoholics Anonymous.

20. 'Remedial Yoga: How Yoga Cured an Alcoholic', *Yoga and Life* (Summer
1977), p. 25.

> With humility I ask will you help?
> I need your suggestions, your
> ideas, your unity.
> My assets – absolute faith and
> untiring energy.[21]

This appeal reveals an important relationship between faith, lifestyle and healing through yoga. Perkins went on to describe the power of yoga as being its ability to bring 'contentment through the realisation of unity – integration of the physical, mental and spiritual self'. This was something, Perkins claimed, no drug could offer.[22]

A suitable property for a residential yoga centre was found the next year: Ickwell Bury, a manor house in rural Bedfordshire; although £8,000 had been raised, Howard Kent had to mortgage his home to secure a lease on the property.[23] The centre could sleep up to thirty in double rooms and Kent soon organised residential courses, most lasting five days, from Sunday to Friday, for £65, starting that same year, 1978.[24] There was a resident nurse present on all courses, and the yoga instructors had experience of the special requirements. Many courses were run for people with specific problems, but others were open for any kind of ability or disability.[25] A 1997 retrospective on the centre reported that up to 1,500 people stayed residentially every year looking for help with conditions including MS, Parkinson's, motor neurone disease, diabetes, asthma, heart disease, ME and arthritis. The centre also offered training for already-qualified yoga teachers who wanted to learn more about dealing with medical conditions. Over time, the Yoga for Health Foundation made international connections in 23 different countries and played host to visiting yoga instructors as well as international groups in pursuit of yoga instruction for specific medical conditions.[26]

21. *Yoga and Life,* Summer 1977, p. 24.

22. 'Remedial Yoga: How Yoga Cured an Alcoholic', *Yoga and Life* (Summer 1977), p. 25.

23. Ibid.

24. *Yoga and Life,* Winter/Spring 1977/1978, p. 20.

25. Kent, 'Acceptance is the Name of the Game', *Yoga and Life* 1 (October 1977), p. 22. See also *The Yoga for Health Foundation Residential Centre, Ickwell Bury, Bedfordshire: A national Yoga Centre Specialising in Remedial, Therapeutic and Relaxation Activities.* The Yoga for Health Foundation, Ickwell Bury, Northill, Bedfordshire, 1978. Pamphlet in the British Library.

26. Kent, 'Acceptance is the Name of the Game', *Yoga and Life* 1 (October 1977).

The Yoga for Health Foundation approach was that yoga was not a therapy; rather, it had 'therapeutic benefits'.[27] The Foundation emphasised the difference between their approach to health and illness and that of the medical profession. An early promotional article stated:

> The start of a new life can begin with 'The Ickwell Concept.' In the world of treatments and prescription, the new Yoga for Health Foundation Remedial Centre . . . will stand as a beacon of sanity. We do not have a National Health Service: we have a National Sickness Service . . .[28]

In contrast to doctors, whose focus was disease and illness, Ickwell Bury offered an oasis of 'peace and quiet' for those seeking to address stress-affected conditions and a supportive environment to 'develop awareness' that would give strength and hope. The Ickwell retreat environment, both physical and psychological, was experienced by many to be healing.

To further the 'Ickwell experience' Kent developed a Yoga for Health Foundation teacher-training programme. This course had much in common with the Yoga for Health Clubs approach, but Kent designed the course with the goal of helping yoga teachers integrate all ranges of ability, including those with severe 'disabilities', into a yoga class. About fifteen to twenty students would meet monthly, with a few residential weekends at Ickwell Bury. Claire Buckingham, who took the course and later became a personal assistant to Howard Kent, referred to the large amount of reading required on the course and its focus on 'personal growth' through yoga.[29] This inclusive approach for personal betterment was the essence of the Yoga for Health Foundation:

> because in every yoga class you get perhaps one person who is healthy – ordinary, healthy, young people don't go to yoga classes.
>
> . . . By not treating disabled people differently, by treating them the same as everybody else, we got a lot of people in wheelchairs, a lot of people who were highly disabled practising yoga. Before we did that, I think that people thought that it couldn't be done.

27. Personal interview with Claire Buckingham (14 September 2006).
28. *Yoga and Life*, Winter/Spring 1977/1978, p. 20.
29. Personal Interview with Claire Buckingham (14 September 2006).

... if you read the descriptions, the essence of yoga is to be still. The
physical practice of yoga is necessary to enable us to become still.[30]

At the Yoga for Health Foundation, the essence of this approach
was encouraging stillness through breath and gentle movements.
The Foundation taught that those with 'disabilities' could participate in such activity just as well as those with full mobility.

So Kent promoted yoga practice to improve quality of life that
was appropriate even for those with severe physical limitations,
such as being confined to a wheelchair. In his book *Yoga for the Disabled*, he states that his focus is on 'human energy and its development through breath' (Kent 1985: 25).[31] He gave numerous public
demonstrations illustrating the improved strength that resulted
from directing calm, full breaths to weakened areas.[32] Because every
human being suffers from stress and strain at some point, the Yoga
For Health Foundation believed it could benefit everyone. *Yoga for
the Disabled* makes it clear that some movement with breath can
be practised even by those with limited mobility. While physical
postures and breathing were featured, relaxation and energising
breathing within the limits of one's ability remained the focus.

Yoga for Health was founded to help people of all abilities with
relaxation, positive thinking, more effective breathing and improved
mobility. Kent wrote:

> In summary, we are all handicapped – physically, mentally, and emo-
> tionally – some more than others, but even that changes with ageing.
> Man is consciously and unconsciously seeking deep satisfaction. The
> value of yoga for 'handicapped' people lies in its tendency to relax
> and energize the body and calm the mind. Yoga can transform atti-
> tudes, habits, and outlooks from negative to positive, thus permitting
> the individual more of a freedom to enjoy life in a relaxed and healthy
> manner.[33]

By improving ability and empowering individuals, Kent and
those involved in the Yoga for Health Foundation believed that they
were addressing not only physical but also mental and emotional
health. Practitioners of all levels of mobility attributed improved

30. Personal Interview with Claire Buckingham (14 September 2006).

31.

32. Promotional video for the Yoga for Health Foundation in the possession of
Claire Buckingham; and personal interview with Claire Buckingham (14 September
2006).

33. *Yoga and Life*, Winter/Spring 1977/1978, p. 20.

feelings of 'well-being' to their yoga. This self-empowered improvement and disability management was seen to have a spiritual significance. In many respects a belief that human limitations, both
mental and physical, can be reduced was the most important aspect
of the Yoga for Health Foundation's approach.

This approach was based on the assumption that many conditions were caused or adversely affected by psychosomatic stresses.
A 'mind–body' approach to yoga would 'establish a harmonious
and peaceful basis to life and to help the body's immune system
to overcome a wide range of illness'. The yoga it taught was not
'therapy' or a 'clinical' response to illness but a 'linking of mind
and body to achieve both basic health and happiness, with that
greatest boon of all – peace of mind'.[34] Peace of mind was assumed
to be related to better health and synonymous with a feeling of
'well-being' – a subjective feeling that was the Foundation's focus
rather than an empirically verifiable improvement of a diagnosed
medical condition, which placed it a different category to that of
medical interventions. As Dr Brosnan, who was affiliated with the
Foundation, explained:

> The purpose of yoga for the physically handicapped is identical with
> the aim and purpose of yoga for anybody. The secondary beneficial
> results which may be achieved – or may not – remains secondary.
> Yoga for them is not an alternative form of physio-therapy, a work or
> a modified PT. It is a form of life, a philosophy of living.[35]

Kent avoided making claims about 'curing' medical conditions, but
rather promoted a belief in positive change and improved levels of
health and happiness, whatever the basic level of health and ability.

By developing yoga teacher-training courses and further skills
training for established teachers, the Yoga for Health Foundation
professionalised the teaching of yoga to those with medical conditions. Its certificates implied the kinds of credentials expected
of other recognised professions, such as medicine or law, but in
emphasising the 'therapeutic benefits' of yoga rather than yoga as
therapy, the Yoga for Health Foundation maintained a separate
sphere of expertise from that of the medical profession – in fact, the

34. *The Yoga for Health Foundation Residential Centre*, 1978. Pamphlet in the British
Library.
35. Brosnan, 'Yoga for the Disabled', *Yoga and Life* 8, p. 13. Yoga for Health Foundation newspaper clippings.

Foundation's teachers bordered between 'expert' and 'professional' forms of authority. Yet by emphasising the personal over the professional aspect of their yoga programmes for specific illnesses and disabilities, the Yoga for Health Foundation avoided conflict with other realms of society.

B.K.S. Iyengar and Remedial Yoga

As we have seen, B.K.S. Iyengar was a sickly and poor child; it was his brother-in-law's expertise in yoga that offered an affordable way to deal with his ill-health. Iyengar's early reputation as a yoga teacher was attained partially by successful treatment of referrals from Pune's doctors (Manos 1987: 360). All 202 asanas described in *Light on Yoga* (1966) are accompanied by claims for health benefits and medical counter-indications. As a child, Iyengar's eldest daughter, Geeta, returned from a month in a nursing home still with a serious case of nephritis and a long list of medications that the Iyengars, at that time, could not afford. According to Geeta, her father told her: 'from tomorrow onwards no more medicines. Either you practise Yoga or get prepared to die.' Geeta's health improved under her father's attentions and Geeta eventually dedicated herself to teaching yoga (G. Iyengar 1990: 3–4).

Iyengar's response to the health problems his students presented was an intense and personal one. Geeta Iyengar explained that her father's approach changed with each patient according to their ability:

> The *āsanas* prescribed vary from person to person according to their constitution . . . old and infirm patients are made to perform [standing] *āsanas* like *Trikoṇāsana* and *Pārśvakoṇāsana* in lying down positions to create movement in the legs. He has made women in advanced stages of pregnancy perform specific *āsanas* after noting their responses and putting them in comfortable positions (G. Iyengar 1978: 183–4).

She goes on to explain, 'There are positive effects by practising asanas correctly and adverse effects by their wrong practices' (G. Iyengar 1978: 184). Therefore, Iyengar's approach to 'yoga therapeutics' relied on his yoga-teaching skill and experience. Iyengar taught 'remedial yoga' in a way that recalled Henrik Ling's medical gymnastics (Fletcher 1984: 83). The idea behind 'remedial yoga' was that therapeutic exercise could stimulate the body into healing itself, correcting posture and improving strength.

An example is the case of 'Robert', who was severely injured when a golf ball hit his head when he was fourteen. According to his carer, Marian Garfinkel, Robert 'survived two major brain operations, but the left side of his body remained partially paralysed and he lost the use of his left arm and hand' (Garfinkel 1987: 389). Although doctors and therapists had given him regular treatment, fifteen years later calcium deposits formed on his left shoulder, elbow and wrist. In the 1970s, Robert was treated by Iyengar during a lecture demonstration in the United States and eventually spent two months taking daily lessons with Iyengar in India. During this time, his carer writes that:

> Through the force of his personality and determination, Mr Iyengar was able to encourage Robert to face the physical pain he had to work through in bringing back to life limbs frozen by many years of inactivity . . . As he worked with Robert, he devised mechanical aids which solved particular problems as they developed. Iyengar treated whatever reactive symptoms appeared . . . Robert progressed enough to stop his medication completely (Garfinkel 1987: 391).

Marian Garfinkel also writes, 'Many times Iyengar demanded that Robert face excruciating pain in order to loosen the calcium deposits so that he would feel new mobility in his limbs' (Garfinkel 1987: 392). Iyengar sometimes pushed people beyond what they thought their limits were and showed them new possibilities. His approach was individual and intensive, and its success required trust on the part of his students. It was radically different from the one taken by Howard Kent and the Yoga for Health Foundation.

Although many people went to Iyengar with physical problems, a particular attraction of yoga as therapy was the way some teachers connected mind and body. A Franco-British Cambridge resident, Janet Downs Tourniere, had suffered a 'nervous breakdown' in the 1970s before travelling to Pune to take yoga lessons from Iyengar. She later self-published her diaries of her first visit, in which she recalled the physical and mental challenges of the classes:

> '*Ardhachandrāsana.* Lift the left hip more . . . left upper arm moves up, right one down . . . open groin of carrying leg!

> I was bewildered, ears heard one instruction, arms and legs carried out another. Eyes confused.

> 'I'm trying.'

'Trying means you are living in the future. With aim. Just do.'

What . . . ? Oh, I see. No, I don't . . . yes, I do.

Incoherence of mind and body exposed (Tourniere 2002: 48).

When Tourniere returned to Cambridge, her friends did not recognise her and she reported that she had felt better than ever before. She later wondered, 'How could physical stretches and postures alter the personality as well as the body?' (Tourniere 2002: 129. Tourniere found sufficient support from Iyengar's instruction to train as a yoga teacher herself and for many subsequent years returned to Pune annually.

Iyengar himself had no bureaucratic or professional qualifications; his institutional learning had ended before he achieved his school leaving certificate (Iyengar n.d.: 3). However, his asana instruction was recognised by local Pune doctors as having therapeutic effects for a range of conditions (Iyengar 1988a: 36–41). Although he was trained in Krishnamacharya's yoga shala, Iyengar's authority in using yoga therapeutically falls firmly in the 'expert' category. Like other forms of yoga therapy, Iyengar's work was an autonomous arrangement between himself and a client. Although he had no 'formal' school-based training, Iyengar spent several years practising asana daily in Mysore and further taught himself by exploring asana after he arrived in Pune. Thus, Iyengar's yoga therapy fits somewhere between the vocational and professional categories of work.

Iyengar's personal charisma and knowledge appears to have had a healing effect for some students, but Iyengar also sought to systemise his teaching so that students could achieve similar results all over the world. In the 1960s, he personally selected students with the required expertise to deal with health problems in his absence and, until the mid-1970s, Diana Clifton and Silva Mehta were the primary students invested with such authority. These early delegates wrote to him regularly for advice about their students' problems. A 1970 response from Iyengar to Diana Clifton reads:

I think you and Silva know more of these things than the others . . . People who get hot . . . flushing, breathlessness, heaviness in the head should be made to do *uttānāsana*, dog pose and *pashimotānāsana* before attempting headbalance.[36]

36. Letter from B.K.S. Iyengar to Diana Clifton, 30 November 1970.

Iyengar used specific asanas for specific conditions, but also adjusted his programme according to the individual. In 1967 Clifton received the following reply in response to a request for advice about a student with cancer:

> Go slow. Give deep breathing. Forward bendings with no strain on the throat. In some cases, the practise of yoga do aggravate the disease. Because the malifant blood is drawn to the other cells. If he enjoys give him mild poses. No standing poses and no inverted poses.[37]

By practising certain postures and actions, Iyengar and his teachers believed that they could control and improve a variety of illnesses and physical conditions. The majority of Iyengar's teachers, in adult-education institutes, however, were expected to instruct those with serious health issues that group classes were not appropriate for their conditions.[38] This policy represents a major difference between the approach of Iyengar's pupils and that of the Yoga for Health Foundation.

By offering specific programmes for individuals with particular medical conditions, the Iyengar approach competed more directly with biomedical treatment models than that of the Yoga for Health Foundation. For example, when asked how to use yoga to work with emotionally disturbed people, Iyengar explained that:

> As I said, or as Patañjali puts it, *avidyā* – want of spiritual understanding is the mother of all ailments . . . Various means or methods are given by Patañjali to quieten the distracted mind . . .
>
> On the practical side . . . there are certain postures where the subconscious mind is lifted and fed with a tremendous energy, like *viparīta dandāsana, setubandha sarvāṅgāsana* . . . This is how we work practically to bring the individual with emotional upheavals to the level of stability.[39]

Here, Iyengar presents a completely different model for thinking about emotional problems than that used by biomedicine. 'Feeding the subconscious' with energy and quieting 'the distracted

37. Letter from B.K.S. Iyengar to Diana Clifton, October 1967 in the archives of the Iyengar Yoga Institute, Maida Vale, London.
38. Letter from B.K.S. Iyengar to Diana Clifton, 29 October 1971. Iyengar writes: 'I think no pupil should accept complicated cases in the class. It is better that the teachers who are recruited pass the difficult cases to people like you and Silva. Let them not go to teach when they do not know.'
39. *Dipika* 12 (Spring 1985), pp. 1–2.

mind' have little in common with biomedical models of chemical imbalance leading to emotional conditions. Iyengar never had, nor claimed to have had, any medical expertise outside of his experience of the curative effects of yoga.

But the relationship between Iyengar yoga and biomedicine was more complex than that. Instead of directly challenging the medical model with his alternative epistemology, Iyengar consistently deferred to biomedical concepts and methods of determining successful clinical outcomes. As a young man in Pune, the doctors who recommended medical cases to him continued to monitor their patients and observe for improvement (Iyengar 1988b: 20–21). Iyengar encouraged medically trained students to test his system with their knowledge and explain his yoga in biomedical terms. In 1989 a long-term physician-student of Iyengar, Dr S.V. Karandikar, established his own clinic for therapeutic yoga in Pune (Alter 2004a: 129–60). In 1984 Iyengar had his breathing tested by biomedical physicians and reported that he asked them 'Please let me know how long I am going to stay on this earth . . .'. He delighted at the response that his lungs were like 'that of a 23–25 year old boy'.[40] The testing of yogic claims by biomedical means has an established tradition, perhaps best exemplified by Swami Kuvalayananda's long engagement with biomedical tests at his centre in Lonavla outside Bombay (established in 1924) (see Alter 2004a; Newcombe 2017).[41] Iyengar's deference to biomedical assessment and opinion means that Iyengar Yoga is positioned as complementary to standard medical treatment rather than as an alternative.

Another reason why Iyengar's therapeutic yoga did not represent a challenge to biomedicine was that it professionalised largely in response to the LEA evening-class environment. In the context of the LEA structure, any medical benefits were an added bonus, but medical counter-indications were the primary concerns. The 1969 ILEA report noted that:

> Many claims have been made for the benefits of Yoga to those suffering from minor and even major disorders. The beneficial effects of increased mobility of the joint complexes, controlled breathing, improved neuro-muscular co-ordination and the reduction of mental

---

40. Story repeated in *Dipika* 12 (Spring 1985), p. 3.
41. See Alter (2004) and Newcombe (2017).

and physical tension are difficult to gauge but may be considerable for some individuals.[42]

The ILEA 'Medical Advisor' considered that those suffering from 'five types of disorder' (unnamed in the report) be excluded as unsuitable from general ILEA yoga classes.[43] With these exemptions, the ILEA officials approved Iyengar's teaching of yoga without directly engaging with the medical and therapeutic claims for asana. In McIntosh's assessment, the public health benefits of encouraging fitness justified the inclusion of the subject; those yoga teachers trained under Iyengar's method were deemed unlikely to cause harm through faulty technique or limited understanding.

As Iyengar teachers became more established in the LEA adult-education system, Iyengar's advice for injury prevention became more formalised, restricting the asanas new teachers were authorised to use and specifying that only certain postures were to be taught to beginners. In the early 1970s, it was reported to Iyengar that two people in Oxford were 'taken to hospital from yoga classes', having reportedly been taught by Wheel of British Yoga members. As a result of this, Iyengar's pupil Diana Clifton was asked to conduct three teacher-training classes at the Oxford College of Further Education. She designed syllabuses with 'an emphasis on safety' and sent it to Iyengar for approval. The course involved observing a beginners' class and, later, the teachers would learn, under Clifton's guidance, 'to assist so as to get an understanding of how to teach beginners'.[44]

42. ILEA Further and Higher Education Sub-committee 'Report 25.11.69 by Education Officer', London Metropolitan Archives ILEA/CL/PRE/16/24.

43. Ibid. The only record of these conditions I have found is a undated letter probably from the 1980s from the Ravensbourne Institute of Adult Education in North Lewisham, London, entitled 'YOGA DECLARATION FORM: Attention to all Hatha Yoga Students', which states: 'It is unwise for students to join Hatha Yoga classes if they suffer from any of the following: 1. Detached retina, 2. Diabetes, 3. Epilepsy, including petit mal, which may be aggravated by deep breathing or hyperventilation of the lungs in any posture, 4. Hypertension or raised blood pressure, other conditions associated with heart disease, 5. Menier's disease or any similar condition in which there is disturbance of balance control of the body, 6. Severe physical handicaps. N.B. Please inform your tutor before beginning classes if you have had any serious illness, operations or broken bones. Letter in Archive of the Iyengar Yoga Institute, Maida Vale.

44. Letter to B.K.S. Iyengar from Diana Clifton, 19 October 1975. Archive of the Iyengar Yoga Institute, Maida Vale.

This method of observing and correcting physical action in asana was always an important aspect of the Iyengar teaching method in Britain, the underlying assumption being that correct physical actions can both improve health and prevent future injury – inside and outside of the yoga class.[45] Qualifications were further formalised by specifying the level of experience required to teach each asana: a detailed system with the aim of preventing injury in large classes. Only the more experienced teachers and students could engage with postures that were considered more likely to cause injury.[46]

When an Iyengar Yoga Institute opened in London in 1984, it had a regular 'remedial' class in its timetable, taught by Silva Mehta. Mehta, who had run the first yoga teacher-training programme in the ILEA, had first come to Iyengar's classes with a serious spinal injury due to a fall. She was living in Bombay at this time and had had twice-weekly lessons from Iyengar for 'over two years' between 1957 and 1960. She later reflected on this period: 'Mr Iyengar's lessons made me feel a new person at a time when I was in agonies with a fractured spine'.[47] According to her daughter, Iyengar gave Silva 'some poses', the practice of which 'kept her mobile and enabled her to lead a normal life'.[48] She moved to London in 1960 and continued to attend classes with Iyengar during his annual visits. While developing the London Iyengar Yoga Institute during the 1980s, Silva Mehta and her two children Shyam and Mira wrote a book called *Yoga the Iyengar Way* at the end of which you would find specific 'Remedial Programs' for a variety of common complaints (Mehta, Mehta and Mehta 1990: 185–7). While treating medical conditions has been an important part of Iyengar's yoga tradition, the key focus of Iyengar Yoga in Britain has been popularising and professionalising weekly group asana classes, which has meant that, generally speaking, the professional training of Iyengar Yoga teachers in Britain has not been specifically focused on therapeutic yoga.

45. Increasingly, the prevention of injury has been connected to issues of legal liability and insurance. However, this subject belongs to a later time period.

46. 'We consider, however, that teaching of intermediate and advanced work is outside the scope of ordinary adult education classes.' *B.K.S. Iyengar Teacher's Association Newsletter*, June 1978, p. 1.

47. Mehta, 'The Story of a Dream', *Dipika: The Journal of the Iyengar Yoga Institute* 16 (1987), p. 25.

48. Personal communication with Mira Mehta (16 March 2007).

Yoga Biomedical Trust

A third important organisation exploring the uses of yoga for improving health was the Yoga Biomedical Trust, established in 1983 by Dr Robin Monro, who originally trained as molecular biologist. During the 1970s, Monro held a variety of academic appointments and had a long-standing interest in Eastern religion, meditation and philosophy. When visiting a university friend in Bombay in 1962, Monro was introduced to B.K.S. Iyengar and sometimes took classes from him during his early visits to London; he incorporated some home asana practice into his daily routine, always with an interest in its therapeutic potential. In the 1970s, Monro's childhood asthma came back in the form of bronchitis and Dr Parchure, personal physician to J. Krishnamurti, taught him some breathing exercises which revolutionised his health and intensified his interest in exploring the potential for healing outside of standard biomedicine.[49]

Monro obtained funding for research into the contemporary situation regarding what he and his co-author termed 'treatment paradigms' that were 'complementary' to standard biomedical ones, including 'acupuncture, anthroposophy, chiropractic, healing, herbalism, homeopathy, hypnotherapy, naturopathy, osteopathy and others' (Munro and Fulder 1981: 80), although yoga did not feature as a recognised alternative or complementary therapy in this research. Monro estimated that tens of thousands of people practised yoga regularly in Britain and anecdotal reports suggested that it had a positive effect on health. Yoga, being largely self-help, was notably also a very economical way of improving personal health. In the winter of 1981–82, Monro travelled to India and noted that therapeutic research into yoga was growing in that country. On his return to Britain, it struck him as curious that such little research was being done into the therapeutic benefits of yoga in this country and decided to try to remedy this lacuna.[50]

After initial discussions with Howard Kent and the Yoga for Health Foundation, Monro surveyed around 2,000 yoga teachers in Britain, through Yoga for Health Foundation networks, about their experiences of how yoga may have affected a list of around twenty specific health conditions. After this pilot, all yoga organisations in Britain were approached to distribute the questionnaire, with over

---

49. Personal interview with Robin Monro (20 November 2005).
50. *Yoga Biomedical Bulletin* 1/1 (1984), p. 2.

10,000 being distributed and around 3,000 returned. In 1983, Monro founded a charity as an independent body to fund and promote exploration of health benefits to yoga, the Yoga Biomedical Trust (YBT), which was initially based in Cambridge.[51]

From its founding, the YBT wanted to remain independent, collaborating with any interested yoga organisations without becoming affiliated to any one faction and thus remaining 'unencumbered by sectarian divisions', raising standards, and mobilising further interest and official support.[52] It sought to be scientific, but not reductionist, noting that:

> We do not advocate 'allopathic yoga' – the exclusive application of specific exercises to particular disorders. Yoga is essentially wholistic, and aims for the integration of a person at all levels from physical to spiritual . . . For instance one cannot relax deeply at a physical level unless one is relaxed mentally; and mental relaxation is affected by one's spiritual attitudes . . . The tailoring of yoga routines to suit individual needs is a highly skilled art and science, which must involve the growing sensitivity of the student as well as the teacher's insight.[53]

In the first few years, the YBT applied to medical research funding bodies for 'over a dozen grants' to further explore the therapeutic potential of yoga; none of the funding applications was successful. Perhaps the trust's holistic approach was somewhat at odds with the reductionism of biomedical understanding at this time.

In the first few years, Monro directed YBT work towards expanding an analysis of survey research, promoting formal trials, and compiling a bibliography of extant research on yoga as therapy. He initially financed the Trust through personal loans in the hope of obtaining larger grants, but in practice it would rely on small grants and donations. Small trials (30 individuals) began at Addenbrooke's Hospital in Cambridge with some funding from Cancer Research Campaign and local health funds. As large grants proved hard to secure, the YBT focused on networking yoga teachers with those seeking therapy and more carefully recording the results of interventions and 'Information Exchange Groups' to facilitate discussion between yoga teachers on the therapeutic applications of

51. *Yoga Biomedical Bulletin* 1/1 (1984), p. 4. See also Robin Monro, 'Relax and keep taking the yoga/Focus on research into yoga therapy', *The Guardian* (London), 8 May 1985.
52. *Yoga Biomedical Bulletin* 1/1 (1984), p. 4.
53. *Yoga Biomedical Bulletin* 1/1 (1984), pp. 4–5.

yoga. Explorations into the potential benefits – and limitations – of yoga for diabetes sufferers was also a focus of research.[54]

In 1987 the YBT created a training course for yoga therapists with practitioners from the Hindu spiritual organisation Vivekananda Kendra in Bangalore, which began through a chance connection between Monro and an Indian affiliate of the Kendra whom he one day found himself working next to at a computer lab in Cambridge.[55] The affiliation between the Kendra and the YBT's Yoga Therapy Diploma lasted three years, after which the YBT offered the diploma independently. These courses were available to qualified yoga teachers and aimed to provide a nurse's-level biomedical understanding of the human body (omitting acute conditions but expanding on yoga's physiological effects), as well as exploring in case studies and project work how yoga might affect particular conditions such as asthma and premenstrual symptoms, as well as yoga for prison inmates. The YBT also served as a hub for networking, comparing notes on best practice and encouraging critical thinking and research on the therapeutic applications of yoga.[56] It also offered intelligent comment as journalists became aware that some were injuring themselves in yoga classes; not all applications of yoga are therapeutic.[57]

An important member of this network was Paul Harvey, who established a centre for yoga in Bath, based on the teachings of his guru, T.K.V. Desikachar. Harvey and Desikachar's approach emphasised a practice that met the needs of the individual, a tradition that follows Krishnamacharya's teaching after his 1952 move from Mysore to Madras, where he became better known for a more individualised, gentle approach to asana and a greater emphasis on pranayama, chanting and other lifestyle changes in pursuit of greater health and well-being. Having been first introduced to Desikachar by European students, Harvey trained intensively in Madras with Desikachar and Krishnamacharya in the late 1970s. Harvey served within the British Wheel of Yoga and taught

54. *Yoga Biomedical Trust Newsletter*, 1986; see also Catherine Stevens, 'Putting a yoga twist on diabetes: Catherine Steven on the therapy that may be a boon to sufferers of "maturity onset" diabetes', *The Guardian* (London), 15 March 1991.

55. Personal interview with Robin Monro (20 November 2003). For more on the Vivekananda Kendra's yoga teaching, see Beckerlegge (2014).

56. *YBT Newsletter* 14 (May 1991), pp. 5–6.

57. Liz Hodgkinson, 'No gain, just pain', *The Times* (London), 10 April 1992.

therapeutic applications of yoga in this tradition in Bath from 1981. In the pages of the *YBT Newsletter*, Harvey stressed the importance of relationships and individuality in establishing a therapeutic application of yoga, as well as the influence of Ayurvedic ways of thinking about imbalance as a cause of ill-health.[58] The Desikachar approach to 'yoga therapy' was both directly and indirectly influential on therapeutic applications of yoga in Britain.

The YBT moved from Cambridge to London around 1994 to facilitate its growing yoga therapy training programme. After a short period in south London, the centre worked out of a few rooms in the Royal Homeopathic Hospital in central London for several years in the mid-1990s, conducting research on yoga as a therapeutic intervention for asthma, and trialling a specific therapeutic programme to treat back pain under the guidance of Dr Dayanand Dongaonkar, an orthopaedic surgeon.[59] From 2002–14, the YBT operated a Therapy Centre on Pentonville Road near King's Cross where it offered diploma courses, other training courses for yoga teachers, as well as therapy for those suffering from a variety of conditions that might be helped by yoga; it continues to offer training programmes and therapy out of various smaller premises. In 2005, Monro described the approach as 'Still holistic, new routine for each individual, but oriented around the physical condition and personal capacities'.[60] Recommended practices often involved breathing and relaxation exercises as well as asana appropriate to the individual concerned. Over the years, eschewing the general introductory yoga class, the YBT has focused on addressing the problems presented by those seeking therapeutic yoga: finding practices that the individual can do at home which might alleviate pain and promote both physical and mental well-being.

Conclusion

The therapeutic benefits of yoga were presented and applied in very different ways by the Yoga for Health Foundation and the teachers who followed B.K.S. Iyengar. However, both organisations were more interested in teaching yoga than presenting themselves as

58. *YBT Newsletter* 14 (May 1991), pp. 8–9.

59. Judy Jones (1995) 'Yoga Guru Offers to Breathe Life Into Asthmatics' *The Observer* (London), 25 February.

60. Personal interview with Robin Monro (20 November 2005).

therapists. Neither group claimed any medical expertise or challenged the authority of physicians; teachers and practitioners did not conceive of their discipline as an alternative medical model. Both organisations have largely sidestepped alternative medicine by teaching techniques the benefits of which could not be confined to a description of specific physical, physiological or emotional effects.

In contrast, the Yoga Biomedical Trust attempted to apply biomedical research methods to a non-sectarian breadth of practices aimed at alleviating specific physical conditions, rather than offering a general introduction to a yoga system. The emphasis of the YBT has been on ensuring safety within biomedical understandings of health as a prerequisite to the therapeutic application of yoga. The treatment of medical conditions within yoga has usually relied largely on personal testimony and anecdotal evidence. Challenging this tendency, the YBT attempted to build a more robust evidence base to therapeutic benefit based on a broad understanding of yoga and its applications for promoting health. While offering diplomas in yoga therapy, the YBT has not achieved a monopoly in this type of qualification, with many other teaching lineages offering their own qualifications and certifications in relation to work with specific ailments.

Although in many cases yoga groups did not work directly together, the training programmes they each established added an educational, bureaucratic aspect to the otherwise 'expert' authority of teaching yoga. The development of qualifications in this model accorded the use of yoga for medical conditions with social credibility and moved yoga towards professional employment by maintaining elements of the vocational type of work, even as bureaucratic models were being developed to professionalise the practice of yoga as therapy. By largely avoiding any specific claims for cures, yoga organisations in Britain sidestepped potential charges of 'quackery' or offering false hope.

While all understood as therapeutic yoga, the types offered by these organisations looked very different. A diversity of theoretical models and qualifications are by no means unique to yoga, however; for example, osteopaths had several competing professional organisations until the formation of the General Osteopathic Council in 1993 (Fulder 1992: 181). But, unlike osteopaths, British yoga teachers do not all claim to be addressing illnesses: the majority would see it first of all as a much broader subject, the therapeutic benefits of which might constitute part of its appeal and drive certain applications of its practice. Yoga teachers in Britain have not sought to replace biomedical models of health and wellness with their own models but instead have promoted therapeutic benefits through a system of physical culture and spirituality. In Britain, public discourse about yoga as therapy has stressed self-care in a regular programme of exercises, a change in mental attitude, and a focus on individual responsibility. This has largely allowed yoga instructors to avoid the medical professionalisation model while maintaining a popular promise about improving health and well-being.

Chapter Eight

Diversity of Practice and Practitioners

Have yoga practitioners been in the vanguard of a 'spiritual revolution' in a secular culture? (see e.g. Heelas, Woodhead et al. 2005; Campbell 1999, 2007; Partridge 2005a,b). This chapter will explore yoga practitioners' beliefs and their understanding of the relationship between the physical and spiritual. Practitioners often describe the experience of greater integration, relaxation and concentration as being essential elements of yoga. This experience is sometimes, but not always, perceived as relating to the divine. Most often, these elements are associated with ideas of health and happiness, and not aligned with any specific theology. While most presentations of yoga insist that spiritual beliefs are not a prerequisite, many practitioners believe their practice to comprise more than just the physical aspect. For the majority who engage with yoga, religious doctrine or descriptions of the divine are largely matters for the individual.

The 1960s onwards saw an increase in more sectarian presentations of yoga, attracting small numbers of very dedicated followers. Many of these groups have been studied with regard to their beliefs and practices.[1] Yoga has also been a dominant theme in many British pagan and magickal organisations.[2] However, many people drift between teachings and teachers over time; additionally, those fully committed to a sectarian yoga movement at any given

---

1. The main presenters of more doctrinally defined forms of yoga – what de Michelis (2004: 188) terms 'Modern Denominational Yoga' – include Yogi Bhajan/3HO (see Deslippe 2012; Jacobsh 2008), Ananda Marga (Voix 2008, 2010; Crovetto 2008), the Brahma Kumaris (Walliss 2002), the Divine Light Mission/Elan Vital/Prem Rawat (Geaves 2004, 2007, 2009), ISKCON (Dwyer and Cole 2007), Osho (aka Rajneesh) (Goldman 1999; Palmer and Sharma 1993), Siddha Yoga (Altglas 2014; Healy 2010), Sahaja Yoga (Coney 1999), the School of Economic Science, Sri Chinmoy and Transcendental Meditation (Mason 1994, 2015) and, more recently, Sri Sri Ravi Shankar's Art of Living Foundation (Jacobs 2015).

2. Personal Interview with Geraldine Beskin (12 January 2007) and Djurdjevic (2014).

time are likely to number in their thousands, while those who have had at least some contact with yoga teachers and classes in Britain are in their millions. This chapter concerns the beliefs of the general population: those who may have attended classes of the two main popularisers of yoga in Britain – the Wheel of Yoga and Iyengar Yoga teachers – or drifted between more sectarian presentations of yoga and more general classes. When we look at the lifetimes of the majority of those who have had contact with the yogic milieu in Britain, we see a general 'seekership' attitude, in tandem with private explorations of ideology outside the yoga class.

The increasing individualisation of religious beliefs has been a theme of many secularisation theories which have noted how religious (as well as other authorities) were challenged in the 1960s, with church attendances continuing to fall markedly in Western Europe (Berger 1990 [1967]; McLeod 2007; Parsons 1974; Wilson and Barker 2005). In the 1970s, Colin Campbell used a model 'mystical religion' to describe the British religious landscape in which people drifted between spiritual teachers (Campbell 1978).[3] Those looking for spiritual inspiration outside organised religion have also been described as 'seekers', which, as Steven Sutcliffe points out, accurately describes an important aspect of alternative religious and spiritual culture in post-1960s Britain (Sutcliffe 1997, 2000). Paul Heelas has argued that a focus on an essential component of the 'self' is a defining feature of the New Age movement, considers 'self-spirituality' the defining feature of the New Age and neo-Pagan movements in Britain. In this, Heelas is referring to a deification or sanctification of an 'inner essence' of the human as distinct from social roles and superficial personality (Heelas 1996). For those popularising yoga in Britain, belief was a private concern. This is particularly true for those associated with the British Wheel of Yoga and the Iyengar practitioners, who were the most influential into the 1990s.

The Yoga Path of the Early Wheel: A 'Soft' Orthodoxy

The Wheel presented yoga as something that could offer both better health and spiritual liberation. In the 1960s Wilfred Clark produced a small A5 *Yoga Handbook* (British Wheel of Yoga 1973) intended: 'to give newcomers to Yoga a straightforward insight into the more

---

3. I previously used Campbell's framework in a sociological analysis of Iyengar Yoga practitioners (Hasselle-Newcombe 2005).

important aspects of Yoga as a science of good, healthy and ethical living'. This phrasing emphasised the secular appeal of yoga for health and moral living. The same handbook expresses wishes for practitioners: 'May they through Yoga find sound health, increasing awareness and happiness supreme by following the Yoga Path which leads to Contentment.' For the Wheel, the physical and emotional benefits were united with the 'higher goals' of yoga through self-realisation and self-knowledge. The *Yoga Handbook* explained:

> The study as well as the physical practice of Yoga brings to every normal receptive person greater tolerance towards people and events, supreme calm and in all this self-realization is the keynote (British Wheel of Yoga 1973: 2).

This 'greater tolerance' and 'supreme calm' through 'self-realisation' was a kind of well-being that can be understood in both physical and 'higher' terms. Health, increasing awareness and 'happiness supreme' did not require overt religious belief or contradict liberal interpretations of most religions. Although those attending a yoga class were not compelled to attach spiritual meaning to their activity, it is clear that Wheel members whose words appeared in the Wheel's journal *Yoga* understood that yoga should be spiritual.

In Wheel literature, the overtly secular goals of 'ultimate' health and happiness were understood to necessitate a spiritual framework in order to be fully realised. The Wheel saw this as the important characteristic that made yoga different from other forms of exercise and relaxation. Wilfred Clark often complained in *Yoga* that yoga in LEA classes was in danger of being reduced to 'Keep Fit' or even a kind of therapy. For example, in 1972 he wrote:

> . . . If one takes up physical Yoga merely for therapeutic purposes, one is in a sense 'cheating'; certainly one is depriving oneself of True Yoga; one may as well join a gymnastic club or Keep Fit class.

> To say one is practicing Yoga and stopping at the physical is akin to joining a church choir for the joy of singing without any thought for Christianity, or kidding oneself that one is learning mathematics and going no farther than the twelve times table!

> What to do about it? What will happen? As within the orbit of the Wheel, no teacher must be considered qualified to teach until he or she thoroughly understands the true implications of Yoga; further education authorities must insist that True Yoga is taught; if any would-be students do not like this, then they must transfer to Keep Fit!

> No education authority would tolerate shortcomings in other subjects; the trouble is that most general educationists know what is required in other subjects; all they know about Yoga is that there is a physical aspect but they are completely ignorant of Yoga's real nature.[4]

Clark was concerned that the means of achieving 'union', e.g. the physical postures that were experienced as improving health, had become mistaken for the ends. It was clear to Wheel members that the 'general public' understood yoga to be: '"postures" – which are said to help tone up and replenish the nervous system when it feels depleted by the demands of modern urban life'. However, in Clark's opinion, 'Yoga is not Yoga if such factors as meditation and short philosophical talks are omitted'.[5] These meditations and philosophical talks are where the physical practices were connected to the 'real nature' of yoga, which was understood as union with the divine.

Sometimes, Wheel literature described physical and spiritual aspects of yoga as separable and hierarchical, but elsewhere described the physical aspects and 'ultimate goals' of yoga as inseparable. The Wheel's *Yoga Handbook* stated that yoga means 'union' and that 'this unity is nothing less than that of the Individual Spirit with the Divine Source of Life, that is to say, the unity of the finite with the infinite' (British Wheel of Yoga 1973: 2). The handbook also explained that:

> By whatever name one calls it however, self-realisation does mean happiness and nowadays many people seek an intermediate goal such as better health or relief from mental tension – happiness (British Wheel of Yoga 1973: 2).

This statement implies that the immediate benefits of yoga practice can be understood as an intermediate stage of the 'higher goal' of yoga, i.e. 'the unity of the finite with the infinite' (British Wheel of Yoga 1973: 2). Though not synonymous, better health and ultimate self-realisation are connected in this interpretation.

While insisting on the importance of yoga's 'higher goals', the Wheel nonetheless felt it necessary to distinguish between yoga and religion.[6] Jim Pym, a practising Buddhist and Quaker, explained in the opening issue of *Yoga*:

4. W. Clark, 'Means Better Than the End?', *Yoga* 11 (Spring 1972), p. 12.
5. Ibid.
6. *Yoga* 13 (1972), p. 11.

> Whenever a soul begins to approach the philosophical aspects of Yoga and to practice meditation, the question always arises, 'Is Yoga, then, a religion?' Though the answer may be that Yoga is not a religion, but is the basis behind all religious systems, those who are Christian by choice may feel some dismay at the predominance of Hindu terms employed.[7]

In *Yoga*, there was an emphasis on individual experience of the divine, without an explicit, prescriptive definition. Although the Wheel promoted an idea of ultimate truth, this truth was to be found in experience and not in a religious label or dogma. A member of the Anglican clergy told a Wheel member in 1972 that she was providing 'a technique and a vocabulary that is really going to help people get through to God'.[8] This was interpreted by the Wheel as a significant approval of its yogic path.

Yoga was addressed to practitioners who may or may not have been teachers. It is probably safe to assume that those who wrote into the magazine were more committed practitioners, many of whom, although certainly not all, would have also been teachers. Additionally, yoga teachers would also consider themselves practitioners. As has been documented in previous chapters, regardless of expertise, prospective yoga teachers in LEA venues were increasingly being asked to complete a training course. While the Wheel urged its teachers to educate their students about the 'supreme goal', each individual was allowed to choose his/her own way along the 'yoga path', a position that allowed for a 'soft orthodoxy' in interpreting the aims of yoga. As the *Yoga Handbook* explained: 'Yoga teaches us that all people are One, that all are One with God and that all religions are true in that they are varying Paths towards the same Goal' (British Wheel of Yoga 1973: 13). If something was 'not filling you with energy', the Wheel advised, 'perhaps you are not following the right Path, for it is not apparently "Enlightening" your Way'.[9] As long as this underlying assumption was maintained, a variety of sources could be interpreted by an individual as offering insight into their personal 'yoga path'.

Rather than using conventional representations of God as per mainstream religions, the pages of *Yoga* depicted experiences of the divine in nature and a greater appreciation of the beauty of life.

7. J. Pym, 'Yoga and Christianity', *Yoga* 1 (1969).
8. 'Working with the Church', *Yoga* 13 (1972), p. 11.
9. 'Attitudes', *Yoga* 19 (1974), p. 7.

The *Yoga Handbook* explained that: 'A teacher of spiritual and ethical Yoga need not be a living person – the sky, the stars, the sea, the wind and so on can all inspire us; the best teacher of course is experience' (British Wheel of Yoga 1973: 2). Sir Paul Dukes's autobiographical *The Unending Quest* (1950: 260) ended with the biblical maxim 'the Kingdom of God is within', an important concept in Wheel ideology and in popular yoga literature. The question 'Who am I?' was taught as a spiritual practice by Ramana Maharshi (1879–1950), who was popularised in the writings of Paul Brunton. Ramana Maharshi was an important inspiration to Wilfred Clark and many other people involved with the Wheel (Brunton 1934).[10] The Wheel's vision of yoga at this time was that of a personal, experiential path that was expected to eventually lead to a single understanding of truth.

Readers wrote in with poetry or favourite phrases from other authors which they felt embodied their experience of the divine. Such expressions of 'the divine' in the pages of *Yoga* were likely to be drawn from British and European culture and often drew on Romantic ideals of a deified nature. In summer 1971, *Yoga* quoted John Donne's 'No man is an island entire of itself' and concluded that it was 'surely pure Yoga . . . a thoughtful essay on Universal Oneness'.[11] William Blake and the sentiments expressed in 'To see the world in a grain of sand' was also seen as a 'true yogist'.[12]

The breadth of the personal searches within the Wheel's 'yoga path' is implied by a letter published in *Yoga* by an anonymous 'gentleman from the Midlands':

> After reading a book called 'Mysticism' by a certain Evelyn Underhill, I felt the need to read more on theosophical matters and hence turned towards Yoga, the first book about which I read being 'Yoga and Relaxation' by Tony Crisp. After that followed 'The Politics of Experience' by R.D. Laing.
>
> From an acquaintance I was able to borrow 'The Bhagavad-Gita' which I found the most remarkable of all. Other works which have come to my notice are: 'Yoga' by Ernest Wood; and 'Buddhism' and 'Zen, a way of life' both by Christmas Humphreys.
>
> With each book I read it seems as if I am fitting the pieces of a puzzle together – I feel that with sufficient time, sufficient patience and

10. See also personal interview with Jim Pym (7 July 2005).
11. 'John Dunne on Universal Oneness', *Yoga* 7 (1971), p. 8.
12. *Yoga* 9 (1971), p. 8.

sufficient thought through meditation, that I shall eventually have a
picture of life as it is in reality . . .

I think it is this which gives me energy to go on and on – I feel I must
read more and more of theosophical works as to enable me to perhaps
glimpse that joy again. But I feel unable to explain any more – I know
no more myself . . . what I seek is a rather vague goal – perhaps a form
of enlightenment, though knowledge and good living – a Karma Yoga
of my own perhaps.[13]

This eclectic mixture is part of the path identified as 'true yoga' by
Wilfred Clark. Although Clark introduced this letter with a declaration that one must 'first wipe clean the slate on which is inscribed
orthodox Western thinking and start afresh with 6000 year-old
wisdom which Mother India has given us', the letter's reading list
implies that traditions other than 'Mother India' are at work. The
correspondent's sources include the (anti-)psychiatrist R.D. Laing,
the explanations of Buddhism by Christmas Humphreys, 'theosophical works' as well as the *Bhagavad Gīta*. While reference to
the ancient origins of yoga was an important part of the Wheel's
self-justification, the idea of yoga as 'the basis behind all religious
systems' also allowed for inspiration from poetry, psychology,
world religions and the Western esoteric traditions.[14]

Individual teachers associated with the Wheel had their own
explanations of the 'yoga path.' One example is Indar Nath, aka
Swami Indrananda Ji (1923–2007), an Indian-born civil servant
who began studying yoga while living in London in the late 1960s.
His introduction to yoga was when Ma Yoga Shakti, a disciple of
Swami Satyananda, visited the Hindu Centre in Chalk Farm, London, where Nath was acting as secretary to maintain contact with
his homeland.[15] Ma Yoga Shakti Saraswati (1927–2015) first came to
London partially through connections with the then Indian High
Commissioner, Apa Pant. Ma Yoga Shakti was also influential in
bringing Swami Satyananda to teach in Britain, which led to the
establishment of the Bihar School of Yoga in London in 1978. A
native of Benares, she became a 'sannyasin' in 1961, renouncing
ties to family life, and eventually opened ashrams in both India and

---

13. 'Yoga Reveals Real Life', *Yoga* 7 (1981), p. 6.
14. For an explanation of the Western esoteric traditions and a cogent placement
of the New Age movement within these, see Hanegraaff (1998).
15. Personal interview with Indra Nath (18 August 2005).

the United States; during the 1970s she was a frequent traveller to Britain.

Under Ma Yoga Shakti's encouragement, Nath began teaching yoga classes at the Hindu Centre and also where he worked at the Post Office headquarters as a typist. In 1972, the yoga instruction he was providing from these and other venues went under the name of the Yoga Centre of North London. By the late 1970s, Nath had renamed his teaching the Patañjali Yoga Centre 'to reflect its dedication to traditional Yoga' (Nath 2001) and formally registered it as a charity in 1980. Nath also dedicated his retirement to living and teaching yoga.[16] During the early 1980s Nath was very active lecturing and teaching at Wheel events.[17]

According to Nath, progress in yoga relies on two key points: discipline and concentration. Translating the first two of Patañjali's *Yoga Sūtras* and using them as his reference, Nath explained that:

> It is the first sloka, *atha yogānuśāsanam*, it means now I am going to explain to you the discipline of yoga, so the first thing any student of yoga is required is the discipline. In his or her life. If it is out of the way, whenever you want, you have a time, you sit for meditation, whenever you have time you go to the yoga class – that is not it. That discipline is from the beginning to the end, whatever you may say.
>
> *Yogaḥ cittavṛtti nirodhaḥ* – the cessation of the fluctuations of the mind. . . . You sit for meditation, you think of something else as well. [If] even one thought creeps in, you have gone away from your path . . .[18]

These two concepts formed the basis of Nath's personal practice as well as his teaching. He regularly taught asana and pranayama during retreats as internal cleansing exercises (*shatkarma*). Nath taught *shatkarma* over the course of a week's residential workshop in which water is flushed through the digestive tract and the colon is believed to become thoroughly cleansed. According to Nath: 'If you want to progress on the path of yoga, you can't do without *shatkarma*. [The] body must be kept clean in every aspect.'[19]

---

16. The Patañjali Yoga Centre was registered on 5 October 1980 (No. 281312) and personal interview with Indra Nath (18 August 2005).

17. See e.g. *Spectrum* Summer 1980, Autumn 1981, Summer 1982, Spring 1985, Summer 1985, Summer 1989 and Winter 1992, and personal interview with Indra Nath (18 August 2005).

18. Personal interview with Indra Nath (18 August 2005).

19. Ibid.

In Nath's teaching, this was typically followed by two more weeks of intensive study, the first on improving posture work and the second on concentration and pranayama. Nath acquired a loyal following of several hundred supporters, but his courses were most popular in the early 1980s when he was invited to many Wheel events.[20] This was also his understanding of how to progress in yoga:

> only one has to do it for ourselves. I can't give you anything, you can't give me anything. The teachers are going to guide it that's all. Nothing else. They are not going to practice it for me or for you.[21]

For Nath, yoga was an all-encompassing discipline of life that guided all his actions. He also practised an hour-and-a-half of chanting, pranayama and concentration daily.[22] An important part of Nath's lasting influence has been inspiration through personal example. In this way the Wheel's spiritual approach to yoga was a continuation of its autodidactic roots with an emphasis on individual exploration and self-discipline.

Orthopraxy: Iyengar's Tradition of Yoga

It was the impression of many during the 1970s that the students of Iyengar were not interested in anything other than the physical performance of asanas. For example, Stephen Annett wrote in his 1976 *Many Ways of Being* that:

> ... while the Wheel says that the physical practice of yoga and the study of the philosophy from which it emerged are inseparable, Iyengar holds that Western man's spiritual development is as yet too slight for him to be able to grasp the subtleties of spiritual enlightenment. Indeed, some members of Iyengar go so far as to claim that anything beyond postures and basic breathing exercises is dangerous, but nonetheless, Iyengar teachers include some philosophy with their physical exercises ... (Annett 1976: 91–2).

Annett contacted all the groups described in his book directly for information, but it is likely that he found contacting Iyengar practitioners difficult as he complained that Iyengar teachers were

---

20. Ibid. For an example of a speaking engagement, see Nath as lecturer at the 'Fifth International Yoga Festival at Crystal Palace', *Spectrum* 1982, special insert.
21. Personal Interview with Indra Nath (18 August 2005).
22. Ibid.

'. . . very poorly organised. There is no central address to write to and there are no full-time workers specifically to handle correspondence. Added to this, they issue no publications, lists or guides' (Annett 1976: 92). On the positive side, he wrote that 'individually, the followers of Iyengar have a full grasp of the basic postures and breathing exercises that make up hatha yoga, and an Iyengar-based class is highly recommended' (Annett 1976: 92). These generalisations showed the Iyengar teachers in an unfavourable light compared to the Wheel, which was well organised for national and international correspondence, had a quarterly magazine and actively explained its beliefs in print during the 1970s.

However, looking at the Iyengar movement and its publications more carefully, it is unlikely that Iyengar taught that the physical practice of asana and philosophy of yoga could be disconnected. During an early demonstration in London, Iyengar's knowledge of Indian scripture was evidenced by his giving quotes as he performed asana.[23] In addition, Iyengar had written in *Light on Yoga* that the physical aspect of yoga asana was intimately connected to the greater aims of yoga:

> Haṭha Yoga and Rāja Yoga complement each other and form a single approach towards Liberation. As a mountaineer needs ladders, ropes and crampons as well as physical fitness and discipline to climb the icy peaks of the Himālayas, so does the Yoga aspirant need the knowledge and discipline of the Haṭha Yoga of Swātmārāma to reach the heights of Rāja Yoga dealt with by Patañjāli (Iyengar 1966: 24-5).

In *Light on Yoga*, Iyengar outlined the eight limbs of Ashtanga Yoga as well as the different paths (mārgas) of *karma, bhakti*, and *jñāna* which the Wheel also discussed in *Yoga* (Iyengar 1966: 24). Although the Inner London Education Authority had declared that the physical aspect of Hatha Yoga could be taught apart from yoga philosophy, Iyengar understood himself as teaching from within a traditional lineage of yoga teachers whose aim was mokṣa as expressed by Patañjali, but also a mokṣa that was compatible with the aims of many different religious traditions (Iyengar 1988: 14-15). However, Iyengar's approach in practice was very different from that of the Wheel.

---

23. *Daily Mail,* 16 June 1961, clipping in the archives of the Iyengar Yoga Institute, Maida Vale. 'Working for Health', *Hampstead and Highgate Express and Hampstead Garden Suburb and Golders Green News,* 7 July 1961, p. 4.

Although his books referred to Patañjali's *Yoga Sūtras* as the basis for his teaching, he did not require his students to believe anything in particular, allowing them to explore their own metaphysical interests and understandings. For example, Iyengar teacher Clara Buck, who donated her books to the Iyengar Yoga Institute in Maida Vale upon her death, had a collection that included Hari Prashad Shastri of the Shanti Sadan, Deepak Chopra, Benjamin Creme and several translations of the Upaniṣads and *Bhagavad Gītā*. She also donated some anatomy books and a few about Rāmānuja, whose Viśiṣṭādvaita philosophy formed the basis of Iyengar's personal metaphysical understanding. The Iyengars, a caste of Kannaḍa and Tamil-speaking Brahmins, are associated with the teachings of Rāmānuja (c. 1077–1157), founder of the philosophical school of Viśiṣṭādvaita; this is a qualified non-dualism, based on a critique of Śaṅkara's non-dualistic theology combined with Śrī Vaiṣṇavism, the worship of the divine in the form of Viṣṇu/Nārāyaṇa. Although Iyengar's teaching in Britain focused almost completely on instruction in asana, Iyengar has upheld his traditional family form of worship on a personal level. The idea of surrendering to God is an important element of Viśiṣṭādvaita philosophy, and Iyengar chose to focus his personal devotional practice on Patañjali and Hanumān, the 'monkey god', a popular devotional figure for all those associated with physical culture, often found in *akhāṛa*s (the gymnasiums for training Indian wrestlers).[24] Iyengar included a shrine to Hanumān on the top of his Institute in Pune (completed in 1976), and in 2004 installed what he claims is the 'world's first' temple dedicated to Patañjali in the village of his birth, Belur in Karnataka.[25] However, when presenting his translation of Patañjali's *Yoga Sūtras*, Iyengar wrote, 'I am neither a learned pundit nor a scholarly academician . . .' (Iyengar 1993a: xx). Iyengar has presented himself primarily as an artist and practitioner and taught from this understanding.

Iyengar further explained his personal relationship between texts and practice in the introduction to his 1985 book *The Art of Yoga*:

> Throughout my life, I have tried to blend my yogic practices with the study of the writings of our ancient sages and their experiences of

24. For more on Hanumān, see Lutgendorf (2007)
25. 'Inauguration of the World's First "Sage Patañjali" Temple at Bellur, Karnataka, India', http://www.bksiyengar.com/modules/Institut/Yogini/temple.htm, accessed 17 June 2007.

yoga, in particular those of Patañjali. With determined effort I infused their thoughts into my lifestyle to capture the essence of their teaching and to grasp the meaning behind the concise statements of the *Yoga Sutras* and other yoga texts. Yet the work is my own. As a musician plays his instrument, or a sculptor chisels a statue, I have tried to use my body and mind as instruments and to refine them. I have attempted to expand my consciousness from the personal to the universal (Iyengar 1993b: xiv).

Iyengar explained that there is a refinement and serenity in his presentation and experience of asana that is hard for him to convey in words. And so Iyengar attempted to teach an embodied experience of concentration and unity of body, breath, mind and soul.

Although his personal religious heritage undoubtedly informed his teaching, Iyengar asked his students to find their own way in their own religious traditions rather than imitate his own. One student recalls that he pointed her to the Bible:

'Here' said BKS Iyengar, and handed me a Bible. 'Look for yourself, you will find it . . . I don't know where it is. These are not my Scriptures, they are yours . . . Look it up. Your Paul said, 'Glorify God in your body' (Perez 1978: 129).[26]

In effect, the direct theological instruction was not so different from that of the Wheel, although the focus on psychosomatic details of experience within asana and pranayama was very different. Being asked to find their own beliefs and understanding gave Iyengar's students a very different idea of asana practice from those associated with the Wheel.

Rather than a 'soft orthodoxy' of belief, as promoted by Wheel of Yoga members, Iyengar presented an orthopraxy. Iyengar focused on the teaching of asana while teaching a method accessing all the different aspects of yoga within this single limb. Beatrice Harthan quoted Iyengar's comment about why he accepted the ILEA's proscription of philosophical instruction:

Truth is the same. Better life can be taught without using religious words. Meditation is of two types, active and passive. I took the active side of meditation by making students totally absorbed in the poses.[27]

26. The verse Iyengar refers to is 1 Corinthians 6:20: 'For you were bought with a price. So glorify God in your body.'

27. Beatrice Harthan, 'The Beginning of the Iyengar Movement in England', Iyengar Yoga Institute, Maida Vale. See also Iyengar (1988b: 148): 'Through the

Iyengar later expanded this idea further. He explained that:

> In my method of teaching, because I take you through a lot of poses,
> I keep you for two or three hours, or sometimes four hours, without
> allowing your mind to go elsewhere . . . do the pupils know that four
> hours have passed? No. So I have kept them in a spiritual state for
> four hours . . .

> Suppose I were to ask you to do a meditation, to close your eyes and
> remain in silence, and suppose I also were to close my eyes. Could
> I know what was going on in your mind? Perhaps you would call
> that spiritual, but I would say there is no spirituality there because
> your mind will be wandering elsewhere. That is not my method of
> teaching . . .

> So I do not need a certificate to say whether this is physical yoga or
> spiritual yoga. When I am teaching I know that for four hours your
> mind has not been allowed to wander. And when I teach I make you
> fully aware of your body, your mind, your senses and your intelli-
> gence (Iyengar 1988b: 161).

Iyengar taught meditation and concentration within the absorption
of the practice of asana. For the beginner, he explained, the first
practice he taught was 'awareness of the various parts of the body':
for example, 'look at the foot, then come to the ankle, connect the
ankle with the foot . . .'. He described this as 'working on the surface
level of the physical body' (Iyengar 1988b: 150).

As Iyengar students became more experienced at this level of
awareness, he attempted to give them a more integrated understanding of the movement of the mind. Eventually, a unity of
mind and intelligence within the somatic experience, according to
Iyengar, can lead to a direct experience of *ātman,* a concept that is
often interchangeable with 'soul' in Iyengar's terminology. Iyengar
explained that:

> When the intelligence feels the oneness between the flesh and the skin,
> it introduces the self . . . the body is forgotten in that moment because
> everything is flowing at the same speed and in the same direction.
> Patañjali says in the third chapter that the yogi's body should move as
> fast as the speed of his soul.

---

performance of asanas, I become totally involved and find oneness of body, mind
and soul. For me this is active meditation.'

But if you forget the body before you go through the earlier stages, you will never reach that point. That is the problem. Until the finite is known, how can we touch the infinite? (Iyengar 1988b: 150–1).

Iyengar taught that, by expanding proprioception using correct bodily alignment, deep peace of mind could be experienced. He aimed to bring his students to an experience of the infinite.

Occasionally, students collected of Iyengar's 'sutras': pithy statements imparted during asana classes that reflected his teaching. These included:

To say 'Ugh' is to abuse God. Say God!

Analytical intelligence is easy to acquire. Practical intelligence is not easy.

The job of the Master is to create disappointment, to teach humility, or there can be no progress.

When the mind says you have had enough in a posture, there is duality somewhere. Only the body must say it.

A preacher is not a teacher. A preacher is a propagandist. [28]

In these quotes, Iyengar parallels the Wheel's search for personal understanding and experience. Iyengar pointed towards the student's personal experience but did not offer any ideological content for that experience. However, he did examine the physical details of his students' performances with exactitude. His 'sutras' are also full of instructions for physical postures:

See the buttocks are parallel.

Don't clench the skin to straighten, the bones are for that purpose.

The frontal part of the nose must be parallel to the ground.

If the toe is dead, the heel is dead.

If eyes become red, person is resting on forehead or arms (in headstand).[29]

This kind of attention to physical detail had no parallel in the Wheel's teaching. In comparison, there certainly appears to be a physical emphasis to Iyengar's instruction.

28. 'The Sutras of Iyengar', untitled document in the archives of the Iyengar Yoga Institute, Maida Vale.
29. Ibid.

Iyengar's students (or at least those who continued to be taught by him for some time) believed that they were experiencing what Iyengar described, at least according to one, who recalled:

> He never warned us or prepared us for special experiences. He simply led us, all unawares, into an altered state of consciousness and then called our attention to it *when we were already there* . . . my mind had been like a deep pool, unruffled by random thoughts and fancies. If I had the slightest expectation that he was going to lead us into that sort of experience, I would have been so greedy for it that I would have missed it altogether (Jackson 1978: 145).

Being led into this experience by Iyengar personally was a real possibility for a British yoga practitioner in the 1960s and '70s, when Iyengar made his annual month-long teaching visits to England. However, the majority of yoga students in LEA classes would have had only an indirect exposure through their local teacher. Although Iyengar attempted to systematise his method, his charismatic personality was a significant influence in the development of yoga in Britain before 1980.

It was difficult for Iyengar and his students to articulate their yoga experience. At times, Iyengar complained that many of the teachers he trained 'are teaching without practice' (Iyengar 1988b: 162). It is also clear that many did not share Iyengar's understanding of his intentions when they attended his classes. During the 1970s, when there were more yoga teachers around to compare him with, complaints abounded about Iyengar's techniques and his harshness of manner. One student remembers being told that 'He is a terror . . . People are shocked by his methods – shouting at students and knocking them around' (Jackson 1978: 142). When effective, Iyengar's methods made for powerful experiences and loyal pupils. But it was in stark contrast to the emphasis of other British yoga groups on gentle relaxing and stretching.

Iyengar hoped to guide his students along the entire yogic 'path' of Patañjali through discipline of the physical body. Later in life, Iyengar reflected that:

> Most people practice yoga within the parameters of the first and second *niyama* which are cleanliness and contentment. They get the immediate payoff of yoga practice (going to a class, doing a bit at home) from the fact that there is increasing health, which is cleanliness, and a deep health, an organic health, a mental clarity, well-being

and repose, an ability to relax and rest, to nourish themselves from better breathing. So this brings an improvement in cleanliness, in deep health and concomitantly there is a greater contentment, integration with the environment, in our ability to handle its ups and downs. These are two circles in which most people are living yoga. It is a quick and wonderful reward . . . (Iyengar, Evans and Abrams 2005: 260).

This quote demonstrates the importance of well-being, feelings of health and greater contentment in Iyengar's students' practice. In this passage, Iyengar acknowledges what the Wheel journal *Yoga* also discusses: that many yoga students stop at a level at which certain physical and mental benefits are attained. However, Iyengar consistently taught that practising even part of the large yoga tradition was a positive action, if not a comprehensive understanding of his yoga teachings.

Individual Navigation of the Yogic Milieu

The religiosity of yoga practitioners can be described as a personalisation of spiritual ideas along with a rejection of ecclesiastical-led authority. Many practitioners reacted against being told what to do or believe, but still wanted to find a greater meaning to life. In this context, techniques and activities that gave feelings of well-being and 'peace of mind' were attractive. Importantly, yoga was an embodied practice that gave experiential benefits, not an institution with affiliation based on belief. John Claxton, a long-time teacher in the Iyengar method, reflected:

I think for a lot of our generation the desire was for a more universal kind of spirituality, not compartmentalised, not institutionalised, more personal and more universal spirituality, but not things that put divisions between people.

One of the things that drew me to yoga really was that here was this technique, a physical technique which led people towards their spiritual selves without dogma, without creed, without ritual. And that's how I stayed really. I meditate. I do my practice. I don't belong to any church, subscribe to any creed or religion.[30]

Claxton's sentiments, emphasising personal practice in opposition to institutional dogma, are echoed by Paul McCartney's reflection on the appeal of the Maharishi to the Beatles in 1968. McCartney

30. Personal interview with John Claxton (5 December 2004).

described the wide variety of ideas circulating in popular culture at the time, as well as the appeal of a personal practice that gave an experience of peace and fulfilment:

> . . . and you started to hear of the *Bhagavad Gita* and stuff like that. And it was all a little bit hazy because it wasn't like official religion, you were chucking in bits of Khalil Gibran and this sort of stuff, *Siddhartha,* which wasn't necessarily to do with it, but all seemed the same kind of thing. We'd all been brought up as Sunday school kids or whatever, traditional religious beliefs, and it hadn't really worked for us because we'd say, 'why is there then suffering in the world?' and the vicar said 'Just because,' and we say ' Oh yeah . . . that's a great answer.' So none of us had been able to be totally convinced in prayer until meditation. Then you started to get the idea: one note, one concentrating, one lessening of stress, one reaching of a sort of new level did seem to get you in contact with a better part of yourself. It was a very hectic world one was living in and this inner peace seemed to be a better thing. If nothing else, what Maharishi was suggesting was a pleasant relief from all that in order to recharge your batteries – that basically was all he said (Green 1988: 160).

Much of the popular practices of yoga and meditation were presented as a technology of the body, free from the dogma of institutional religion. This was true for the British Wheel of Yoga, Iyengar Yoga and many independent teachers. Yoga practitioners experienced what they considered physical, psychological and sometimes 'spiritual' benefits, but they were not required to align their experience to 'irrational' belief and could define for themselves the metaphysical significances of their practices. Additionally, yoga practitioners post-war were no longer obligated to local church networks; much of the social support that churches traditionally provided in the case of illness or accident were now met by the welfare state. They could now explore their religious identities free from any commitment to a local church.

The ideas of relaxing, 'inner peace' and 'recharging your batteries' were important elements of British yoga practitioners' spirituality. Relaxation for a moment of 'inner peace' was an important aspect of Sunita Cabral's teaching at the popular series of yoga classes at the Birmingham Athletic Institute between 1962 and 1970. In a manual she self-published in 1965, Cabral explained that 'One is not born with worry, one grows into it, then passes it on' (Cabral 1965). According to Cabral, worry creates tension and 'tension tends to tighten the system over a period of years, leaving the system vulnerable to mental or physical disorders' (Cabral 1971 [2002]: 11). Cabral explained that methods of relaxation in her 'Pranayama Yoga' allowed one to choose between 'Heaven – permanent health' and 'Hell – permanent tension' (Cabral 1971 [2002]: 11). Kailash Puri, who taught yoga with her husband in Liverpool from the late 1960s, also emphasised the importance of relaxation in yoga and its profound and beneficial effects on her students' lives.[31] The back cover of Dr Gopal Puri's self-published yoga book describes him as a 'Yoga Relaxation Consultant' and includes quotes from students who attribute better health, happiness and 'self-realisation' to the practice of pranayama and relaxation (Puri 1974). These Indian-born teachers equated relaxation with 'self-realisation' and did not discuss their personal religious beliefs as part of their yoga teaching.

Mark Singleton has argued that the emphasis on relaxation in yoga is a 'relatively new and composite phenomenon' and that the 'theological and ideological frameworks that underpin them tend to remain permeated by assumptions of New Age religion and indigenous Western esotericism' (Singleton 2005: 289, 290). Religious and scientific exchange between India, Britain and the United States has been a complex phenomenon for centuries and it is unlikely that a concept such as 'relaxation' can ever have a definitive genealogy.[32] In any case, the idea of 'salvation through relaxation'[33] was important for British yoga practitioners in the 1960s and '70s. This idea united an empirical experience of relaxation with both better health and greater spiritual understanding.

During the 1970s there was no shortage of Indian swamis and gurus visiting the British Isles, as evidenced by the notices in the pages of *Yoga & Health* and the Wheel's journal *Yoga*. However, very few yoga practitioners locked themselves into following any one guru or tradition, but most were happy to learn from whomever was available. Alongside the well-documented expansion of new religions in the 1970s, yoga ashrams also appeared in Britain at this time. In 1970, Swami Satchidananda of the Bihar School of Yoga toured the country; this included an appearance on Midlands

31. Personal interview with Kailash Puri (25 May 2007).
32. However, some pieces of the puzzle are found in de Michelis (2004), Alter (2004a) and Singleton (2010).
33. A phrase Singleton adapts from William James (1983 [1899]).

ATV.[34] The Kundalini Yoga of Yogi Bhajan and the Happy Healthy Holy Order (3HO) was often featured in *Yoga & Health* during the 1970s in articles by Vikram Singh, aka Victor Harvey Briggs. After its impromptu beginnings, the Sivananda Yoga Vedanta Centre was more formally established in London in 1972. The Satyananda Yoga Centre in London was founded in 1978. However, the numbers of practitioners taking sannyasin vows, adopting Indian names and joining a monastic order were always dwarfed by the number practising yoga in LEA supervised classes or exposed to yoga on television. For most, yoga was not about dedicating life to a guru but rather about finding what they as individuals needed in order to have a less stressful and more satisfying life. Scepticism towards external sources of authority might help explain the pick-and-choose element of what Colin Campbell characterised as the 'cultic milieu' (Campbell 1972).

Some of these organisations encouraged exclusive membership and did find a limited number of converts, but the population by and large remained distantly curious. Among the high-commitment groups most successful in gaining members during the 1970s was the International Society for Krishna Consciousness (ISKCON). 'Core membership' of ISKCON in Britain, meaning temple residents and others with 'full-time devotional engagement', rose from less than ten in 1969 to almost 250 in 1983. Since 1983, ISKCON's 'core membership' has remained constant but its 'congregational membership' has increased as ISKCON has integrated with the Indian immigrant community (Ross 2007: 54–9). A late 1970s ISKCON leaflet claimed that 1,500 individuals attended Bhaktidevanta Manor near Watford every Sunday and 'hundreds of other people had come into contact with the movement at the time of its annual processions throughout the streets of London, Leicester and Birmingham'. The growing Indian diaspora were increasingly among those attending ISKCON temples.

Other highly visible guru figures in Britain included the young boy, Prem Pal Singh Rawat (b. 1957), who was introduced to Britain at age of thirteen at the Glastonbury free festival of June 1971. By the summer of 1973, the movement around Rawat, known as the Divine Light Mission, claimed to have 8,000 devotees (called 'premies') and about 40 designated premie households in Britain (Price 1979: 281).

34. *Yoga* 2 (1970), p. 1.

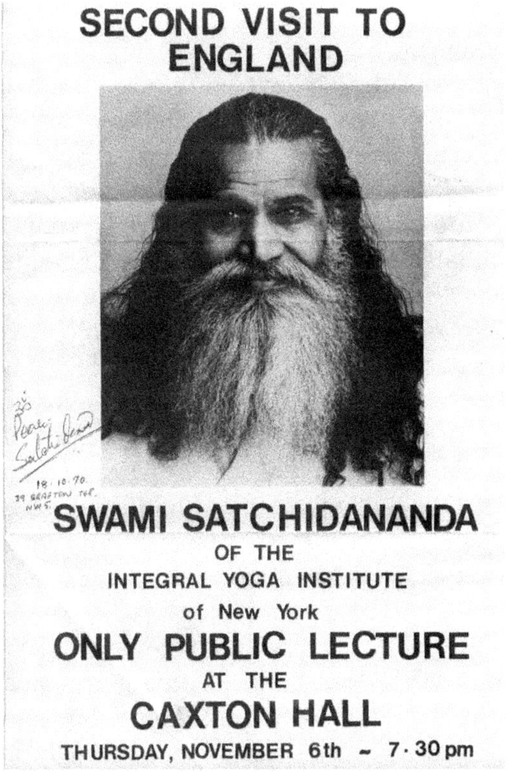

SECOND VISIT TO
ENGLAND

Fig. 8.1 Flyer for an
appearance by Swami
Sachidananda in London in
1972. Photograph courtesy of
Ken Thompson.

SWAMI SATCHIDANANDA
OF THE
INTEGRAL YOGA INSTITUTE
of New York
ONLY PUBLIC LECTURE
AT THE
CAXTON HALL
THURSDAY, NOVEMBER 6th - 7.30 pm

The group was always much more successful in the United States, and in 1973 the group claimed global membership figures as high as 50,000 with branches in Australasia, Canada, South America and Japan as well as many countries in Europe (Geaves 2009: 23). Rawat's father, Shri Hans Maharaj Ji (1900–1966), had gained a large following in north India, teaching what he called 'the Knowledge of the Divine Light and Holy Name', formally establishing the Divine Light Mission in 1960; the leadership of the organisation passed to his young son after his death in 1966. The tradition combines Sant Mat with Advaita Vedānta non-dualist soteriology which emphasises divinity without attributes and focuses on promoting transformative experiential understanding through meditative techniques. In the 1970s, a series of internal problems and negative publicity led to Rawat closing all his ashrams in 1982 and reconvening his global followers under the banner of Elan Vital (1984–2010). By the late 1980s, the Elan Vital movement could claim 1,420 committed supporters, who pledged £5 a month to Rawat (now known as Maharaji), with 5,000 on the mailing list and 7,000 practising his techniques called 'The Knowledge' (Barker 1989: 178).[35] Since 2010, Prem Rawat has been teaching 'The Knowledge' under his own name to audiences of 2,000–3,000 on visits to Britain, now largely drawn from the diasporic north Indian population.

Another highly visible Indian-based group in Britain comprised the followers of Bhagwan Shree Rajneesh (1931–1990), later known as Osho. Eileen Barker estimated that, in the early 1980s, these initiates, known as sannyasins, 'numbered 3–4,000; they belonged to what was possibly the most fashionable and fastest-growing alternative spiritual/religious movement in Britain' (Barker 1989: 203). Sri Chinmoy (1931–2007) also attracted large crowds in Britain during the 1970s, largely due to his associations with British jazz musician John McLaughlin (b. 1942) and Mexican-American guitar legend Carlos Santana (b. 1947), who both became high-profile devotees of Chinmoy during the 1970s. In 1973, they released an album together entitled *Love Devotion Surrender* intended as a tribute to Chinmoy and John Coltrane.

There were several other numerically small Indian-inspired sectarian organisations during the 1970s such as Ananda Marga and the Brahma Kumaris, and many people explored the teachings of the silent teacher Meher Baba, whose popularity relied much on his association with Pete Townshend, who dedicated his 1969 'rock opera' *Tommy* to his guru. Taken together, the committed members of any of these Indian 'new religions' probably numbered only a few tens of thousands at their peak, but it would be a mistake to measure their influence on British society only by these numbers. Those others who casually attended a single lecture or leafed through the ubiquitous ISKCON edition of the *Bhagavad Gītā* were much more numerous and would have included many yoga practitioners.

When considering the influence of gurus in 1960s and '70s Britain, it is worth remembering that many within the 1970s counter-culture were vehemently anti-guru. Scepticism for authority figures did not exclude those offering exotic knowledge from abroad. Sue Miles, who was deeply involved in promoting the 'beat culture' in 1960s Britain, later explained that:

35. For more on the later transformations of Prem Rawat's teaching, see Geaves (2004, 2007, 2009).

There were all these Indian travelling salesmen, all these gurus who packed up their suitcases and rushed over to England. The first Hare Krishnas were sent to [Barry] Miles and me . . . put them in touch with a load of Pakistanis in Ealing, quite sensibly. People who knew how to eat cauliflower cheese with their fingers or chopsticks – 'cos we didn't and we didn't want to learn (Green 1988: 232).

Geraldine Beskin of the Atlantis Bookshop also recalled a generally negative attitude towards those who attached themselves strongly to a single group or leader. In reference to Bhagwan Shree Rajneesh, she commented that some 'used to call him Guru Bagwash because everyone was in orange and things' and she had a feeling that those who joined were 'often just escaping things'. Beskin, like many of her generation would not accept any person or organisation with an attitude of 'only because you say so it must be true'.[36] A combination of scepticism and credulity was behind the majority trend of individuals investigating a number guru figures before settling on one, or none.

The presence of Indian spiritual teachers encouraged many to find their own guru. This process did not necessarily involve rejecting all other spiritual teachers or staying with a single teacher for a long period of time. An example of how a particular individual navigated the yoga courses on offer during the 1970s is that of yoga teacher Ernest Coates. Coates primarily drew inspiration from Swami Gitananda, whom he found only after exploring several other yoga teachers in the London area: Sir Paul Dukes's pupil Stella Cherfas and Iyengar-trained Silva Mehta. He also practised Siddha Yoga mediation for many years.[37] Siddha Yoga was popularised by Swami Muktananda (1908–1982) who initiated many American and European disciples; its main practices are meditation, chanting, *seva, dakshina, satsang* and *darśhan*, rather than asana and pranayama (Caldwell 2001; Altglas 2005a,b; Jain 2012, 2014a).

Coates claimed that all these experiences informed his understanding of yoga but Swami Gitananda's tradition had been his primary focus. He remembered attending a retreat Swami Gitananda was running in Wales some time in the 1970s:

I met Swami Gitananda after being involved in the Wheel and Iyengar, and I thought at long last I've found a real yoga teacher. He

36. Personal interview Geraldine Beskin (12 January 2007).
37. Personal Interview with Ernest Coates (19 December 2004).

had studied yoga from a boy, had a guru and his lineage was true. That lineage knew so much about yoga – more than any of the others I have come across. And I went to his ashram in the south of India. So I then found a real proper guru to study with. So that was the direction I went.[38]

Coates began teaching when the regular LEA teacher left unexpectedly and a replacement could not be found. He acknowledges an Iyengar influence in his teaching of standing postures, which he presented in the same sequence each week so that students could easily remember the practice outside of class. Coates emphasised the pragmatics of teaching from personal experience and seeing what 'worked' for his students.

> Obviously, all teachers, whoever they are, teaching whatever subject, bring to it their own experience. So I am bringing to my yoga classes many many years of experience . . . I have found out what worked. I have seen over the years the different groups I have done, up in London, weekends, holidays abroad and stuff . . . the biggest thrill I have ever had in teaching is seeing people change and understand. And they do not grow and understand by doing Keep Fit – they don't. But when they work on the emotional level and, if you like, spiritual level, the energy level, they do change.[39]

Coates considered yoga to be a subject consisting of the specific techniques of asana, pranayama, *bhanda*, *kriyā* and meditation as well-being: 'a spiritual teaching of the Vedas, the Upaniṣads, and more concerned with the spiritual life than the physical life'. *Bandha* are energy and muscular 'locks' performed at the bottom, middle and top of the torso. *Kriyā* roughly translates as 'action', but refers to quite different practices depending on the type of yoga transmission. Ernest defined *kriyā* in Gitananda's method as 'to do with the mind and the way the energy flows . . .' and consists of specific mental practices that settle the mind within the somatic experience.[40] For Coates all these aspects are a necessary part of yoga: 'if you want to develop yourself in yoga that's it. Otherwise just do Keep Fit classes but don't call it yoga.'[41] Although his path was based on personal experience rather than being developed within an organisation,

38. Ibid.
39. Ibid.
40. Ibid.
41. Ibid.

Coates's opinions on the essence of yoga parallels those expressed in the British Wheel's journal *Yoga* in the 1970s.

The importance of a personal journey towards wholeness and a greater sense of being was cited by other people involved with yoga in Britain. Kathleen Pepper, a Friends of Yoga (FRYOG) yoga teacher, explained how she understood her role:

> I encourage them [the students] to find their own way and I don't make them join anything. And when they finish here, many of them come back, but many of them don't. And I don't look on myself as a guru. I look on myself as somebody who gives people freedom to be themselves.[42]

Pepper explained that 'whatever a person's spiritual journey is, it is fine, whether they are a born-again Christian or move to Glastonbury, doesn't matter, what matters is their spirituality'.[43] Pepper unambiguously positioned the authority for defining how this spiritual quest manifests itself as internal rather than external to the individual. This internal placement of spiritual authority has been important for many British yoga practitioners.

Mina Semyon (b. 1938) took a very different path towards teaching yoga, seeing it as freedom from pain, worry and suffering. Semyon was introduced to yoga by her therapist, R.D. Laing, in 1969, within the first six months of her therapy: 'The feeling was that it wasn't enough to just talk . . .'.[44] At that time, Laing himself was beginning his personal exploration of yoga and Buddhism. Challenging the traditional power relationship and doctor–patient boundaries in the mental health field, Laing became friends with Semyon and they studied asana from B.K.S. Iyengar's *Light on Yoga* while they and their families were on holiday together in Italy:

> We started doing yoga together. He didn't have much experience with yoga postures but he certainly deeply understood the philosophy of yoga - practising with mindfulness, unifying mind–body–breath and releasing the emotional patterns held in mind–body, which obscure the wholeness of being.[45]

---

42. Personal interview with Kathleen and Roy Pepper (12 July 2005).
43. Ibid.
44. Personal interview with Mina Semyon (16 August 2006). For more details on Semyon's experience, see Semyon (2003, 2004).
45. Personal Interview with Mina Semyon (16 August 2006).

Semyon said that Laing gave her a manuscript of Patañjali's *Yoga Sūtras* which he had copied out in his own hand as a practice. Laing warned her not to read the commentaries, 'but of course I had to read [some commentaries] to see what he means . . .'.[46] She found that

> The yoga sutras spoke to me directly. It felt like you didn't need any special education to understand them, whereas the commentaries were more academic and conceptual, taking me away from the direct perception . . . so I thought that's what he must have meant.[47]

In March 1971, Laing departed for Sri Lanka and India where he would spend a year in search of wisdom under traditional teachers and practising mediation (Laing 1994: 150–9). Both before and after this trip, Laing showed a keen interest in Buddhism, and Semyon remembered him often discussing the Four Noble Truths and the importance of alleviating suffering. Laing, Semyon and her husband had daily yoga lessons with one of Iyengar's close pupils, Dona Holleman. Semyon also took lessons with Iyengar during his visits to London in the early 1970s.[48] She continued her practice and by the mid-1970s was beginning to teach.

Semyon's yoga practice, however, was not embedded within either an Orientalist India or an image of a traditional guru figure. When asked if she encountered other guru figures in the 1970s, she reflected that 'through Ronnie Laing I was introduced to Timothy Leary and Allen Watts'.[49] She found that the practice of yoga postures made her more aware of feeling 'disconnected' and described feeling a need 'to become whole'. For Semyon, yoga is an understanding of awareness, of letting go of habits, of opening up to the present moment. This is what she hoped to convey to her students. In her book, *The Distracted Centipede,* Semyon wrote:

> This is what I consider my own practice to be and this is what I
> am inspired to teach:
> Effort towards concentration on
> The breath,
> Being present
> Recognising how we disconnect

46. Ibid.
47. Ibid.
48. Ibid.
49. Ibid.

Letting go of thoughts or emotional reactions
Connecting to gravity and letting the body release from the
ground upwards.
Making a connection between feelings and the breath (Semyon
2004: 24).

Semyon's yoga is rooted in an experience of Patañjali's *Yoga Sūtras*, Buddhism's Four Noble Truths, human potential psychology and the group of people who spent their lives around R.D. Laing. In this emphasis on an internal experience of unity and wholeness in opposition to dogma and institutional authority, Semyon's understanding of yoga had much in common with that of other yoga practitioners during this period.

A Soteriology of Well-being?

Many yoga practitioners found meaning and spiritual purpose in their lives through a relatively uncontroversial physical practice. The gains of stress reduction, exercise, relaxation and better health were self-evident. Although some might have committed themselves to a sectarian organisation with specific metaphysical beliefs, the majority continued to learn eclectically from different teachers, assessing techniques and explanations within their guidelines of their own experience. Yoga practitioners' individualised, metaphysical understanding within a certain cultural context has parallels with the New Age movement, with its healing and spiritual practices, which was also developing during this period (Hanegraaff 1999; Heelas 1996). While there was overlap between the two, yoga could also offer a distinctly defined set of practices and an ideology.

Although yoga was routinely presented as 'something more' than physical, there was no requirement to subscribe to a particular set of beliefs regarding the 'something more', with the emphasis on personal experience and private metaphysical beliefs. Practitioners were encouraged to connect the well-being benefits of yoga to the 'ultimate goal' – however an individual chose to define it. The improved 'well-being' experienced through these techniques became a kind of 'elastic soteriology' – a practitioner could embrace a theological understanding of yoga or ignore any such interpretation. Religious and spiritual beliefs remained a private concern. The opportunity to improve one's well-being on a secular or spiritual basis depending on personal preferences or social context made yoga a practice that fitted comfortably between secularism and religiosity.

The doctrines of both the British Wheel and Iyengar pointed towards an imminent experiential rather than distant divine. The Wheel presented a normative goal of yoga as 'union with the divine' and recognised a variety of paths leading towards an experience of the numinous. Experience of an imminent divine was also the ideology behind Iyengar's practice:

> As we perfect asana, we will come to understand the true nature of our embodiment, of our being, and of the divinity that animates us. And when we are free from physical disabilities, emotional disturbances, and mental distractions, we open the gates to our soul (*ātman*) (Iyengar, Evans and Abrams 2005: 22–3).

However, it is far from clear that the doctrine of imminence was a defining feature of the experience and practice of yoga for the majority in the post-war period. As has been demonstrated throughout this book, yoga teachers were often silent about metaphysical aspects, although this might simply imply an awareness that spiritual experiences might not sit well with secular teaching contexts or understandings of traditional, institutional religiosity. However, it is hard to measure the importance of unarticulated experiences to those who continue to practise.

Religion as a subject for personal conscience rather than public discussion was a fundamental characteristic of the metaphysical positioning of yoga in post-war Britain. The public value of yoga was in its presumed salubrious effects, which was a subject open for public debate. The values implicit in this position include those of individual responsibility to an educated and healthy citizen. No less important was an often-implicit doctrine that mothers are responsible for their family's educational and physical well-being. While mothers have not necessarily encouraged the whole family to practise yoga, they have often found the practice supportive of the wider goal of responsible citizenry. As one woman explained in 1980:

> I am into my third year of yoga now, and this well-being and calm has been an important benefit for me. Like most women today I work as well as looking after two small children and running a home. This can play havoc with your nerves . . . any doctor will tell you a high

percentage of young mothers take Valium. I am these days much better able to cope with life's daily crises.[50]

As part of his argument about the 'Easternisation' of the West, Colin Campbell claimed that:

In the early postwar years those who wished to persuade Westerners of the merits of yoga usually had to play down its spiritual significance, now if anything the tendency is rather opposite (Campbell 2007: 35; see also Hamilton 2002).

In contrast, this book has found no evidence that the 'spiritual significance' of yoga became more important as the post-war period progressed; throughout this period there has been a constant tension between spiritual and secular presentations of yoga. Celebrity interest in Indian spirituality in the late 1960s probably increased the public's association of yoga with spirituality, but the avoidance of metaphysics was normalised by both LEA adult education and public-service television broadcasting – from Sir Paul Dukes in 1950 through to Lyn Marshall in 1984. The LEA evening classes may have encouraged reflection on the numinous, but metaphysical doctrine was not appropriate in the adult-education culture.

The 'spiritual significance' was not always downplayed in the early post-war years. The interviewer in the first BBC *Woman's Hour* feature on yoga in 1958 assumed that yoga was something to do with 'Eastern religion', and interviewed a Swami from the Ramakrishna Vedānta Centre and a 'Mr Nandi', who taught yoga in Hampstead and claimed to have been 'a Hindu priest in a silent order'.[51] The audience response to Sir Paul Dukes's 1950 BBC programme included a significant minority requesting more information on the 'doctrinal aspects of Yoga'.[52] Simply, the forms of yoga that became most popular were those in which religious and spiritual beliefs were private matters. Yoga bloomed by following, rather than challenging, the mainstream establishment agendas of improving health, education and contentment. Yoga thrived because it supported British cultural values that prevailed in the post-war period.

50. M. Lodge, 'One Satisfied Customer', *Dipika: The Journal of the Iyengar Yoga Institute* (Spring 1980), p. 7.
51. Script of *Woman's Hour*, 'Yoga', by Stephen Black, broadcast 20 November 1958, 2–3 pm, BBC Written Archive Centre.
52. TV Talks, 'Yoga', 1948–1950, T32/367, BBC Written Archives Centre.

Despite yoga's focus on somatic experience and private religious thought, women in post-war Britain did not describe their motivations as including a rejection of their roles as wives and mothers: they reported yoga courses helping them to perform their 'life as' roles with more calmness and effectiveness.[53] Eileen Williams interviewed on BBC *Woman's Hour* for Leeds reported that she:

> enjoyed the relaxation period. After a busy day with the family chores, this was sheer bliss. I was taught how to relax completely ... my friends made remarks about the change that had come over me both physically and mentally ... I didn't shout at the children any more, and they seemed to me to become better behaved.[54]

Sunita Cabral encouraged her students to 'slip a second' in order to 'give completely' to the demands of the world (Cabral 1972 [2002]: 14). So, while yoga practitioners might have been turning their attention towards their subjective experiences, there was an important connection between this and the performance of socially expected roles.

Health and education became increasingly subject to government regulation and direction, and yoga practitioners were able to attain semi-professional status through their independent labour and the need for specialised knowledge in the physical techniques of asana, pranayama and meditation. During the 1960s and '70s, the British Wheel of Yoga positioned itself as an educational authority on the different types of yoga, arguing that the job of the yoga teacher was to offer a thorough introduction to all the branches of the subject to facilitate students' personal exploration. Iyengar's yoga became standardised through the development of syllabuses to prevent injury in the context of LEA classes. The professional authority claimed by both these groups was primarily in the area of education and health.

The British government has long supported policies that educate the population about connections between behaviour and health, encourage personal responsibility, and provide access to facilities to enable such choices – an ideal that was taken up by many involved in the adult-education sector in post-war Britain. Lester Burney,

53. E.g. Maria Teresa Martinez de Vilar, 'Housewife Syndrome', *Yoga* 27 (Spring 1976), p. 7.

54. Transcript of *Woman's Hour*, 'Healthy and Happy: Eileen Williams on Yoga, Tuesday from Leeds', 10 December 1970, BBC Written Archives Centre.

principal of the College of Adult Education in Manchester, reflected on 35 years of managing the school in 1980:

> We defined adult education as the provision of educational facilities for all sorts and conditions . . . and paid regard to the very much under-rated aspect of adult education as therapy. We thought that it was not so much what we know but what we *are* that counts and the aim of adult education is to make us better and happier people by our knowing. So, at the one end we had graduates but at the other end of our provision were adult illiterates; most of us enjoyed good health but there were disabled people who badly needed help; there were the young, the middle-aged and the old and we tried to do something for as many different needs as possible . . .[55]

The ideal of a healthy citizenry overlapped with the ideal of continuing adult education. This principal's vision of 'better and happier people by our knowing' – liberal self-development for greater public health – was supported by yoga as presented in post-war Britain.

In sum, yoga in post-war Britain supported rather than challenged government policy and public opinion on religion, morality, education and public health. It aligned with the moral agenda of better public health and adult educational development, while simultaneously inviting private spiritual exploration, rather than a public identification with religious dogma.

---

55. E. Lester Burney, 'Looking Back', *Ventre*, 1980, *p.* 11, archives of the College of Adult Education, Manchester Central Library, M698/1/12003/35, Box 13 (emphasis in original).

Postscript

Yoga in Britain after the 1980s

Yoga in Britain has not developed in a linear manner. Rather, old and new co-exist, adapting to suit the specific needs of a particular time and place. Throughout the twentieth century, yoga was many different things to different people. In the first half of the twentieth century, it could be found in the pages of *Health & Strength* as well as in the practices of esoteric secret societies, and as a philosophy of the Shanti Sadan. Each of these layers developed and changed, and new transformations manifested themselves.

A first generation of yoga gurus and teachers founded new religious movements which developed and changed from the early twentieth century into the present, including the monks of the Ramakrishna Vedānta Centre, Hari Prashad Shastri's Shanti Sadan and several other groups which have faded from memory. There were also a number of more esoteric proponents who incorporated yoga into their teachings, such as Aleister Crowley, Dion Fortune, Rollo Ahmed, Kenneth Grant and Dadaji (aka Shri Gurudev Mahendranath) (Djurdjevic 2014).[1] The early physical culture influences of Sir Paul Dukes and Desmond Dunne, who ran a postal school of Yogism in the 1940s, helped make a secular yoga form more acceptable in the initial post-war period (Dunne 1951).

A new generation of gurus promoting yoga became influential among the youth in the late 1960s and early '70s. The Maharishi Mahesh Yogi and the School of Economic Science continue to promote mantra-based meditation practices into the twenty-first century. ISKCON went through a variety of challenges after the death of Prabhupada in 1977, but by the mid-1990s had emerged again as a strong social movement promoting Bhakti Yoga in Britain, this time supported by both families of Indian origin as well as some

1. For Ahmed in 1930s Britain, see Josiffe (2017) and personal correspondence with William Breeze (11 August 2017).

ethnically British (Dwyer and Cole 2007; Knott 1986; Rochford 2007). The Divine Light Mission under Prem Rawat attracted audiences of tens of thousands for public teachings in the 1970s (Price 1979; Geaves 2004). New generations of gurus became popular in Britain, particularly among the second and third generations of the Indian diaspora. These included Sri Sri Ravi Shankar (b. 1956) (Ališausk-ienė 2009; Jacobs 2015), Sadhguru (born Jaggi Vasudev in 1957) and, perhaps the most important, Swami Ramdev (b. 1965, 1968 or 1975) (Pathak-Narain 2017).

Alongside continuity of groups and teachers, there were also large changes. One of the key changes in the social structure of Britain during the 1980s involved the neoliberal reforms of Margaret Thatcher, prime minister from 1979 to 1990. In 1987, she famously declared that 'There is no such thing as society', a quote that has come to epitomise her philosophy of small government and the primacy of the individual actor in the economic marketplace (Thatcher 1987). Under this administration, much of the government funding for adult education was cut: the journal *Adult Education* reported in 1982 that enrolments in inner-London adult education provision from outer-London addresses had fallen from 32,000 to 8,300 in the previous year; this may have been in part because those claiming unemployment benefits were having their benefits cut if they attended courses (the government's argument being that attending educational courses made them unavailable for employment).[2] While it was probably always the middle classes deriving the most benefit from the physical education classes, adult-education providers had to scramble to provide services for much less money in the 1980s.

This meant that yoga classes were gradually to be found in other venues. Ever flexible, practices under the name of yoga adapted into the neoliberal-flavoured private marketplace. Peter McIntosh's vision of physical discipline underpinning a stronger and fitter citizenry was not entirely lost to those who had the resources to develop themselves. The gyms of the 1980s[3] did not initially include yoga classes, but the latter did not disappear from those venues still offering adult physical education.

2. *Adult Education* 55 (1982), pp. 114–16.
3. Anecdotal reports suggest that yoga did not become a common feature in private gyms until the late 1990s.

Initially, new forms of fitness rose to prominence in the 1980s: Jane Fonda's popular fitness classes and aerobics provided secular exercise for women. But there was still quite a lot of crossover in women's physical culture. Fonda opened 'The Workout' studio in Beverly Hills in 1979 as a way to fund a non-profit founded by her then-husband Tom Hayden, a left-leaning politician in California: the Campaign for Economic Democracy (CED) promoted solar energy, environmental protection and renters' rights, among other ideas. The Workout originally had three studio rooms and a bathroom, and offered 'Pregnancy, Birth and Recovery Workout', 'ballet, jazz and stretch classes' as well as a signature 'The Workout' routine (Fonda 2005: 390–1). She also made what is probably the first 'workout' video for home viewing: *Jane Fonda's Workout* (1982), on the new VHS technology. In some ways Fonda's exercise programme catered for a huge new market; in other ways, it was a more modern way of packaging exercises that would have been familiar to those attending a Women's League of Health and Beauty class in 1940s Britain. Fonda recalled in her autobiography:

> Letters began coming in by the basketful from women who were 'doing Jane,' as they called it, all over the world ... these women poured their hearts out, about weight they had lost, self-esteem they had gained, how they were finally able to stand up to their boss or recover form a mastectomy, asthma, respiratory failure, diabetes ... (Fonda 2005: 394 .

Certainly, many of the reported benefits echoed those attributed to yoga classes in the 1960s. And the model of the multi-roomed studio would become more prevalent for yoga as the new millennium approached.

By the end of the twentieth century, private venues had overtaken publicly funded programmes as the primary yoga providers. These ranged from individuals with relatively small circles of students who relied on word-of-mouth, to classes in church halls, to larger charities like the Iyengar Yoga movement and the British Wheel of Yoga. Both organisations continued to network among their affiliated teachers, providing training and certification, and increasingly becoming focused on sports qualifications and educational standards. The British Wheel of Yoga was recognised by the Sports Council (now Sports England) as having 'National Governing Body' status over yoga in 1993 (Tittley 1993: 3). This accreditation signified a kind of privatisation of yoga teaching as physical culture outside of the adult-education framework.

When the Sports Council was looking for a governing body to oversee yoga as a 'sports activity' in 1991, it considered the two most numerically significant yoga organisations in Britain at that time: the British Wheel of Yoga and the Iyengar Yoga Association. However, perhaps it did not fully appreciate the ideological differences that many of the smaller groups teaching and exploring things called yoga had with both the Wheel and the Iyengar approach. An Iyengar representative at the discussions explained a central ideological impasse that halted negotiations:

> In our submission we challenged the assumption made by the Sports Council that Yoga was a single activity, on which basis discussions had proceeded . . . it would have been helpful to have raised the questions as to whether Yoga is one or more activities prior to the series of discussions (Tittley 1993: 4).

The idea of yoga being certified as a 'sport' has always been controversial for those deeply invested in yoga. There has always been a close relationship between Keep Fit, physical culture and yoga practices in Britain but the idea that any one organisation could be responsible for governing or certifying yoga instructors based on the criterion of physical exercise alone is not widely accepted and has attracted criticism from a number of yoga enthusiasts (see e.g. Witts 2013). The Sports Council, like local authorities before it, sought to ensure minimum standards of safety and to standardise students' expectations – at least in contexts such as fitness centres, sports clubs or adult physical education classes. The British Wheel was eventually certified by Sports England as its accrediting body; it was the largest membership-based organisation, produced its own yoga teacher-training programmes as well as being willing to accredit a variety of other training programmes.

This diversity of interpretations soon led to an increase in self-accrediting organisations of yoga teachers. The Independent Yoga Network (IYN) was set up in 2004 in response to fears that yoga in Britain would become overly defined and regulated by the fitness industry,[4] and that its spiritual aims might be lost or minimised

4. 'History', Independent Yoga Network, https://www.independentyoganetwork.org/about/history. Personal interview with Ernest Coates (19 December 2004).

because of the Wheel affiliation. Yoga Alliance was established in 2006 as a more commercially minded accreditation body for ensuring minimum standards in yoga teacher-training. Although somewhat modelled on the US yoga accreditation organisation of the same name, the two organisations were not affiliated, and the UK organisation relaunched as Yoga Alliance Professionals in 2016.[5] Other yoga organisations also offer their own forms of qualification and insurance coverage. Fears that yoga will become overly defined by the fitness industry periodically recur whenever there is a new initiative towards standardisation or regulation of yoga teaching (Curtis 2016; Saner 2016).

Another important motivation for accreditation bodies in the post-1990s period has been an increasing need for liability insurance against injury in order to teach yoga in either a privately owned commercial 'yoga centre', a gym or sports studio, or a charitable educational venue. The accreditation bodies uphold public standards of training and act as brokers for group discounts on insurance policies. Although yoga maintains its reputation as a safe form of exercise, like in any other physical activity there are occasional injuries (Broad 2012; Remski 2016).

From the 1990s onwards, a new style of yoga enjoyed increasing popularity and visibility in Britain: Ashtanga Vinyasa Yoga. In contrast to 1960s and '70s yoga classes largely populated by middle-aged women, Ashtanga Vinyasa classes attracted younger, more ambitious students and more men. In fact, Ashtanga Vinyasa classes were not new but based on what B.K.S. Iyengar's guru Krishnamacharya had been teaching to young men in the 1930s. The practice involves long series of increasingly complex asana, framed through a flowing sun salutation sequence, which had been taught by Krishnamacharya's student Pattabhi Jois in Mysore from 1937 onwards. A Belgian yoga enthusiast André Van Lysbeth discovered Jois's Mysore classes in the 1960s and mentions the 'Astanga Yoga Nilayam de Mysore' in his *J'apprends le Yoga* (1968), along with the ashram of Swami Sivananda in Rishikesh, Vishwayatan Yogashram in Delhi, the teachings of Dhirendra Brahmachari and the Kaivalyadhama Samhiti of Lonavla, as places where he studied yoga during his previous five years in India (Van Lysbeth 1968: 15).

---

5. 'About Us', Yoga Alliance Professionals, https://www. yogaallianceprofessionals.org/aboutus.

However, the English edition of this work, *Yoga Self-taught* (1971) does more to promote Van Lysbeth's synchronistic, Brussels-based Yoga Institute than any Indian source.[6] However, Van Lysbeth ended his *Yoga Self-taught* with a quote from Swami Sivananda: 'An ounce of practice is worth several tons of theory'; a variation of this mantra would help define the more physical practice–focused yoga of Jois's Ashtanga Vinyasa sequences (Van Lysbeth 1971: 26, 1968: 321).

The American David Williams discovered Pattabhi Jois's yoga around the same time: while undertaking a yoga teacher-training programme at Swami Gitananda's ashram in Pondicherry, Tamil Nadu, in 1972, he encountered Jois's son K.P. Manju demonstrating the 'primary series sequence'. Inspired by Manju, Williams travelled to Mysore the following year, studied intensely with Pattabhi Jois and became certified by Jois to teach others. In 1975, he helped facilitate Manju and Jois's teaching in Encinitas, California, before moving to the island of Maui, Hawaii. Hawaii, with its temperate climate, was a focus of counter-cultural activity in the 1970s, and many were taught yoga by Williams.

A particularly influential student was Danny Paradise, who discovered this system of yoga accidentally while on a layover in Hawaii in the 1970s. Paradise travelled to Britain in the 1980s, teaching yoga as well as playing guitar in clubs.[7] On one such visit he became acquainted with Dominic Miller, a British guitarist, and taught him yoga, a connection that led to the British pop musician Sting who also became a Paradise student around 1990.[8] In 1993, a feature article in *Esquire* magazine entitled 'Yoga with Sting at the Ritz'[9] had a huge impact on the attention being paid to Jois's Ashtanga system, as did Sting's comments about yoga improving his sexual stamina. Paradise attracted more celebrity followers and his class sizes grew as he travelled around the world. Another celebrity influence at the turn of the twenty-first century was American pop

6. An 'adept of Ashtanga Yoga Nilayam of Mysore' is shown in a photograph demonstrating Jalandhara Bandha in Van Lysbeth's *Pranayama* (1983 [1979]: 135).

7. One interviewee remembers first encountering Ashtanga Vinyasa Yoga when Danny Paradise was teaching in Clapham Town Hall in south London in 1984.

8. K. Shattuck, 'Yoga Teacher to Stars Tries Becoming One', *New York Times*, 24 September 2000, Section 9, p. 1.

9. D. Stanton, 'Yoga with Sting at the Ritz', *Esquire Magazine*, March 1993.

singer Madonna, who announced her conversion to yoga on the popular television show *Oprah* in 1988.

Much of the global popularity of Jois's sequence was on account of American enthusiasts, but there was an important, charismatic populariser of these teachings in Britain: the Brighton-born Derek Ireland (1949–1988). Ireland came to yoga from a background in sports and music: he had promoted punk bands on the south coast in the mid-1970s. After his involvement in rock'n'roll, he and his partner Radha Warrell travelled to India, first studying Sivananda Yoga, then being introduced to Jois's sequences. Having studied with Jois in Mysore in the early 1980s, Ireland and Warrell taught the sequences in New York City's central park as well as in Britain, eventually opening a yoga retreat centre on Crete in 1991 (Guttridge 1998). The Mediterranean was a popular holiday destination for the British, and Ireland's charismatic athleticism inspired many to try the practice. A 1997 article in the *Independent* described Ireland's yoga at the Practice Place using a modified version of the quote often used to describe Jois's yoga:

> It's a yoga without dogmas or meditation – 99 per cent practice, 1 per cent theory, 100 per cent sweat (Guttridge 1997).

The intensity of the practice suited the lifestyles of the more affluent and career-focused, but who were also seeking both fitness and inner calm in their lives. Before founding his own centre, Ireland had taught yoga at the Skyros Centre, which had been founded by British people interested in personal development and the human potential movement, and which opened its doors on the Greek island of Skyros in 1979.

It was here, in the successful counter-culture holiday for those who had participated in mainstream culture enough to afford it, that John Scott encountered Ireland teaching Ashtanga Vinyasa Yoga in 1987. Ireland encouraged Scott to learn from Jois directly in Mysore, and the native New Zealander would go on to further popularise this form of intensive practice in Britain, teaching workshops throughout Britain from the 1990s onwards, including early-morning sessions in London which were popular with young working professionals. Scott produced a number of successful practice manuals for Jois's sequences and eventually settled in

Penzance, Cornwall, where he continues to work intensively with small groups of practitioners.[10]

The community of practitioners inspired by Jois's Ashtanga Vinyasa Yoga enjoy committing to an intense physical practice, usually done first thing in the morning. But often these practitioners are also interested in psychological transformations, personal ethics and in reading and developing the spiritual aspects of their understanding of yoga (Burger 2006; Byrne 2014; Smith 2007, 2008). Variants of the Ashtanga Vinyasa practice, where the sequences are broken down into teaching points, are sometimes described as 'Power Yoga' or 'Dynamic Yoga' on the 'drop-in' class lists of commercial yoga studios which became more prevalent in cities during the second half of the 1990s.[11]

The model of multiple classes in yoga studio premises also represented a continuity of older trends. The drop-in model perhaps began in the 1960s in Britain with Centre House and Gandalf's Garden. However, these early initiatives also recalled the eclecticism of the Theosophical Society and the Society for Psychical Research in the early years of the twentieth century. The overlap with other activities was also nothing new: yoga was offered as one of many activities in counter-cultural venues in the 1960s and '70s; Centre House was listed in the *Aquarian Guide to Occult, Mystical, Religious, Magical London and Around* (1970) as offering:

> HOMEOPATHY STUDY GROUP – SANSKRIT and JNANA YOGA GROUP – HATHA YOGA – EXPLORATIONS IN MEDITATION AND AWARENESS – MANTRA YOGA – DHYANA YOGA – GUNA YOGA – ZAZEN – RADIAESTHESIA – NATURAL HEALING (Strachan 1970: 25).

Multiple approaches to personal development were very much a part of the human potential movement and 'cultic milieu' of the 1970s, which Colin Campbell (1972) defined by fluid networks of seekers rather than adherence to any particular group. This later developed into the New Age movement and into various 'holistic' milieux in the twenty-first century (Hanegraaff 1998, 1999; Heelas

10. 'John Scott: Interview', UK Yoga People, 2001. 'About', John Scott, http://johnscottyoga.com/about.

11. For example, the yoga teaching of Godfrey Deveroux (1998, 2001), who was a manager at the Life Centre in the late 1990s, helping pioneer the schedule of all-day yoga classes that eventually led to a successful business model.

1996). While some yoga practitioners have overlapped with these social networks, yoga milieux also existed in other networks.

In many ways, however, the multi-style, drop-in, commercial yoga centre of the 1990s was a new development. One of the first manifestations was the Life Centre in Notting Hill, London, which opened its doors in 1993.[12] However, financial viability was a problem; it only really turned a profit after a change of ownership in the early twenty-first century.[13] Just before the turn of the century, two centres opened in London providing studio space for teachers of many different, often 'branded', yoga techniques: triyoga in Primrose Hill opened in 1999 and the Yoga Place in Bethnal Green in 2001.[14] Over time, their business model has proved sustainable, and several of the more successful centres have expanded into multiple premises.

To some extent, yoga teachers have always been entrepreneurs. However, from the mid-1990s onwards 'brands' and 'styles' of yoga began to vie for market share, particularly in the new yoga studios where you could try everything on offer. The inauguration of the 'Yoga Show' as an annual event in 2005 – an exhibition-hall fair of yoga styles, products and teachers – exemplifies this trend.[15] However, many of the most successful 'brands' had connections with earlier models, either through a continuity of the student–teacher exchange or through the adult-education context.

In this environment of commerciality and multiple branding, some contemporary British yoga practitioners in the early twenty-first century, who number hundreds of thousands in total, have anxieties and confusions about the authenticity of their practice. A evening symposium in November 2016 at triyoga on the subject of 'Authenticity in Yoga', aimed at yoga teachers and serious

12. 'About Us', The Life Centre, http://www.thelifecentre.com/welcome/about-us. Personal interview with Jonathan Sattin (19 June 2013).

13. The Life Centre Education Limited, company number 04375834, annual accounts and registration documents at Companies House, https://beta.companieshouse.gov.uk/company/04375834.

14. Personal interview with Jonathan Sattin (19 June 2013). Yoga Place E2 Limited, company number 04330372, annual accounts and registration documents at Companies House, https://beta.companieshouse.gov.uk/company/04330372.

15. OM Yoga Show, http://www.omyogashow.com. 'Listings', Time Out, 14 September 2005, p. 53.

practitioners, attracted an audience of 175.[16] Some in the Indian diaspora have also voiced concern about a lack of respect paid to the fact that yoga is experienced as the heart of Indian spirituality for many. The commercialisation, secularisation and sexualisation of contemporary yoga practices is also seen as disrespectful and morally repugnant to some committed yoga practitioners from other ethnic backgrounds as well.[17] Although an ongoing discussion, this narrative in Britain has not been as influential, nor received as much media coverage, as the Take Back Yoga campaign run by the Hindu American Foundation from 2008–14.[18] However, with Narendra Modi's election as prime minister of India, yoga has become closely associated with more political expressions of Indian nationalism. Also subject to debate is the extent to which yoga should be associated with political Hinduism, who can 'own' yoga, and the extent to which contemporary practitioners might be complicit in advancing Hindutva agendas (see Jain 2014b; McCartney 2017). The popularisation of yoga in Britain demonstrates how essentialist understandings of yoga are not based on historical evidence (see also Newcombe 2018). The popularisers of yoga in Britain included many individuals of Indian and British origin, the majority of whom interpreted yoga somewhat idiosyncratically while genuinely striving to promote a greater well-being for both individuals and society.

A further layer of complexity is added to the development of yoga in Britain by the slow establishment of a community of academics studying yoga from within European intellectual traditions. Some of the first work in this area included Joseph Alter's anthropological exploration of the development of yoga in India, alongside his other long-standing interests in Mahatma Gandhi and Indian wrestling traditions. In 2004, Alter's monograph *Yoga in Modern India* and Elizabeth de Michelis's *A History of Modern Yoga* both appeared, marking a seminal moment in the establishment of 'yoga studies'.

16. Triyoga, 'Authenticity in Yoga: A Discussion', 18 November 2016, https://www.youtube.com/watch?v=UPpZlX3w3lI. Triyoga, 'Cultural Appropriation in Yoga', 9 September 2017, https://soundcloud.com/triyogauk/04-cultural-appropriation-in-yoga. Personal communication with Genny Wilkinson-Priest (5 April 2017).

17. Keep Yoga Free, 2017, http://www.keepyogafree.co.uk. National Council of Hindu Temples (2016).

18. Hindu American Foundation, 'Take Back Yoga: Bringing to Light Yoga's Hindu Roots', https://www.hafsite.org/media/pr/takeyogaback.

The Dharam Hinduja Institute of Indic Research (in existence from 1995 to 2004) played a major role in initiating the study of modern yoga from an academic perspective. Based at the Faculty of Divinity at the University of Cambridge, this institute was an early leader in yoga studies and hosted an international conference on 'Yoga: The Indian Tradition' in 1988. Under the directorship of Elizabeth de Michelis (between 2000 and 2004), Cambridge became a focus for the establishment of this new subject. The initial stages of the research for this book was undertaken in this environment, as a doctoral study in the Faculty of History at Cambridge (2003–2007). Mark Singleton, who undertook his PhD under de Michelis's supervision at Cambridge during this period, published *Yoga Body* (2010), which explored the extent to which the contemporary postural practice of asana was influenced by European forms of physical culture in early-twentieth-century India. Singleton's book has triggered much discussion among yoga practitioners who feel both challenged and intrigued by the suggestion that some elements of contemporary posture-based yoga practice might have very recent, European influences (Remski 2015). With its increasing visibility and mainstream popularity, yoga has increasingly been explored by scholars of other disciplines including history, sociology, psychology, sports studies and religious studies.

A second intellectual tradition of yoga study in Britain has focused on philology and the translation of Sanskrit texts. Exemplifying this discipline in Britain are James Mallinson (2010) and Jason Birch (2011) who have been translating the Sanskrit haṭha texts, expanding our understanding of the Indian traditions of postural yoga. Based at the School of Oriental and African Studies (SOAS), University of London, Mallinson has headed a larger team under the Haṭha Yoga Project (HYP), a five-year European Research Council–funded project (2015–20). This project will build on Singleton and Mallinson's collaboration *Roots of Yoga* (Mallinson and Singleton 2017) which has brought new excerpts from historical yogic texts into the hands of contemporary practitioners. The HYP (2015–20) will combine research on the history of postural yoga practices in Sanskrit texts with artistic and architectural evidence, as well as an element of contemporary ethnography to better chart the history of physical yoga practices.[19] Related to this initiative was the establish-

19. Haṭha Yoga Project, http://hyp.soas.ac.uk.

ment of the Master of Arts in Traditions of Yoga and Meditation and the founding of a Centre of Yoga Studies at the SOAS in May 2018; both of these initiatives draw on a large population of committed yoga practitioners interested in learning more about the history and context of their contemporary practices.

A second European Research Council–funded project, Entangled Histories of Yoga, Ayurveda and Alchemy in South Asia (Ayuryog) (2015–20), seeks to explore historical traditions of yoga in a different framework by exploring overlaps and entanglements of yoga with the Indian medical and alchemical traditions (Ayurveda and *rasaśāstra*) from the tenth century to the present, focusing on the disciplines' health, rejuvenation and longevity practices.[20] The later part of the research on this book was supported by my being employed on this research project, which was primarily based at the University of Vienna. The growth of academic study and the integration of this knowledge into the communities of yoga practitioners is likely to have a profoundly transformative effect on the self-understandings of yoga practitioners in the twenty-first century.

Some have criticised modern forms of yoga for applying a sticking plaster over the uncertainties of modern life, allowing people to tolerate insecure working environments and growing income inequality, rather than aiming for deep personal transformation or radical social change (Schnäbele 2010). Others, however, have emphasised overlaps with various charitable and environmental projects, and the space yoga practice gives for non-normative bodies and minds to find peace and become more self-established (Klein and Guest-Jelley 2014; Wong 2017). Yoga has also shown itself to be subject to the same moral and at times criminal abuses of authority that have surfaced in a variety of new and established religious movements.[21] It is clear that yoga has been a useful tool for many people suffering from chronic pain; even where it cannot replace the biomedical model, it can offer some a new relationship with their body which enables them to transform their experience in positive ways (Garrett 2001).

20. 'Entangled Histories of Yoga, Ayurveda and Alchemy in South Asia', Ayuryog, http://ayuryog.org.
21. See Remski (2019), Lucia (2018), Caldwell (2001), Crovetto (2008), Dwyer and Cole (2007), Deslippe (2012) and Voix (2008), among other literature dealing with criminal and ethical problems in yoga groups.

The practice of yoga is not entirely without risk of harm. But people continue to practise it because it works for them on many different levels. For most yoga practitioners, it is the embodied, personal experience and not an ideology or dogma that attracts them. The experience of practising yoga in Britain sits ambiguously between an apparent dichotomy between the secular and the religious, the physical and the spiritual. Some contemporary practitioners find meaning and new understandings of themselves in relation to others from the most physical of practices; others prefer to focus on yoga as a philosophy or mental discipline. Yoga is not one thing to all people – and, even for the individual, it often defies simple categorisation or intellectual explanation.

Perhaps this book can offer insights into the authority and legitimacy of the yoga tradition in Britain today. Its fundamental contribution, I would argue, is to highlight what a complicated and multi-layered phenomenon yoga is. Authority for teaching these practices might derive from a variety of sources: teaching lineages, personal experience, or an ability to place the practices into a historical and sociological context. Understanding and appreciating the variety of meanings and approaches to yoga there has been in Britain is one way of being respectful to both yoga's roots in the Indian subcontinent and the complexity of its current forms.

Bibliography

Archival Sources

Allen & Unwin Archive, University of Reading
Birmingham Central Library
BBC Written Archives Centre, University of Reading
British Film Institute Archive
General Register Office
Iyengar Yoga Institute (Maida Vale), London
Lexis-Nexis Newspaper Archive
London Metropolitan Archive
Manchester Archives and Local Studies, Manchester Central Library
Mary Ward Centre, London
Penguin Archives, University of Bristol Special Collections
Ramamani Iyengar Memorial Yoga Institute (RIMYI), Pune, India
Staffordshire Record Office
Ken Thompson's personal collection
Warburg Institute, University of London
William Salt Local Studies Library, Stafford

Newspapers, Magazines and Journals

Adult Education (1955–89)
Bhavan's Journal
Bulletin of the Yoga Research Centre (Department of Anthropology, Durham University, 1979)
Cosmopolitan (1972–80)
Floodlight (London: LCC) (1955–95)
Gandalf's Garden (1969–71)
Health & Strength
International Psychic Gazette (1910–20)
Shanti-Sadan Bulletin (1935–41)
Shanti Sevak: A Quarterly Magazine (1942–49)
She (1970–90)
Spectrum: Journal of the British Wheel of Yoga (1979–present)
The Times Digital Archive (1785–1985)
Vedanta For East and West (1952–61)
Yoga Awareness: Quarterly Journal of Yococen (1977)
Yoga & Health (1971–75)
Yoga: Journal of the British Wheel of Yoga (1969–79)
Yoga Today (1976–89) continued as *Yoga and Health* (1990–present)

272 *Yoga in Britain*

Published Sources

Akhtar, M. and S. Humphries (2001). *The Fifties and Sixties: A Lifestyle Revolution*. London: Boxtree.

Alain (Max Alain Schwendiman) (1957). *Yoga for Perfect Health*. London: Thorsons.

Albanese, C. (2007). *A Republic of Mind and Spirit: A Cultural History of American Metaphysical Religion*. New Haven, CN: Yale University Press.

Aldrich, Auretta Roys (1904). *Life and How to Live It*. London: Gale & Polden.

Ališauskienė, M. (2009). 'Spirituality and Religiosity in the Art of Living Foundation in Lithuania and Denmark: Meanings, Contexts and Relationships', 339–64 in C. Williams et al. (eds.), *Subcultures and New Religious Movements in Russia and East-Central Europe*. London: Peter Lang.

Alston. A.J. (1980–89). *A Śaṅkara Source-Book*, vols. 1–6. London: Shanti Sadan.

Alter, J. (2000). *Gandhi's Body: Sex, Diet, and the Politics of Nationalism*. Philadelphia, PA: University of Pennsylvania Press.

– (2004a). *Yoga in Modern India: The Body between Science and Philosophy*. Princeton, NJ: Princeton University Press.

– (2004b). 'Indian Clubs and Colonialism: Hindu Masculinity and Muscular Christianity'. *Comparative Studies in Society and History* 46: 497–534.

Altglas, V. (2005a). 'Neo-Hinduism in the West between Religion and Psychology. The Innerworldly Reinterpretation of a Religious Path'. Paper presented at Recherches Epistémologiques et Historiques sur les Sciences (REHSEIS) Conférence (15 February).

– (2005b). *Le nouvel hindouisme occidental*. Paris: Éditions du CNRS.

– (2014). *From Yoga to Kabbalah: Religious Exoticism and the Logics of Bricolage*. Oxford: Oxford University Press.

Anderson, B. (1983). *Imagined Communities: Reflections on the Origin and Spread of Nationalism*. London: Verso.

Anderson, J. (2004). 'Fowler, Eileen Philippa Rose (1906–2000)'. *Oxford Dictionary of National Biography*. Oxford: Oxford University Press.

Annett, S. (1976). *Many Ways of Being A Guide to Spiritual Groups and Growth Centres in Britain*. London: Turnstone Books.

Arnold, M. (1964). *Passages from the Prose Writings of Matthew Arnold: Selected by the Author William E. Buckler*. London: Vision.

Atkinson, P. (1985). 'Strong Minds and Weak Bodies: Sports, Gymnastics and the Medicalization of Women's Education'. *British Journal of Sports History* 2: 62–71.

Avalon, A. (1917). *The Serpent Power Being the Shat-chakra-nirūpana and Pādukā-panchaka*. London: Luzac.

Badman, K. (2000). *Beatles off the Record*. London: Omnibus.

– (2004). *The Beach Boys: The Definitive Diary of the America's Greatest Band on Stage and in the Studio*. Milwaukee, WI: Backbeat Books.

Baier, K. (2009). *Meditation und Moderne. Zur Genese eines Kernbereichs moderner Spiritualität in der Wechselwirkung von Zur Genese eines Kernbereichs moderner Spiritualität in der Wechselwirkung zwischen Westeuropa, Nordamerika und Asien.* [Meditation and Modernity: About the Genesis of a Core Area of

Modern Spirituality and the interactions between Western Europe, North America and Asia], 2 vols. Würzburg: Königshausen & Neumann.

– (2012). 'Mesmeric Yoga and the Development of Meditation within the Theosophical Society'. *Theosophical History: A Quarterly Journal of Research,* 16/3–4: 150–61.

– (2016a). 'Theosophical Orientalism and the Structures of Intercultural Transfer: Annotations on the Appropriation of the Cakras in Early Theosophy', in Julie Chajes and Boaz Huss (eds.), *Theosophical Appropriations: Esotericism, Kabbalah, and the Transformation of Traditions.* Beer Sheva, Ben-Gurion University of the Negev Press.

– (2016b). ' "Das Evangelium der Entspannung": Euroamerikanische Entspannungskultur und die Genese des modernen Yoga' [' "The Gospel of Relaxation": Euro-American Relaxation Culture and the Genesis of Modern Yoga']. *Entspannungsverfahren. Zeitschrift der Deutschen Gesellschaft für Entspannungsverfahren* (DG-E e.V.) 33: 45–63.

– (2018). 'Yoga within Viennese Occultism: Carl Kellner and Co.', 387–438, in *Yoga in Transformation: Historical and Contemporary Perspectives on a Global Phenomenon,* conference proceedings volume in 'Wiener Forum für Theologie und Religionswissenschaft' ('Viennese Forum for Theology and the Study of Religions') series. Göttingen: V&R University Press. Available at: https://www.academia.edu/33373168/Carl_Kellner_on_Yoga

Bainbridge, W.S. (1997). *The Sociology of Religious Movements.* London: Routledge.

Baines, P. (2005). *Penguin by Design: A Cover Story.* London: Allen Lane.

Balaskas, A. (1975). *Every Body Knows: Yoga Demystified.* London: BBC.

– (1977). *Bodylife.* London: Book Club Associates.

Balaskas, A. and J. Balaskas (1979). *New Life: The Book of Exercises for Childbirth.* London: Sidgwick & Jackson.

Banerji, S.C. (1995). *Studies in Origin and Development of Yoga.* Calcutta: Punthi Pustak.

Barker, E. (1989). *New Religious Movements: A Practical Introduction.* London: HMSO.

Barua, A. (2016). 'The British Amnesia of Empire: Reflections on School Curricula in India and the UK'. Self-published essay. Available at: https://www.academia.edu/29708439/The_British_Amnesia_of_Empire_Reflections_on_school_curricula_in_India_and_the_UK

Beatles, The. (2000). *The Beatles Anthology.* London: Cassell & Co.

Beckerlegge, G. (2000). *The Ramakrishna Mission: The Making of a Modern Hindu Movement.* New Delhi: Oxford University Press.

– (2004). 'The Early Spread of Vedanta Societies: An Example of "Imported Localism" '. *Numen* 51: 296–320.

– (2014). 'Eknath Ranade, Gurus and Jivanvratis: Vivekananda Kendra's Promotion of the "Yogic Way of Life" ', 327–50, in Mark Singleton and Ellen Goldberg (eds.), *Gurus of Modern Yoga.* New York: Oxford University Press.

Beckman, S. (1990). 'Professionalization: Borderline Authority and Autonomy in Work', 155–138 in M. Burrage and R. Torstendhal (eds.), *Professions in Theory and History: Rethinking the Study of the Professions.* London: Sage:

Beaman, L.G. and S. Sikka (eds.) (2016). *Constructions of Self and Other in Yoga, Travel and Tourism: A Journey to Elsewhere*. London: Palgrave.

Benson, J. (1997). *Prime Time: A History of the Middle Aged in Twentieth-Century Britain*. London: Longman.

- (2005). *Affluence and Authority: A Social History of Twentieth Century Britain*. London: Hodder Educational.

Berg, V. (1981). *Yoga in Pregnancy*. London: Watkins.

Berger, P. (1990 [1967]). *The Sacred Canopy: Elements of a Sociological Theory of Religion*. New York: Anchor Books.

Berlant, J.L. (1975). *Profession and Monopoly: A Study of Medicine in the United States and Great Britain*. London: University of California Press.

Bernard, T. (1939). *Heaven Lies Within Us: Yoga Gave Me Superior Health*. London: Rider.

- (1941) *Heaven Lies Within Us* [*On Yoga*]. London: Rider.

- (1950). *Hatha Yoga: A Report of a Personal Experience*. London: Rider.

Besant, A. (1908). *Introduction to Yoga. Four Lectures*. London: Theosophical Publishing Society.

Birch, J. (2011). 'The Meaning of Haṭha in Early Haṭhayoga'. *Journal of the American Oriental Society* 131/4: 527–554.

- (2013). 'Rājayoga: The Reincarnations of the King of All Yogas'. *International Journal of Hindu Studies* 17/3: 401–44.

- (2018) 'Premodern Yoga Traditions and Ayurveda'. *History of Science in South Asia* 6: 1-83. https://doi.org/10.18732/hssa.v6i0.25

Bogdan, H. (2006). 'Challenging the Morals of Western Society: The Use of Ritualised Sex in Contemporary Occultism'. *The Pomegranate: The International Journal of Pagan Studies* 8/2: 211–46.

- (2010). 'Introduction', in *Brother Curwen, Brother Crowley: A Correspondence*. York Beach, ME: Teitan Press.

- (2013). 'Reception of Occultism in India: The Case of the Holy Order of Krishna', 177-202, in Gordon Djurdjevic and Henrik Bogdan (eds.), *Occultism in a Global Perspective*. London: Routledge.

Bogdan, H. and Martin P. Starr (eds.) (2012). *Aleister Crowley and Western Esotericism*. New York: Oxford University Press.

Bordas, L. (2011). 'Mircea Eliade as Scholar of Yoga: A Historical Study of His Reception (1936-1954)', in Irina Vainovski-Mihai (ed.), *New Europe College Ştefan Odobleja Program Yearbook 2010-2011*. Bucharest: New Europe College.

- (2016). 'Yoga între magic şi mistic. Reflecţie hermeneutică şi experienţă religioasă la primul Eliade'. *Studii de istorie a filosofiei româneşti* XII. Bucharest: Editura Academiei Române.

Bourque, J. (2010). *Robes of Silk, Feet of Clay*. Self-published, Printing Partners, Lithuania.

Boyd, J. (2005). *White Bicycles: Making Music in the 1960s*. London: Serpent's Tail.

British Wheel of Yoga (1973). *Yoga Handbook 1973*. A5 booklet. British Wheel of Yoga.

Broad, W. (2012). *The Science of Yoga: The Risks and the Rewards*. New York: Simon & Schuster.

Bronkhorst, J. (1981). 'Yoga Seśvara Sāṃkhya'. *Journal of Indian Philosophy* 9: 309–20.

- (1998). *The Two Sources of Indian Asceticism*. 2nd edn. Delhi: Motilal Banarsidass.
Brook, D. (1976). *Naturebirth: Preparing for Natural Birth in an Age of Technology*. London: Penguin.
Brooks, C.W. (1986). *Pettyfoggers and Vipers of the Commonwealth: The 'Lower Branch' of the Legal Profession in Early Modern England*. Cambridge: Cambridge University Press.
Brown, C. (2001). *The Death of Christian Britain*. London: Routledge.
Bruley, S. (1999). *Women in Britain Since 1900*. London: Palgrave.
Brunton, P. (1934). *A Search in Secret India*. London: Rider & Co.
Bucke, R.M. (1901). *Cosmic Consciousness: A Study in the Evolution of the Human Mind*. E.P. Dutton & Company, Inc.
Burger, M. (2006). 'What Price Salvation? The Exchange of Salvation Goods between India and the West'. *Social Compass* 53: 81–95.
- (2013). 'Sāṃkhya Interpretation in a Transnational Perspective: Śrī Anirvāṇa and Lizelle Reymond'. Paper presented at Yoga in Transformation: Historical and Contemporary Perspectives on a Global Phenomenon conference, University of Vienna (20 September).
Burgess, J. (1968). 'Training the Part-time Craft Teacher'. *Adult Education* 41 (July).
Burnham, J.C. (1998). *How the Idea of Profession Changed the Writing of Medical History*. London: Wellcome Institute for the History of Medicine.
Burrage, M. and R. Torstendhal (eds.) (1990). *Professions in Theory and History: Rethinking the Study of Professions*. London: Sage.
Busia, K. (2007). *Iyengar: The Yoga Master*. London: Shambala.
Byrne, J. (2014). ' "Authorized by Sri K. Pattabhi Jois": The Role of Parampara and Lineage in Ashtanga Vinyasa Yoga', in M. Singleton and E. Goldberg (eds.), *Gurus of Modern Yoga*. New York: Oxford University Press.
Cabral, S. (1965). *Pranayama Yoga: The Art of Relaxation*. Walsall: Yoga Relaxation Centre.
- (1971 [2002]). *Pranayama Yoga: The Art of Relaxation*. Repr. of 3rd edn. Eckington: Lotus and the Rose Publishers.
- (2002 [196?]). 'The Art of Relaxation'. Audio cassette. Eckington: Lotus and the Rose Publishers.
- (2012). *Pranayama Yoga: The Art of Relaxation*. 4th edn. Eckington: Lotus and the Rose Publishers.
Caldwell, S. (2001). 'The Heart of the Secret: A Personal and Scholarly Encounter with Shakta Tantrism in Siddha Yoga'. *Nova Religio* 5: 9–51.
Campbell, B.F. (1980). *Ancient Wisdom Revived: A History of the Theosophical Movement*. Berkeley, CA: University of California Press.
Campbell, C. (1972). 'The Cult, the Cultic Milieu and Secularization'. *A Sociological Yearbook of Religion in Britain* 5: 119–36.
- (1978). 'The Secret Religion of the Educated Classes'. *Sociological Analysis* 39: 146–56.
- (1999). 'The Easternization of the West', 35–48, in B. Wilson and J. Cresswell (eds.), *New Religious Movements: Challenge and Response*. London: Routledge.
- (2007). *The Easternization of the West: A Thematic Account of Cultural Change in the Modern Era*. London: Paradigm Publishers.

Cantú, K. (2016a). 'Śrī Sabhāpati Swami: The Forgotten Yogi of Western Eso-tericism'. Paper presented at the American Academy of Religion annual meeting in San Antonio, Texas, November 2016 (with slight revisions).

– (2016b). 'The Essential Image in Sabhapati Swami's Lifework and an Inquiry into its Resemblance to Bengali Yogic Practice'. Paper presented at the Yoga Darśana, Yoga Sādhana: Traditions, Transmissions, Transformations con-ference in Kraków, Poland, 19–21 May 2016.

Carter, M. (2004). 'New Poses for Macho Men'. *The Times* (London), 22 May, Issue 68082: S3, 14.

Chance, J. (1992). *The Lord of the Rings: The Mythology of Power*. New York: Twayne Publishers.

Chitty, C. (2004). *Education Policy in Britain*. Basingstoke: Palgrave Macmillan.

Clark, M. (2017). *The Tawny One: Soma, Haoma and Ayahuasca*. London: Muswell Hill Press.

Clark, P. (2004). *Hope and Glory: Britain 1900–2000*. 2nd edn, London: Penguin.

Clark, W. (n.d.) *History of Yoga in Britain*. Solihull: Wheel of British Yoga.

Clay, J. (1996). *R.D. Laing: A Divided Self. A Biography*. London: Hodder & Stoughton.

Clayson, A. (2001). *George Harrison*. London: Sanctuary.

Cleave, M. (2006 [1966]). ' "How Does a Beatle Live? John Lennon Lives Like This". *Evening Standard* (London), 4 March 1966', 85–91, in J. Skinner Saun-ders (ed.), *Read the Beatles*. London: Penguin.

Cole, B. (1976). *John Coltrane*. London: Collier Macmillan Publishers.

Colebatch, H.K. (1990). *Return of the Heroes: The Lord of the Rings, Star Wars and Contemporary Culture*. Perth: Australian Institute for Public Policy.

Collins, M. (2005). *Osteopathy in Britain: The First Hundred Years*. Charleston, SC: Booksurge.

Coney, J. (1999). *Sahaja Yoga: Socializing Processes in a South Asian New Religious Movement*. Richmond: Curzon Press.

Cook, H. (2005). *The Long Sexual Revolution: English Women, Sex, and Contracep-tion 1800–1975*. Oxford: Oxford University Press.

Crisp, T. (1975 [1976, 1977]). *Yoga and Childbirth*. Wellingborough: Thorsons.

Crovetto, H. (2008). 'Ananda Marga and the Use of Force'. *Nova Religio: The Journal of Alternative and Emergent Religions* 12/1 (August): 26–56.

Crowley, A. (1913). *Book Four*. By Frater Perdurabo (Aleister Crowley) and Soror Virakam (Mary D'este Sturges). London: Wieland & Co..

– (1939). *Eight Lectures on Yoga* [written under the pseudonym Mahatma Guru Sri Paramahansa Shivaji] being *The Equinox* 3/4. London: O.T.O.

Curry, P. (1997). *Defining Middle-Earth: Tolkien, Myth and Modernity*. New York: St Martin's.

Curtis, B. (2016). 'A "National Occupational Standard" for Yoga Teachers?'. *Keep Yoga Free*, 13 November. Available at: http://www.keepyogafree. co.uk/articles_files/national-occupational-standard-yoga.html

Cusack, C. and S. Sutcliffe (2017). *Gurdjieff: A Critical Introduction*. London: Rou-tledge.

Davies, H. (1966). *The New London Spy*. London: Corgi Books.

De Michelis, E. (2004). *A History of Modern Yoga: Patañjali and Western Esoteri-cism*. London: Continuum.

Desikachar, K. (2005). *The Yoga of the Yogi: The Legacy of T. Krishnamacharya.* Chennai, India: Krishnamacharya Yoga Mandiram.

Desikachar, T.K.V. (1998). *Health, Healing and Beyond: Yoga and the Living Tradition of Krishnamacharya.* New York: Aperture.

Deslippe, P. (2011). *The Kybalion: The Definitive Edition.* New York: Jeremy P. Tarcher/Penguin.

– (2012). 'From Maharaj to Mahan Tantric: The Construction of Yogi Bhajan's Kundalini Yoga'. *Sikh Formations* 8: 369–87.

– (2018). 'The Swami Circuit'. *Journal of Yoga Studies* 1: 5–44 (May). Available at: https://journalofyogastudies.org/index.php/JoYS/article/view/2018. v1.Deslippe.TheSwamiCircuit, accessed 22 June 2018.

Desponds, S. (2007) 'L'enseignant de yoga européen entre *adhikāra* et pédagogie: Une analyse de la qualification socio-religieuse des enseignants dans la rencontre entre l'Union européenne de yoga et le lignage de T. Krishnamacharya'. PhD thesis. Université de Lausanne, Faculté des lettres.

Deveroux, G. (1988). *Dynamic Yoga: The Ultimate Workout that Chills Your Mind as it Changes Your Body.* London: Thorsons.

– (2001). *Hatha Yoga: Breath by Breath.* London: Thorsons.

Devi, I. (1955 [USA 1953]). *Forever Young, Forever Healthy.* Blackpool: A. Thomas.

– (1965 [USA 1963]). *Renew Your Life through Yoga.* London: George Allen & Unwin.

Dhyansky, Y. (1987). 'The Indus Valley Origin of a Yoga Practice'. *Artibus Asiae* 48: 89–108.

Diamond, D. (ed.) (2013). *Yoga: The Art of Transformation.* Washington, DC: Freer Gallery of Art and the Arthur M. Sackler Gallery.

Dick-Read, G. (1960). *Childbirth Without Fear.* London: William Heinemann Medical Books.

Dixon, Joy. (2001). *Divine Feminism: Theosophy and Feminism in England.* Baltimore, MD: Johns Hopkins University Press.

Djurdjevic, G. (2012). 'The Great Beast as a Tantric Hero: The Role of Yoga and Tantra in Aleister Crowley's Magick', 107–140, in Henrik Bogdan and Martin P. Starr (eds.), *Aleister Crowley and Western Esotericism.* New York: Oxford University Press.

– (2014). *India and the Occult: The Influence of South Asian Spirituality on Modern Western Occultism.* London: Palgrave.

Dukes, P. (1938). The Story of 'ST 25'. London: Cassell.

– (1940). *An Epic of the Gestapo.* London: Cassell.

– (1947). *Come Hammer, Come Sickle!* London: Cassell.

– (1950). *The Unending Quest: Autobiographical Sketches.* London: Cassell & Co.

– (1953). *Yoga for the Western World.* Parow, South Africa: Cape Times.

– (1960). *The Yoga of Health, Youth and Joy. A Treatise on Hatha Yoga Adapted for the West.* London: Cassell & Co.

Dunne, D. (1951). *Yoga for Everyman: How to Have Long Life and Happiness.* London: Duckworth.

– (1959). *The Manual of Hypnotism.* London: Foulsham & Co.

– (1962). *Yoga Made Easy.* London: Souvenir Press.

Dwyer, G. and R.J. Cole (2007). *The Hare Krishna Movement: Forty Years of Chant and Change.* London: I.B. Tauris.

Eagle, R. (1978). *Alternative Medicine: A Guide to the Medical Underground*. London: BBC.

Eliade, M. (1954). *Yoga, Immortality and Freedom*. Trans. Willard Trask. Princeton, NJ: Princeton University Press.

– (1963). 'Yoga and Modern Philosophy'. *Journal of General Education* 15: 124–37.

Ellwood, R. (2002). *Frodo's Quest: Living the Myth in the Lord of the Rings*. Wheaton, IL: Theosophical Society Publishing House.

Faithfull, M. (1995). *Faithfull*. London: Michael Joseph.

Farnell, K. (2005). *Mystical Vampire: The Life and Works of Mabel Collins*. Oxford: Mandrake.

Fisher, R. (2000). 'Obituary: Peter McIntosh: Historian of the Social Science of Sport'. *The Guardian* (London), 14 August, p. 18

FitzRoy, Almaric (1905) *Report of the Inter-departmental Committee on Physical Deterioration*. London: HMSO.

Fleming, R.P. (1934). *One's Company: A Journey to China*. London: Jonathan Cape.

Fletcher, S. (1984). *Women First: The Female Tradition in English Physical Education 1880–1980*. London: The Athlone Press.

Fonda, J. (2005). *My Life So Far*. London: Ebury Press.

Forsthoefel, T.A. (2005). 'Weaving the Inward Thread to Awakening: The Perennial Appeal of Ramana Maharshi', in T. Forsthoefel and C.A. Humes (eds.), *Gurus in America*. Albany, NY: State University of New York Press (SUNY).

Foxen, A. (2017). *The Biography of a Yogi: Paramahansa Yogananda and the Origins of Modern Yoga*. New York: Oxford University Press.

Fraim, J. (1996). *Spirit Catcher: The Life and Art of John Coltrane*. West Liberty, OH: Greathouse.

Fulder, S. (1992). 'Alternative Therapists in Britain', 166–82, in Mike Saks (ed.), *Alternative Medicine in Britain*. Oxford: Clarendon Press.

Galbraith, J.K. (1958). *The Affluent Society*. London: Hamish Hamilton.

Garfinkel, M. (1987). 'Robert's Story', 388–393, in M. Manos (ed.), *Iyengar: His Life and Work*. Porthill, ID: Timeless Books.

Garrett, C. (2001). 'Transcendental Meditation, Reiki and Yoga: Suffering, Ritual and Self-Transformation'. *Journal of Contemporary Religion* 16: 329–42.

Geaves, R. (2004). 'From Divine Light Mission to Elan Vital and Beyond: An Exploration of Change and Adaptation'. *Nova Religio* 7: 45–62.

– (2007). 'From Totapuri to Prem Rawat: Reflections on a Lineage (*Parampara*)', 265–90, in A. King (ed.), *Indian Religions: Renaissance and Renewal*. London: Equinox.

– (2009). 'Forget Transmitted Memory: The De-traditionalised "Religion" of Prem Rawat'. *Journal of Contemporary Religion* 24: 19–33 .

Gershuny, J. and K. Fisher (2000). 'Leisure', in A.H. Halsey (ed.), *Twentieth Century British Social Trends*. 3rd edn, London Macmillan.

Gilbert, R.A. (2004). 'Watkins, Geoffrey Maurice (1896–1981)'. *Oxford Dictionary of National Biography*. Available at: http://www.oxforddnb.com/view/article/53853

- (2009). 'The Great Chain of Unreason: The Publication and Distribution of the Literature of Rejected Knowledge in England during the Victorian Era'. PhD dissertation, University of London.

Giuliano, G. (1989). *Dark Horse: The Secret Life of George Harrison*. London: Pan.

Godwin, J. (1994). *Theosophical Enlightenment*. Albany, NY: SUNY Press.

Gold, J. (1969). *Yoga for Health and Beauty*. London: Thorsons.

Goldberg, E. (2016). *The Path of Modern Yoga: The History of an Embodied Spiritual Practice*. Rochester, VT: Inner Traditions.

Goldberg, M. (2015). *Goddess Pose: The Audacious Life of Indra Devi, the Woman Who Helped Bring Yoga to the West*. London: Alfred A. Knopf.

Goldman, M. (1999). *Passionate Journeys: Why Successful Women Joined a Cult*. Ann Arbor, MI: University of Michigan Press.

- (2012). *The American Soul Rush: Esalen and the Rise of Spiritual Privilege*. London: New York University Press.

Green, J. (1988). *Days in the Life: Voices from the English Underground, 1961–1971*. London: William Heinemann.

- (1999). *All Dressed Up: The Sixties and the Counter Culture*. London: Pimlico.

Greene, J.M. (2005). *Here Comes the Sun: The Spiritual and Musical Journey of George Harrison*. John Wiley & Sons, Inc., Hoboken, NJ.

Greer, G. (1970). *The Female Eunuch*. London: MacGibbon & Key.

Guttridge, P. (1997). 'Sun, Sea And Sweat: Yoga with a Kick'. *The Independent*, 9 February. Available at: http://www.independent.co.uk/money/sun-sea-and-sweat-yoga-with-a-kick-1277659.html

- (1998). 'Obituary: Derek Ireland'. *The Independent*, 27 September. Available at: http://www.independent.co.uk/arts-entertainment/obituary-derek-ireland-1201093.html

Hackett, P. (2012). *Theos Bernard, the White Lama: Tibet, Yoga, and American Religious Life*. New York: Columbia University Press.

Hall, Charles A. (1903a). *The Art of Being Happy*. Paisley: Alexander Gardner.

- (1903b). *The Art of Being Healthy*. Paisley: Alexander Gardner.

- (1908). *The Manly Life and How to Live It*. London: Simpkin, Marshall, Hamilton, Kent & Co.

Hamilton, M. (2002). 'The Easternization Thesis: Critical Reflections'. *Religion* 32: 243–58.

Hamlin, C. (1994). 'State Medicine in Great Britain', 132–64, in D. Porter (ed.), *History of Public Health and the Modern State*. Amsterdam: Rodopi.

Hanegraaff, W. (1998). *New Age Religion and Western Culture: Esotericism in the Mirror of Secular Thought*. Albany, NY: State University of New York Press.

- (1999). 'New Age Spiritualities as Secular Religion'. *Social Compass* 46: 145–60.

Hargreaves, J. (1993). *Sporting Females: Critical Issues in the History and Sociology of Women's Sport*. London: Routledge.

Harris, J. (1961). 'The Development of the Keep Fit Association of England and Wales'. *Physical Education* 53: 38–43

Harrison, G. (2002 [1980]). *I Me Mine*. London: Phoenix.

Hasselle-Newcombe, S. (2005). 'Spirituality and 'Mystical Religion', 305–21, in Contemporary Society: A Case Study of British Practitioners of the Iyengar Method of Yoga'. *Journal of Contemporary Religion* 20.

Hauser, B. (ed.) (2013). *Yoga Traveling: Bodily Practice in Transcultural Perspective*. London: Springer.

Healy, J. (2010). *Yearning to Belong: Discovering a New Religious Movement*. Aldershot: Ashgate.

Heelas, P. (1996). *The New Age Movement: The Celebration of the Self and the Sacralization of Modernity*. Blackwell, London.

Heelas, P., L. Woodhead et al. (2005). *The Spiritual Revolution: Why Religion Is Giving Way to Spirituality*. London: Blackwell.

Hennock, E.P. (1987). *British Social Reform and German Precedents: The Case of Social Insurance 1880–1914*. Oxford: Clarendon Press.

Herlihy, D. (2004). *Bicycle: The History*. New Haven, CT: Yale University Press.

Hill, T. and M. Clayton (2000). *The Beatles Unseen Archives*. London: Parragon.

Hills, C. (1977 [1968]). *Nuclear Evolution: Discovery of the Rainbow Body*. Planetary Publishing Company.

Hittleman, R. (1962). *Be Young with Yoga*. Englewood Cliffs, NJ: Prentice Hall.

– (1964). *Yoga for Physical Fitness*. Preston: A. Thomas & Co.

Hoare, S. (1985). *Yoga and Pregnancy*. London: Unwin Paperbacks.

Hobsbawm, E. (1994). *Age of Extremes: The Short Twentieth Century 1914–1991*. London: Abacus.

Hopkins, J. (2000). *Ginsberg in London*. London: Andrew Sclanders.

Horton, C. and R. Harvey (2012). *21st Century Yoga: Culture, Politics, and Practice*. Chicago: Kleio Books.

Huggins, M. (2001). 'Walking in the Footsteps of a Pioneer. Peter McIntosh: Trail-blazer in the History of Sport'. *International Journal of the History of Sport* 18: 136–47.

Hughes, M. (1973). 'Educating Women'. *Adult Education* 46.

Humes, C.A. (2005). 'Maharishi Mahesh Yogi: Beyond the TM Technique', in T. Forsthoefel and C.A. Humes (eds.), *Gurus in America*. Albany, NY: State University of New York Press.

Humphries, J. (2000). 'Women and Paid Work', in J. Purvis (ed.), *Women's History: Britain 1850–1945*. London: University College London Press.

Hurst, K.T. (1989). *Paul Brunton: A Personal View*. New York: Burdett.

Huxley, A. (1942). *The Perennial Philosophy*. New York: Harper Brothers.

– (1962). *Island*. London: Chatto & Windus.

Ingham, M. (1981). *Now We Are Thirty: Women of the Breakthrough Generation*. London: Eyre Methuen.

Inglis, B. (1964). *Fringe Medicine*. London: Faber & Faber.

– (1979). *Natural Medicine*. London: Collins.

International Society for Krishna Consciousness (ISKCON) (1982). *Chant and Be Happy… The Story of the Hare Krishna Mantra Based on the Teachings of His Divine Grace A.C. Bhaktivedanta Swami Prabhupaada. New Exclusive George Harrison Interview*. London: The Bhaktivedanta Book Trust.

Iyengar, B.K.S. (1966). *Light on Yoga*. London: George Allen & Unwin.

– (1988a). 'My Yogic Journey: A Talk given by Guruji on his 70th Birthday 14 December 1988 at Tilak Smarak Mandir, Pune'. Archives of the Iyengar Yoga Institute, Maida Vale, London.

– (1988b). *Yoga Vṛkṣa: Tree of Yoga*. Ed. Daniel Rivers-Moore. Oxford: Fine Line Books.

- (1993a). *Light on the Yoga Sutras of Patañjali*. London: Aquarius Books.
- (1993b). *The Art of Yoga*. London: HarperCollins.
- (n.d.) Typewritten autobiographical manuscript (an account from birth to 1954, but only written after 1958) in the archives of Maida Vale Iyengar Yoga Institute, London.
Iyengar, B.K.S., J.J. Evans and D. Abrams (2005). *Light on Life: The Yoga Journey to Wholeness, Inner Peace, and Ultimate Freedom*. London: Rodale Books.
Iyengar, G. (1978). 'Yoga Therapeutics', 183–4, in BKS Iyengar 60th Anniversary Celebration Committee (ed.), *Yoga the Shrine, Body thy Light*. Bombay: B.I. Taraporewala.
- (1990). *Yoga: A Gem for Women*. Palo Alto, CA: Timeless Books.
Jackson, C.T. (1975). 'New Thought Movement and the Nineteenth Century Discovery of Oriental Philosophy'. *Journal of Popular Culture* 9: 523–48.
- (1981). *Oriental Religions in American Thought: Nineteenth Century Explorations*. Westport, CN: Greenwood Press.
Jackson, I. (1978). 'Running', 136–46, in BKS Iyengar 60th Birthday Celebration Committee (ed.), *Body the Shrine, Yoga thy Light*. Bombay: B.I. Taraporewala.
Jacobs, S. (2015). *The Art of Living Foundation: Spirituality and Wellbeing in the Global Context*. Aldershot: Ashgate.
Jacobsh, D. (2008). '3HO/Sikh Dharma of the Western Hemisphere: The "Forgotten" New Religious Movement?'. *Religion Compass* 2: 385–408. doi: 10.1111/j.1749-8171.2008.00068.x
Jain, A. (2012). 'Branding Yoga: The Cases of Iyengar Yoga, Siddha Yoga, and Anusara Yoga'. *Approaching Religion* 2: 3–17.
- (2014a). 'Muktananda: Entrepreneurial Godman, Tantric Hero', in E. Goldeberg and M. Singleton (eds.), *Gurus of Modern Yoga*. New York: Oxford University Press.
- (2014b). 'Who Is to Say Modern Yoga Practitioners Have It All Wrong? On Hindu Origins and Yogaphobia'. *Journal of the American Academy of Religion* 82: 427–71.
- (2015). *Selling Yoga: From Counterculture to Pop Culture*. New York: Oxford University Press.
James, W. (1983 [1899]). *Talks to Teachers on Psychology and to Students on Some of Life's Ideals*. Harvard, MA: Harvard University Press.
Jarvis, Alaice-Azania (2014) 'Is Modern Yoga Dominated by a Culture of Backbiting?' *The Independent*, 21 August. Available at: https://www.independent.co.uk/life-style/health-and-families/features/bks-iyengar-one-of-the-founders-of-modern-yoga-has-died-at-the-age-of-95-9684537.html
Johnson, F.J.M. (1966). 'Sport in the Field'. *Adult Education* 39: 156.
Jones, H. (2001). 'Health and Reproduction', 86–101, in I. Zweiniger-Bargielowska (ed.), *Women in Twentieth-century Britain*. London: Longman.
Josiffe, C. (2017). 'Rollo Ahmed: London's Black Magician'. Talk given at Treadwell's Books, London WC1, 10 August.
Kent, H. (1974). *Day by Day Yoga*. London: Hamlyn.
- (1985). *Yoga for the Disabled*. Ickwell Bury: Yoga for Health Foundation.
Kirk, H. (1976). *Portrait of a Profession: A History of the Solicitor's Profession, 1100 to the Present*. London: Oyez Publishing.

Kitzinger, S. (1967 [1962]). *The Experience of Childbirth*. 2nd edn, London: Pelican.

- (1972). *An Approach to Antenatal Teaching*. London: The National Childbirth Trust.

Klein, M. and A. Guest-Jelley (2014). *Yoga and Body Image: 25 Personal Stories about Beauty, Bravery and Loving*. Woodbury, MN: Llewellyn Publications.

Knott, K. (1986). *My Sweet Lord: The Hare Krishna Movement*. Wellingborough: Aquarian Press.

Kofsky, F. (1970). *Black Nationalism and the Revolution in Music*. London: Pathfinder.

Kripal, J.J. (2007). *Esalen: America and the Religion of No Religion*. London: University of Chicago Press.

Krishna, G. (1995). *The Yogi: Portraits of Swami Vishnu-devananda*. St Paul, MN: Yes International Publishers.

Krishnamurti, J. (1929). 'The Truth is a Pathless Land' (3 August). Text available at: https://www.jkrishnamurti.org/about-dissolution-speech

- (1954). *The First and Last Freedom*. London: Victor Gollancz.

- (1970). *The Krishnamurti Reader*. London: Penguin.

Kureishi, H. (1990). *The Buddha of Suburbia*. London: Faber & Faber.

Kynaston, D. (2007). *Austerity Britain 1945–1951*. London: Bloomsbury.

Laing, A. (1994). *R.D. Laing: A Life*. London: HarperCollins.

Laing, R.D. (1959). *The Divided Self*. London: Tavistock.

Lane, A. (1966). 'A.S.B. Glover: Obituary'. *The Times*, 8 January, p. 10, col. G. Accessed at *The Times Digital Archive 1785–1985*.

Lapham, L. (2005). *With the Beatles*. New York: Melville House Publishing.

- (1979 [1978]). *Inner Beauty, Inner Light*. London: Collins.

-(1997 [1976]). *Loving Hands: The Traditional Art of Baby Massage*. New York: Newmarket Press.

- (2002 [1975]). *Birth without Violence*. Rev. edn, Rochester, VT: Healing Arts Press.

Leslie, A. (1973). 'Start Saving for a Trip to Unforgettable India'. *Cosmopolitan* (February).

Lewis, J. (2005). *Penguin Special: The Life and Times of Allen Lane*. London: Viking.

Lister, D. (1999). 'Genius who Spread his Gift to the Youth of the World'. *The Independent* (London), 13 March, p. 3.

Lock, S. (1997). 'Medicine in the Second Half of the Twentieth Century', 123–46, in I. Loudon (ed.), *Western Medicine: An Illustrated History*. Oxford: Oxford University Press.

Love, R. (2010). *The Great Oom: The Mysterious Origins of America's First Yogi*. New York: Penguin.

Lowe, R. (1970). 'The North Staffordshire Miners Higher Education Movement'. *Educational Review* 22: 263–77.

- (1988). *Education in the Post-War Years: A Social History*. London: Routledge.

- (1997). *Schooling and Social Change 1964–1990*. London: Routledge.

Lucia, A. (2018). 'Guru Sex: Charisma, Proxemic Desire, and the Haptic Logics of the Guru–Disciple Relationship'. *Journal of the American Academy of Religion* 86/4 (December): 953–88. doi:10.1093/jaarel/lfy025

Lutgendorf, P. (2007). *Hanuman's Tale: The Messages of a Divine Monkey*. Oxford: Oxford University Press.

Lutyens, M. (1990). *The Life and Death of Krishnamurti.* London: John Murray.

Maas, P. (2013). 'A Concise Historiography of Classical Yoga Philosophy', 53–90, in Eli Franco (ed.), *Periodization and Historiography of Indian Philosophy.* Publications of the De Nobili Research Library, 37. Vienna: Sammlung de Nobili, Institut für Südasien-, Tibet- und Buddhismuskunde der Universität Wien.

Macdonald, I. (2005). *Revolution in the Head.* Rev. 2nd edn, London: Pimlico.

Maclure, J.S. (1990). *A History of Education in London 1870–1990.* London: Allen Lane/Penguin.

Magidoff, R. (1973). *Yehudi Menuhin: The Story of the Man and the Musician.* London: Robert Hale & Company.

Maimaris, D. (2006). 'Meeting Diana Clifton, One of Britain's First and Most Senior Yoga Teachers and Honorary Member of NELIYI and IYA(UK)'. *North East London Iyengar Yoga Institute News* 38 (Autumn): 6–11.

Mallinson, J. (2004). *The Gheranda Samhita in the Original Sanskrit and an English Translation.* Woodstock, NY: YogaVidya.com.

– (2010). *The Kecharīvidyā of Ādinātha: A Critical Edition and Annotated Translation of an Early Text of Haṭhayoga.* London: Routledge.

Mallinson, J. and M. Singleton (2017). *The Roots of Yoga.* London: Penguin.

Mangan, J.A. and J. Walvin (eds.) (1987). *Manliness and Morality: Middle-Class Masculinity in Britain and America, 1800–1940.* Manchester: Manchester University Press.

Manos, M. (ed.) (1987). *Iyengar: His Life and Work.* Porthill, ID: Timeless Books.

Marnham, P. (2005). *The Road to Katmandu.* London: Tauris.

Marshall, L. (1975). *Wake Up to Yoga.* London: Ward Lock.

– (1976). *Lyn Marshall's Keep Up with Yoga.* London: Ward Lock.

– (1978). *Lyn Marshall's Yoga for Your Children.* London: Ward Lock.

– (1982). *Lyn Marshall's Everyday Yoga.* London: BBC.

Martin, L., H. Gutman and P. Hutton (eds.) (1988). *Technologies of the Self: A Seminar with Michel Foucault.* Boston, MA: University of Massachusetts Press.

Marwick, A. (2000). 'Introduction', in A. Aldgate, J. Chapman and A. Marwick (eds.), *Windows on the Sixties: Exploring Key Texts of Media and Culture.* London: I.B. Tauris.

Mascaró, J. (trans.) (1938). *The Himalayas of the Soul.* London: John Murray.

– (trans.) (1962). *Bhagavad Gītā.* London: Pelican.

– (trans.) (1965). *The Upaniṣads.* London: Pelican.

– (1999). *The Creation of Faith.* Calgary: Bayeux Arts.

Maslen, J. (1997). 'The Early Years', in *The Silver Jubilee of the Manchester and District Institute of Iyengar Yoga.* Manchester: MDIIY.

Mason, P. (1994). *The Maharishi: The Biography of the Man Who Gave Transcendental Meditation to the West.* Element Books.

– (2015). *Roots of TM: The Transcendental Meditation of Guru Dev and Maharishi Mahesh Yogi.* Premanand.

Masson, J.M. (1989). *Against Therapy.* Monroe, ME: Common Courage Press.

– (2003 [1993]). *My Father's Guru: A Journey through Spirituality and Disillusion.* New York: Ballantine Books.

Matthews, J.J. (1987). 'Building the Body Beautiful'. *Australian Feminist Studies* 5: 17–34.

Mauss, M. (1979 [1950]). 'Body Techniques', in B. Brewster (trans.), *Sociology and Psychology: Essays*. Boston, MA: Routledge & Kegan Paul.

McCartney, P. (2017). 'Yoga Fundamentalism and the "Vedic Way of Life". Patrick McCartney. Articles'. *Global Ethnographic* (May). Available at: http://oicd.net/ge/wp-content/uploads/Politics-byond-the-Yoga-Mat-P.-McCartney.pdf

McCrone, K.E. (1988). *Sport and the Physical Emancipation of English Women, 1870–1914*. London: Routledge.

McIntosh, P. (1968). *Sport in Society*. London: C.A. Watts & Co.

– (1969 [1957]). *Landmarks in the History of Physical Education*. London: Routledge & Kegan Paul.

– (1972 [1952]). *Physical Education in England Since 1800*. London: G. Bell.

McKibbin, R. (1998). *Classes and Cultures: England 1918–1951*. Oxford: Oxford University Press.

McKeown, T. (1976). *The Role of Medicine: Dream, Mirage, or Nemesis?* London: Nuffield Provincial Hospitals Trust.

McLeod, H. (2007). *The Religious Crisis of the 1960s*. Oxford: Oxford University Press.

McLuhan, M. (2006 [1964]). *Understanding Media*. London: Routledge.

Medau Society (2007). 'Medau History Sheet'.

Mehta, S., S. Mehta and M. Mehta (1990). *Yoga the Iyengar Way*. London: Dorling Kindersley.

Melton, J.G. (1992). 'New Thought and the New Age', 15–29, in J.R. Lewis and J.G. Melton (eds.), *Perspectives on the New Age*. Albany, NY: State University of New York Press.

Menuhin, Y. (1996). *Unfinished Journey*. London: Methuen.

Miles, B. (2002). *In the Sixties*. London: Jonathan Cape.

– (2004). 'Going Underground', 238–9, in P. Trynka (ed.), *The Beatles: Ten Years That Shook The World*. London: Dorling Kindersley.

Mills, A.C. (1995). 'Death and Taxes: When Famed American Yoga Guru Richard Hittleman Died in Santa Cruz in 1991, he Left his Ex-wife with a Million-dollar Tax Bill, Merciless IRS Agents at the Door and Nowhere to Turn'. *Metro*, 22–29 November. Available at: http://www.metroactive.com/papers/metro/11.22.95/yogi-9547.html

Mishra, R.S. (1972a [1963]). *The Textbook of Yoga Psychology*. London: Lyrebird Press.

– (1972b [1959]). *Fundamentals of Yoga*. London: Lyrebird Press.

Monro, R. and S. Fulder (1981). *The Status of Complementary Medicine in the United Kingdom*. London: Threshold Foundation.

Moore, J. (1991). *Gurdjieff: The Anatomy of a Myth*. London: Element.

Müller, Max. (1879). *The Upanishads, Vol. I*. Oxford: Clarendon Press.

Munrow, D. (1966). 'Sport in the Field', *Adult Education* 39: 156.

Murray, M. (1980). *Seeking the Master: A Guide to the Ashrams of India*. Jersey: Spearman.

Nath, I. (2001). *Yoga: The Classical Way*. 3rd edn, Jane Still, Tower White for the Patañjali Yoga Centre, Battle.

National Council of Hindu Temples (2016). 'Yoga: Not a Part of Hinduism? Dissecting Dharma . . .'. Available at: http://www.nchtuk.org/index.php/extensions/s5-image-and-content-fader/yoga-not-a-part-of-hinduism

Nesbitt, E. with J. Parry (1996). 'Professor Gopal Singh Puri 1915–1995: Scholar and Humanist'. *Sikh Bulletin*.

Newcombe, S. (2007). 'Stretching for Health and Well-Being: Yoga and Women in Britain, 1960–1980'. *Asian Medicine* 3/1: 37–63.

– (2013). 'Magic and Yoga: The Role of Subcultures in Transcultural Exchange', in B. Hauser (ed.), *Yoga Traveling: Bodily Practice in Transcultural Perspective*. London: Springer.

– (2014). 'The Institutionalization of the Yoga Tradition: "Gurus" B.K.S. Iyengar and Yogini Sunita in Britain', 147–67, in Mark Singleton and Ellen Goldberg (eds.), *Gurus of Modern Yoga*. Oxford: Oxford University Press.

– (2017). 'The Yoga Revival in Contemporary India'. *Oxford Research Encyclopaedia* (online). doi: 10.1093/acrefore/9780199340378.013.253

– (2018). 'Spaces of Yoga: Towards a Non-essentialist Understanding of Yoga', 551–73, in Karl Baier, Philipp André Maas and Karin Preisendanz (eds.), *Yoga in Transformation: Historical and Contemporary Perspectives*. Wiener Forum für Theologie und Religionswissenschaft. Göttingen: V&R University Press.

Newman, R. (2006). *Abracadabra! The Complete Story of the Beatles' Revolver*. Self-published, London. Available at: http://www.revolverbook.co.uk/abracadabrav1.0.pdf

Oakley, A. (1974). *Housewife*. London: Allen Lane.

Odent, M. (1976). *Bien Naître*. Paris: Souil.

Offer, A. (2001). 'Body Weight and Self-control in the United States and Britain since the 1950s'. *The Society for the Social History of Medicine* 14: 79–106.

– (2006). *Challenge of Affluence: Self-Control and Well-being in the United States and Britain since 1950*. Oxford: Oxford University Press.

Office of National Statistics (2002). 'Population and Private Households, 1901 to 1996: Social Trends 30'. London: HMSO.

Oliver, P. (2014). *Hinduism in the 1960s*. London: Bloomsbury.

Owen, A. (2004). *The Place of Enchantment: British Occultism and the Culture of the Modern*. London: University of Chicago Press.

– (2006). 'The "Religious Sense" in a Post-war Secular Age'. *Past and Present* Supplement 1: 159–77.

Palmer, Susan J., and Arvind Sharma (eds.) (1993). *The Rajneesh Papers: Studies in a New Religious Movement*. Delhi: Motilal.

Pant, A.B. (1970). *Surya Namaskārs: An Ancient Indian Exercise – by Apa Pant; as explained to . . .* [him by his father] *Bhawanrao Pant Pratinidhi*. Bombay: Orient Longman.

Parsons, T. (1974). 'Religion in Postindustrial America: The Problem of Secularization'. *Social Research* 41: 193–225

Partridge, C. (2005a). *The Re-enchantment of the West, Vol. I*. London: Continuum.

– (2005b). *Alternative Spiritualities, Sacralization, Popular Culture and Occulture, Vol. II*. London: Continuum.

– (2018). *High Culture: Drugs, Mysticism, and the Pursuit of Transcendence in the Modern World*. New York: Oxford University Press.

Pathak-Narain, P. (2017). *Godman to Tycoon: The Untold Story of Baba Ramdev*. New Delhi: Juggernaut.

Paytress, M. (2004). 'A Passage to India', 286–303, in P. Trynka (ed.), *The Beatles: Ten Years That Shook the World*. London: Dorling Kindersley.

Penguin (1960). *Penguins Progress 1935–1960*. London: Penguin.

- (1985). *Fifty Penguin Years*. London: Penguin.

Perez, N.C. (1978). 'Glorify God in Your Body', 129–32, in B.K.S. Iyengar 60th Birthday Celebration Committee (ed.), *Body the Shrine, Yoga thy Light*. Bombay: B.I. Taraporewala.

Phelan, N. and M. Volin (1963). *Yoga for Women*. London: Stanley Paul.

Porter, D. (ed.) (1994). *History of Public Health and the Modern State*. Amsterdam: Rodopi.

- (2000). 'The Healthy Body', 201–16, in R. Cooter and J. Pickstone (eds.), *Medicine in the Twentieth Century*. Amsterdam: Harwood Academic.

Porter, L. (1998). *John Coltrane: His Life and Music*. Ann Arbour, MI: University of Michigan Press.

Porter, R. (2000). *Quacks, Fakers and Charlatans in English Medicine*. London: Stroud.

Porter, R. and D. Porter (1989). *Patient's Progress: Doctors and Doctoring in Eighteenth Century England*. London: Polity Press.

Posse, B.N. (1908). *The Special Kinesiology of Educational Gymnastics*. London: Arthur F. Bird.

Potter, K.H. (ed.) (1981). *Encyclopedia of Indian Philosophies, Vol. 3: Advaita Vedānta up to Śaṅkara and his Pupils*. Princeton, NJ: Princeton University Press.

Power, R.M. (1991). 'The Whole Idea of Medicine: A Critical Evaluation of the Emergence of "Holistic Medicine" in Britain in the Early 1980s'. PhD thesis, Polytechnic of the South Bank.

Prashad, V. (2000). *The Karma of Brown Folk*. University of Minnesota Press.

Pratinidhi, B.P. (1928). *Surya Namaskars (Sun-Adoration) for Health, Efficiency and Longevity*. Aundh: R.K. Kirloskar.

- (1938). *The Ten Point Way to Health Surya Namaskars*. Edited with an introduction by Louise Morgan et al. London: J.M. Dent & Sons.

Price, M. (1979). 'The Divine Light Mission as a Social Organization'. *The Sociological Review* 27: 279–96.

Puri, G.S. (1974). *Yoga–Relaxation–Meditation: A Western-Trained Biologist Takes a New Look at an Age Old Eastern Science*. 3rd edn, self-published, Liverpool.

Puri, K. and E. Nesbitt (2013). *Pool of Life: The Autobiography of a Punjabi Agony Aunt*. Eastbourne: Sussex Academic Press.

Puttick, E. (2000). 'Personal Development: The Spiritualisation and Secularisation of the Human Potential Movement', in S. Sutcliffe and M. Bowman (eds.), *Beyond New Age: Exploring Alternative Spirituality*. Edinburgh: Edinburgh University Press.

Raine, K. (1982). 'Obituary: Geoffrey Watkins'. *Temenos* 2: 272.

Ramacharaka (1903). *The Hindu-Yogi Science of Breath. A Complete Manual of the Oriental Breathing Philosophy of Physical, Mental, Psychic and Spiritual Development*. Palmya, NJ: Yogi Publication Society.

Reck, D.R. (1985). 'Beatles Orientalis: Influences from Asia in a Popular Song Tradition'. *Asian Music* 16: 83–149.

Remski, M. (2015). 'Yoga Body Author Mark Singleton Responds to Critics'. *Yoga International*, 30 October. Available at: https://yogainternational.com/article/view/yoga-body-author-mark-singleton-responds-to-critics-who-didnt-want-to-under

– (2016). 'The Problem with Pain in Yoga'. *Yoga International*, 7 March. Available at: https://yogainternational.com/article/view/the-problem-of-pain-in-yoga

– (2019). *What Are We Actually Doing in Asana?*

Richmond, K. (ed.) (2011). *Aleister Crowley, the Golden Dawn and Buddhism: Reminiscences and Writings of Gerald Yorke*. York Beach, ME: The Teitan Press.

Rinehart, Robin (1999). *One Lifetime, Many Lives: The Experience of Modern Hindu Hagiography*. New York: Oxford University Press.

Roberts, A. (2012). *Albion Dreaming: A Popular History of LSD in Britain*. 2nd edn, Singapore: Marshall Cavendish.

Robertson, J. (2004). 'Help! The End of the Beginning', in P. Trynka (ed.), *The Beatles: Ten Years That Shook the World*. London: Dorling Kindersley.

Robins, J. (1961). 'East or West. There are Some Things Every Woman Wants: Youth and Happiness. Here's a Wife with the Secret of Both'. *Sunday Mercury*, 12 March.

Rochford, B. (2007). *Hare Krishna Transformed*. New York: New York University Press.

Rodrigues, S. (1982). *The Householder Yogi: Life of Shri Yogendra*. Bombay: Yoga Institute.

Rose, J. (2001). *The Intellectual Life of the British Working Classes*. London: Yale Press.

Ross, A. (2007). '(Comment on) Moving into Phase Three: An Analysis of ISKCON Membership in the UK', 54–59, in G. Dwyer and R.J. Cole (eds.), *The Hare Krishna Movement: Forty Years of Chant and Change*. London: I.B. Tauris.

Rowbottom, S. (2001). *Promise of a Dream: Remembering the Sixties*. London: Verso.

Saks, M. (1986). 'Professions and the Public Interest: The Response of the Medical Profession to Acupuncture in Nineteenth and Twentieth Century Britain'. PhD dissertation, London School of Economics and Political Science, University of London.

– (2003). *Orthodox and Alternative Medicine: Politics, Professionalization and Health Care*. London: Continuum.

Salmon, J.W. (ed.) (1984). *Alternative Medicines: Popular and Policy Perspectives*. London: Tavistock.

Samuel, R. (1998a). 'North and South', in R. Samuel (ed.), *Island Stories: Unravelling Britain, Theatres of Memory. Vol. II*. London: Verso.

– (1998b). 'The Voice of Britain', in R. Samuel (ed.), *Island Stories: Unravelling Britain, Theatres of Memory. Vol. II*. London: Verso.

Sandbrook, D. (2005). *Never Had It So Good: A History of Britain from Suez to the Beatles*. London: Little, Brown.

– (2006). *White Heat: A History of Britain in the Swinging Sixties*. London: Little, Brown.

Sandow, E. (1919). *Life is Movement: The Physical Reconstruction and Regeneration of the People (A Disease-less World): The Family Encyclopedia of Health*. Hertford: Simson & Co..

Saner, E. (2016). 'Disharmony in British Yoga Community over Moves to Regulate Teachers'. *The Guardian*, 28 October. Available at: https://www.theguardian.com/lifeandstyle/2016/oct/28/disharmony-in-british-yoga-community-over-moves-to-regulate-teachers

Sarasvati, S. (1970). *Yoga for Vital Beauty*. London: Harrap.

Sarbacker, S. (2005). *Samadhi: The Numinous and Cessative in Indo-Tibetan Yoga*. Albany, NY: State University of New York Press.

– (2008). 'The Numinous and Cessative in Modern Yoga', in M. Singleton and J. Byrne (eds.), *Yoga in the Modern World: Contemporary Perspectives*. London: Routledge.

Satter, B. (1999). *Each Mind a Kingdom: American Women, Sexual Purity, and the New Thought Movement, 1875–1920*. University of California Press.

Saunders, N. (1972). *Alternative London*. 1st edn, self-published, London.

– (n.d.). *Alternative London*. 2nd edn, self-published, London.

Seddon, C. (2012). 'Measuring National Well-being: What we do, 2012'. Office of National Statistics (ONS). Available at: http://webarchive.nationalarchives.gov.uk/20160111031517/http://www.ons.gov.uk/ons/dcp171766_258996.pdf

Semyon, M. (2003). 'Take As Long As It Takes', in B. Mullan (ed.), *R.D. Laing: Creative Destroyer*. London: Sage.

– (2004). *The Distracted Centipede*. Victoria, Canada: Trafford.

Schnäbele, V. (2010). *Yoga in Modern Society*. Hamburg: Verlag Dr Kovač.

Shah, T. (1988 [2011]). *Sorcerer's Apprentice: An Incredible Journey into the World of India's Godmen*. New York: Arcade Publishing.

Shapiro, M. (2002). *All Things Must Pass*. London: Virgin.

Shastri, H.P. (1948). *The Heart of the Eastern Mystical Teaching*. London: Shanti Sadan.

– (1957). *Yoga*. London: Foyles.

– (n.d.). *Scientist and Mahatma: An Account of the Life of Rama Tirtha and Translations from his Writings*. London: Shanti Sadan.

Shringy, R.K. (ed.) (1977). 'The International Yoga Co-ordination Centre Yoga Awareness'. *Quarterly Journal of Yococen* 1 (July).

Siegel, L. (1991). *Net of Magic: Wonders and Deceptions in India*. Chicago: Chicago University Press.

Singleton, M. (2005). 'Salvation through Relaxation: Proprioceptive Therapy and its Relationship to Yoga'. *Journal of Contemporary Religion* 20: 289–304.

– (2007a). 'Yoga, Eugenics and Spiritual Darwinism in the Early Twentieth Century'. *International Journal of Hindu Studies* 11: 125–46.

– (2007b). 'Suggestive Therapeutics: New Thought's Relationship to Modern Yoga'. *Asian Medicine: Tradition and Modernity* 3: 64–84.

– (2010). *Yoga Body: The Origins of Modern Posture Practice*. New York: Oxford University Press.

Singleton, M. and J. Byrne (eds.) (2008). *Yoga in the Modern World: Contemporary perspectives*. London: Routledge.

Singleton, M. and T. Fraser (2014). 'T. Krishnamacharya, Father of Modern Yoga', in M. Singleton and E. Goldberg (eds.), *Gurus of Modern Yoga*. New York: Oxford University Press.

Sjoman, N.E. (1999). *The Yoga Tradition of the Mysore Palace*. 2nd edn, New Delhi: Shakti Malik.

Sloss, R.R. (1991). *Lives in the Shadow with J. Krishnamurti*. London: Bloomsbury.

Smith, B.R. (2007). 'Body, Mind and Spirit? Towards an Analysis of the Practice of Yoga'. *Body & Society* 13: 25–46.

– (2008). '"With Heat Even Iron Will Bend": Discipline and Authority in Astanga Yoga', in M. Singleton and J. Byrne, *Yoga in the Modern World: Contemporary Perspectives*. London: Routledge.

Spencer, N. (2004). 'Eastern Rising', 230–5, in P. Trynka (ed.), *The Beatles: Ten Years That Shook The World*. London: Dorling Kindersley: .

Spock, B. (1974). *Bringing up Children in a Difficult Time: A Philosophy of Parental Leadership and High Ideals and Baby and Childcare*. London: Bodley Head.

Squires, R.J. (1985). *Marginality, Stigma and Conversion in the Context of Medical Knowledge, Professional Practices and Occupational Interests: A Case Study of Professional Homeopathy in Nineteenth Century Britain and the United States*. Leeds: University of Leeds.

Stack, M B. (1931). *Building the Body Beautiful: The Bagot Stack Stretch-and-Swing System*. London: Chapman & Hall.

Stack, P. (1988). *Zest for Life: Mary Bagot Stack and the League of Health and Beauty*. London: Peter Owen.

Stasulane, A. (forthcoming). 'From Imagined Hinduism to the Hindu Diaspora in Latvia', in F. Sardella and K. Jacobsen (eds.), *Hinduism in Europe*. Leiden: Brill.

Strauss, S. (2002a). '"Adapt, Adjust, Accommodate": The Production of Yoga in a Transnational World'. *History and Anthropology* 13: 231–51.

– (2002b). 'The Master's Narrative: Swami Sivananda and the Transnational Production of Yoga'. *Journal of Folklore Research* 39: 217–41.

– (2005). *Positioning Yoga: Balancing Acts Across Cultures*. Oxford: Berg.

Strachan, F. (1970). *Aquarian Guide to Occult, Mystical, Religious, Magical London and Around*. London: Aquarian Press.

Strutt, M. (1976a). *Living Yoga*. London: Centre Community Publications.

– (1976b). *A Stage One Course in Yoga*. London: Centre Community Publications.

– (1977a). *Wholistic Health and Living Yoga*. London: Centre Community Publications.

– (1977b). *A Stage Two Course in Yoga*. London: Centre Community Publications, London.

Strube, J. (2017). 'Occultist Identity Formations between Theosophy and Socialism in Fin-de-Siècle France'. *Numen* 64/5–6: 568–95.

– (forthcoming). 'Hinduism, Western Esotericism and New Age Religion in Europe', in Kunt Jacobsen and Ferdinando Sardella (eds.), *Hinduism in Europe*. Leiden: Brill.

Sundaram, S. (1928). *Yogic Physical Culture or the Secret to Happiness*. Yoga Publishing House.

Sutcliffe, S. (1997). 'Seekers, Networks and "New Age"'. *Scottish Journal of Religious Studies* 15: 97–114.

- (2000). 'Seekers and Gurus in the Modern World,' in S. Sutcliffe and M. Bowman (eds.), *Beyond the New Age: Exploring Alternative Spirituality*. Edinburgh: Edinburgh University Press.

Sutherland, G. (1990). 'Education', in F.M.L. Thompson (ed.), *The Cambridge Social History of Britain 1750–1950. Vol. III*. Cambridge: Cambridge University Press.

Szasz, T. (1956). 'Malingering: "Diagnosis" or Social Condemnation?'. *A.M.A Archives of Neurology and Psychiatry* 76 (October): 432–43.

- (1997 [1970]). *The Manufacture of Madness*. Syracuse, NY: Syracuse University Press.

Szreter, S. (2005). *Health and Wealth: Studies in History and Policy*. Rochester, NY: University of Rochester Press.

Talbot, C.J.C. (ed.) (1852). *Meliora or Better Times to Come*. London: John Parker & Son.

Tangali, D. (2016). '99 Facts about Yoga: The Most Successful Global Phenomenon'. Available at: https://www.dr-discount.nl/blog/english/99-facts-abouts-yoga

Taraporewala, B.I. (1978). 'How "Light on Yoga" was Written', in B.K.S. Iyengar 60th Birthday Celebration Committee (ed.), *Body the Shrine, Yoga thy Light*. Bombay: B.I. Taraporewala.

Taylor, A. (1992). *Annie Besant: A Biography*. New York: Oxford University Press.

Taylor, P.B. (2004). 'Gurdjieff and Prince Ozay'. Self-published at http://www.Gurdjieff-Bibliography.com.

Thatcher, M. (1987). 'Interview for *Woman's Own* ("No Such Thing as Society")', 23 September. Available at: https://www.margaretthatcher.org/document/106689.

Thumim, J. (2004). 'Inventing Television Culture: Men, Women and the Box', in C. Brunsdon and J. Caughie (eds.), *Oxford Television Studies*. Oxford: Oxford University Press.

Tittley, I. (1993). 'Sports Council'. *LOYA News* 14: 3–4.

Tobias, M. (2007). 'Light on B.K.S. Iyengar', 285–91, in K. Busia (ed.), *Iyengar: The Yoga Master*. London: Shambala.

Tourniere, J.D. (2002). *Eating Fox: A Break Through to India*. Self-published, Cambridge.

Tuft, N. (1971). 'Standing on her Head to Face the Day'. *Daily Telegraph*, 31 December. Newspaper clipping in the file Vol 2 at the Ramamani Iyengar Memorial Yoga Institute in Pune, India.

Turner, S. (2006). *The Gospel According to the Beatles*. London: Westminster John Knox Press.

Urban, H. (2001). 'The Omnipotent Oom: Tantra and Its Impact on Modern Western Esotericism', 218–59, in Esoterica, Vol. III [online]. Available at: http://www.esoteric.msu.edu/VolumeIII/HTML/Oom.html, accessed 12 April 2009.

- (2006). *Magia Sexualis: Sex, Magic, and Liberation in Modern Western Esotericism*. Berkeley, CA: University of California Press.

Van Lysbeth, A. (1968). *J'apprends le Yoga*. Brussels: Flammarion.

- (1971). *Yoga Self-taught*. London: Allen & Unwin.

– (1983 [1979]). *Pranayama: The Yoga of Breathing*. London: Allen & Unwin.

Vernon, R.J. (2007). 'The Beginning of Freedom', in Kofi Busia (ed.), *Iyengar: The Yoga Master*. London: Shambala.

Verter, B. (1997). 'Dark Star Rising: The Emergence of Modern Occultism, 1800–1950'. PhD Dissertation, Princeton University, available at the Warberg Institute, London.

Vishnu-devananda, S. (1959a). *The Complete Illustrated Book of Yoga*. New York: Bell Publishing/Julian Press.

– (1959b [USA 1957]). *Yoga Asanas. A Natural Method of Physical and Mental Training*. Introduction and poses by Swami-Vishnoudevananda; photographs by Louis Frédéric; translated from the French by Geoffrey A. Dudley. London: Fowler.

Visram, R. (2002). *Asians in Britain: 400 Years of History*. London: Pluto Press.

Vivekananda, Swami (1896). *Yoga Philosophy: Lectures . . . on Raja Yoga, or Conquering the Internal Nature. Also Patanjali's Yoga Aphorisms, with Commentaries, etc.,* London: Longmans & Co.

Voix, R. (2008). 'Denied Violence, Glorified Fighting: Spiritual Practices and Controversy in a Contemporary Indian Religious Group'. *Nova Religio: The Journal of Alternative and Emergent Religions* 12: 3–25.

– (2010). *Dévotion, ascèse et violence dans l'hindouisme sectaire: Ethnographie d'une secte shivaïte du Bengale*. PhD dissertation, Université de Paris Ouest Nanterre La Défense.

Walliss, J. (2002). *The Brahma Kumaris as a 'Reflexive Tradition': Responding to Late Modernity*. London: Taylor & Francis.

Washington, P. (1993). *Madame Blavatsky's Baboon: Theosophy and the Emergence of the Western Guru*. London: Seeker & Warburg.

Waterman, M.I. (ed.) (1992). *B.A.I.: The Birmingham Athletic Institute Remembered*. Birmingham: Brewin Books.

Watts, A. (1957). *The Way of Zen*. New York: Pantheon Books.

– (1972). *In My Own Way: An Autobiography 1915–1965*. London: Jonathan Cape.

Weber, M. (1947). *The Theory of Social and Economic Organization*. Trans A.M. Henderson and Talcott Parsons; ed. Talcott Parsons. London: Macmillan.

Wegg, W.J. (1973). 'Middle-class Bingo Substitutes'. *Adult Education* 46/3 (September).

Weller, S. (1978). *Easy Pregnancy with Yoga*. Wellingborough: Thorsons.

Wheel of Yoga (1973). *Yoga Handbook*. Wheel of Yoga.

White, D.G. (2012). *Yoga in Practice*. Princeton, NJ: Princeton University Press.

– (2014). *The Yoga Sutra of Patanjali: A Biography*. Princeton, NJ: Princeton University Press.

Whitney, W.D. (1997). *The Roots, Verb-Forms and Primary Derivatives of the Sanskrit Language*. Delhi: Motilal Bandarsidass.

Willard, F. (1985). 'A Wheel within a Wheel: How I Learned to Ride the Bicycle'. Reprinted in S. Twin (ed.), *Out of the Bleachers*. Old Westbury, NY: Feminist Press, 1979.

Williams, R. (2003 [1974]). *Television*. London: Routledge.

Wills, H. and F. Wills (1974). *Yoga for All*. London: BBC.

Wilson, E. (1980). *Only Halfway to Paradise: Women in Postwar Britain 1945–1968*. London: Tavistock.

Wilson, B.R. and E. Barker (2005). 'What Are the New Religious Movements Doing in a Secular Society?', 291–317, in A.F. Heath and D. Gallie (eds.), *Understanding Social Change*. Oxford: Oxford University Press.

Witts, M. (2013). 'Reportage: The British Wheel of Yoga'. Final edn, self-published. Available at: https://docs.yuj.it/_media/method/research/reportage_british_wheel_yoga.pdf

Women's Health London (1993). 'Women's Health, Alternative Medicine, Promoting Good health'. Pamphlet in the British Library.

Wong, K.A. (2017). 'Child's Pose: Children's Yoga and the Complexities of Normalisation'. PhD dissertation, University of Sydney.

Wood, E. (1936). *Is This Theosophy?* London: Rider & Co..

– (1959). *Yoga: An Explanation of the Practices and Philosophy of Indian Yoga, and How They Can Be Applied in the West Today*. London Pelican Books.

Woods, J.H. (1914). *The Yoga-System of Patañjali*. Cambridge, MA: Harvard University Press.

Workers' Educational Association (WEA) Working Party (1960). 'Aspects of Adult Education: A Report Prepared by a Working Party Appointed by the WEA and Presented to the WEA Conference in March 1960'. London: WEA.

Yesudian, Selvarajan, and Elizabeth Haich (1953). *Yoga and Health*. Trans. John P. Robertson. London: Allen & Unwin.

– (2016). '2016 Yoga in America Study Conducted by *Yoga Journal* and Yoga Alliance Reveals Growth and Benefits of the Practice'. *PRNewswire*. Available at: http://www.prnewswire.com/news-releases/2016-yoga-in-america-study-conducted-by-yoga-journal-and-yoga-alliance-reveals-growth-and-benefits-of-the-practice-300203418.html

Yogananda, P. (1994 [1946]). *Autobiography of a Yogi*. Los Angles: Self-Realization Fellowship.

Young, R.J.C. (2006). 'Burdwan in My Life'. Available at: http://www.robertjcyoung.com, accessed 20 June 2007.

Yorke, G. (1935). *China Changes: On Experiences in Contemporary China. With Plates*. London: Jonathan Cape.

Zweiniger-Bargielowska, I. (2001). *Women in Twentieth-century Britain*. London: Longman.

– (2005). 'The Culture of the Abdomen: Obesity and Reducing in Britain, circa 1900–1939'. *Journal of British Studies* 44 (April): 239–73.

– (2006). 'Building a British Superman: Physical Culture in Interwar Britain'. *Journal of Contemporary History* 41: 595–610.

– (2007). 'Raising a Nation of "Good Animals": The New Health Society and Health Education Campaigns in Interwar Britain'. *Social History of Medicine* 20: 73–89.

Index

www.ingramcontent.com/pod-product-compliance
Lightning Source LLC
Chambersburg PA
CBHW071837270326
41929CB00013B/2025